AF443252

QUALITY ASSURANCE IN DIALYSIS
Second Edition

DEVELOPMENTS IN NEPHROLOGY

Volume 39

The titles published in this series are listed at the end of this volume.

Quality Assurance in Dialysis

Second Edition

Edited by

LEE W. HENDERSON
Baxter Healthcare Corporation, McGaw Park, IL, U.S.A.

and

RICHARD S. THUMA
Baxter Healthcare Corporation, Roundlake, IL, U.S.A.

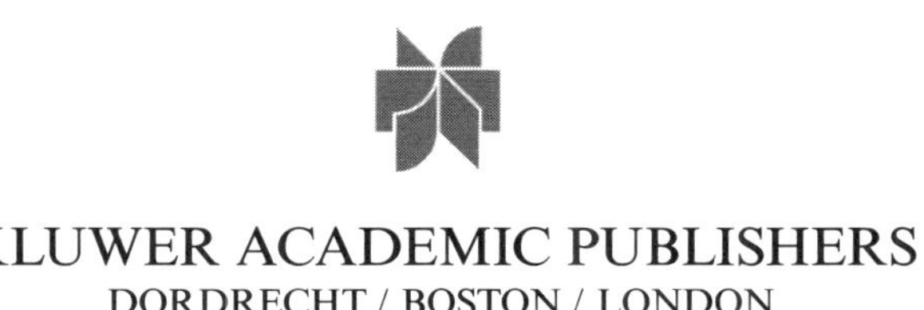

KLUWER ACADEMIC PUBLISHERS
DORDRECHT / BOSTON / LONDON

Library of Congress Cataloging-in-Publication Data is available.

ISBN 0-7923-5281-5

Published by Kluwer Academic Publishers BV,
PO Box 17, 3300 AA Dordrecht, The Netherlands.

Sold and distributed in North, Central and South America
by Kluwer Academic Publishers, PO Box 358,
Accord Station, Hingham, MA 02018-0358, USA

In all other countries, sold and distributed
by Kluwer Academic Publishers, Distribution Center,
PO Box 322, 3300 AH Dordrecht, The Netherlands

Printed on acid-free paper

All Rights Reserved
© 1999 Kluwer Academic Publishers

No part of this publication may be reproduced or utilized in any form or by any means, electronic, mechanical, including photocopying, recording or by any information storage and retrieval system, without written permission from the copyright owner.

Printed and bound in Great Britain by MPG Books, Bodmin, Cornwall.

Table of contents

List of Contributors

R Allen Baxter World Trade Corporation, Renal Therapy Services, Plantation, FL 33324, USA

NS Amin Baxter Healthcare Corporation, Renal Division, Deerfield, IL 60015, USA

CR Blagg Seattle, WA 98122, USA

CA Boyle Director, Clinical Operations, Renal Division, Baxter Healthcare Corporation, McGaw Park, IL 60085, USA

DN Churchill St Joseph's Hospital/McMaster University, Hamilton, Ontario, L8N 4A6, Canada

WR Clark Renal Division, Baxter Healthcare Corporation, McGaw Park, IL 60085, USA

RM Hakim Vanderbilt University Medical Center, Division of Nephrology, Nashville, TN 37232-2372, USA

LW Henderson Baxter Healthcare Corporation, McGaw Park, IL 60085, USA

SF Hoff Regulatory Affairs, Renal Division, MPR-A2E, Baxter Healthcare Corporation, McGaw Park, IL 60085, USA

G Hohner Baxter Healthcare Corporation, McGaw Park, IL 60085, USA

CJ Holmes Renal Division, Baxter Healthcare Corporation, McGaw Park, IL 60085, USA

AA Kaplan Division of Nephrology, University of Connecticut Health Center, Farmington, CT 06030, USA

R Lindsay Victoria Hospital Corporation, London, Ontario, N6A 4G5, Canada

EG Lowrie Cape Neddick, Maine 03902, USA

L Martis Baxter Healthcare Corporation, McGaw Park, IL 60085, USA

PG McDonnell Grayslake, IL 60030, USA

J O'Neill Attorney at Law, Wheeling, IL 60090, USA

BG Pereira New England Medical Center, Boston, MA 02111, USA

BF Prowant Dialysis Clinic Inc, Columbia, MO 65201, USA

RW Steiner UCSD Medical Center, San Diego, CA 92130, USA

J Tattersall   Renal United, Lister Hospital, Stevenage, Herts., SG1 4AB, UK

R Villano   Baxter Healthcare Corporation, Deerfield, IL 60015, USA

E Vonesh   Baxter Healthcare Corporation, Deerfield, IL 60015, USA

Preface

In examining the preface of our first book, it is apparent that the editorial comments made in 1994 are even more pertinent in today's cost-constrained healthcare environment than when first written. We repeat them in part.

This is a time in history when the concept of quality is reaching new highs in terms of public awareness. Articles describing quality, CQI, quality tools, critical success factors, failures, and lessons learned appear in local newspapers, trade journals, scientific periodicals, and professional publications on a daily basis, yet implementation of a quality system in many hospital units is approached with caution and the basic tenants of quality systems and CQI continue to be misunderstood.

In the United States today, the public debate on healthcare issues rages on. The application of strategies, such as cost–benefit analysis as a means for evaluating addition of new technologies to the healthcare cost structure has not succeeded in curbing the rise in costs of healthcare services.

Because of this focused attention by third-party payers, federal and state governments, and insurance companies, healthcare organizations are being pressured to change. One of the strategies for changing involves implementing quality assurance practices. The focus on quality should produce improvements in productivity, innovation and profitability. But, most importantly, the desired outcome of a quality assurance program is self-improvement.

In its drive to become more productive and more competitive, industry looked to such Quality Leaders as W. Edwards Deming, and J.J. Juran for ideas. According to Deming, the way to become competitive is to undergo a top-to-bottom quality-based transformation of the organization. This quality transformation will produce the productivity improvements, innovation and profitability

increases needed. The Deming philosophy emphasizes that quality is never fully achieved: process improvement is never ending.

But, what is quality? Without defining, David Garvin makes the point that "in its original form, quality activities were reactive and inspection-oriented; today. quality related activities have broadened and are seen as essential for strategic success" [1]. How can the broad context of quality be applied to the diverse aspects of ESRD?

Furthermore, although far from a new concept, Continuous Quality Improvement (CQI) has taken its place as a dominant theme in many industries. CQI is more broadly applicable, both in concept and execution, to service as well as manufacturing-based operations. How have the variously described elements of Continuous Quality Improvement been linked to aspects of renal therapy strategies?

Many industries are now concentrating on customer satisfaction as a means for creating competitive advantage. What are the implications of the recent focus on customer satisfaction and meeting customer requirements with respect to the process of caring for patients with end stage renal disease?

How do the concepts of quality in a dialysis unit stack up against the issues of quality of life?

The editors believe that this book will aid in addressing some of those questions. The contents, although quite diverse, attempt to address some aspects of questions posed above.

OVERVIEW OF CONTENTS

As you will note, there are many new chapters added to the present work and many of the original chapters, in areas where changes have occurred, have been rewritten. There are three broad groupings. Chapters 1 and 10 offer either a

L.W. Henderson and R.S. Thuma (eds.), Quality Assurance in Dialysis, 2nd Edition, ix–x.
© 1999 *Kluwer Academic Publishers. Printed in Great Britain*

x

broad overview of the quality process or a description of tools that can be used within that process to improve outcome. For example, David Churchill (Chapter 1) explores evidence-based medicine; whereas Ed Vonesh (Chapter 4) offers insight into choosing the appropriate statistical model for judging clinical outcome.

Chapters 11 and 18 address more patient-related concerns in the arena of hemodialysis. Chapters 19 and 20 examine both hemodialysis and peritoneal dialysis from the stand point of membrane characteristics and judging membrane performance. The remaining chapters address patient-related issues and technical considerations for improving the quality of peritoneal dialysis, transplantation, and acute renal failure.

It should be noted that the authors were selected for their expertise and professional experience in, for example, overseeing a large hemodialysis network or in running a home dialysis program rather than from their written contributions to the quality assurance literature. The authors were instructed simply to create a chapter addressing quality assurance principles from their perspective in the context of their assigned titles. As a result, chapter content ranges broadly from the overtly philosophical to the sharply technical. You will find this diversity makes lively and informative reading.

L.W. Henderson and R.S. Thuma

Reference
1. Garvin D. Managing Quality. New York: The Free Press, 1988.

1. Evidence-based medicine as a strategy for improving the quality of clinical decision making for dialysis patients

DAVID N. CHURCHILL

INTRODUCTION

Traditional clinical decision making has been based on information provided by clinical experts, usually during undergraduate and post graduate training, and then supplemented by formal continuing medical education and informally through consultations. There is an implicit assumption that the need for scientific information is satisfied by this process. However, there is convincing evidence that this assumption is incorrect [1]. The opinion of experts is often inconsistent with scientific evidence [2]. In response to this unsatisfactory situation, the concept of evidence-based medicine has evolved [3].

EVIDENCE-BASED MEDICINE

The concept of evidence-based medicine is considered a paradigm shift [3]. Thomas Kuhn has described a scientific paradigm as a method of addressing problems and the range of evidence which might be applied to that problem [4]. If the existing paradigm is found be defective and requires a new method to address a particular problem, it can be described as a paradigm shift.

The traditional medical paradigm assumes that: (1) unsystematic observation from clinical experience is a valid method to establish and maintain clinical knowledge; (2) the understanding of pathophysiology is a sufficient guide for clinical practice; (3) medical education and common sense are sufficient to evaluate the medical literature and (4) content expertise and clinical experience are sufficient to generate valid guidelines for clinical

research. The new paradigm assumes that an understanding of pathophysiologic principles and clinical experience are necessary but not sufficient for rational clinical practice. In addition, an understanding of certain rules of evidence is essential for the correct interpretation of the medical literature addressing causation, prognosis, diagnostic tests and treatment strategy [3].

The evidence for a particular intervention can be classified according to the methodologic strength of the research design [5]. The classification described by Carruthers et al. [5] has 6 levels of research design strength (Table 1.1). Although important information can be provided by non-randomized clinical trials, they should be considered as hypothesis generating rather than hypothesis testing.

EVIDENCE-BASED MEDICINE AND THE CLINICIAN

Although evidence-based medicine is conceptually attractive, the clinician must know how to access

Table 1.1. Level of evidence

1.	Randomized clinical trial (RCT) with adequate sample size
2.	Randomized clinical trial (RCT) with low statistical power
3.	Cohort study with contemporaneous control group *or* RCT sub-group
4.	Cohort study with historical control group or before and after study
5.	Case series > 10 patients
6.	Case series < 10 patients

Modified from reference [5]

1

L.W. Henderson and R.S. Thuma (eds.), Quality Assurance in Dialysis, 2nd Edition, 1–6.
© 1999 *Kluwer Academic Publishers. Printed in Great Britain*

the information and how to efficiently apply the rules of evidence. The approach to this problem has been described by Oxman and colleagues [6]. The clinician must first pose a question which is focused and answerable. Traditional search strategies such as asking colleagues, use of standard textbooks and personal reprint files have largely been replaced by electronic searches of the medical literature. Clinicians can easily acquire these basic computer skills which are becoming an essential basic skill for practising modern evidence-based medicine [7].

Publications can be divided into primary and integrative studies. The primary studies are divided into those addressing therapy, diagnosis, harm and prognosis; the integrative studies are divided into overviews, practice guidelines, decision analysis and economic analysis (Table 1.2). As the focus of this chapter is on interventions for dialysis patients, the primary studies dealing with therapy and integrative studies dealing with overviews and clinical practice guidelines are of particular interest. For each of the studies retrieved by the electronic literature search, three questions are posed [6]. These are: (1) Are the results of the study valid? (2) What are the results? (3) Will the results help me in caring for my patients? (Table 1.3).

Table 1.2. Study classification

Primary studies	Integrative studies
Therapy	Overview
Diagnosis	Practice guidelines
Harm	Decision analysis
Prognosis	Economic analysis

Modified from reference [6]

Table 1.3. Basic questions

1. Are the results of the study valid?
2. What are the results?
3. Will the results help me in caring for my patients?

In a series of articles entitled "Users Guides to the Medical Literature", two of these articles address evaluation of publications dealing with therapy (i.e. interventions) [8, 9]. The first question

Table 1.4. Validity of study results

Primary guides
1. Was the assignment of patients to treatments randomized?
2. Were all the patients who entered the trial properly accounted for and attributed at the conclusion?

Secondary guides
1. Were patients, health care workers and study personnel blinded to treatment allocation?
2. Were the groups similar at the start of the trial?
3. Aside from the experimental interventions, were the groups treated equally

Modified from reference [8]

deals with the validity of the study results. There are 2 primary and 3 secondary guides (Table 1.4). The first primary guide is: "Was the assignment of patients to treatments randomized?" This is an important guide as research designs which allocate treatment by any method other than randomization tend to show larger treatment effects than do randomized clinical trials. Ineffective therapies may appear beneficial when less rigorous research designs are used [10, 11]. An example is the use of extra cranial-intracranial bypass to prevent strokes in patients with symptomatic cerebrovascular disease. Non-randomized clinical trials indicated that this was an effective procedure but a randomized clinical trial demonstrated that the only effect of surgery was to have worse outcomes in the immediate postoperative period [12]. The second primary guide dealing with the issue of the validity of the study results is: "Were all the patients who entered the trial properly accounted for and attributed at the conclusion?" The greater the number of subjects lost to follow-up, the less credible the results of the study. As patients lost to follow-up may be different from other patients, they may have experienced an undesired outcome. In a trial which showed treatment benefit, assume that all patients lost to follow-up had the undesired outcome and recalculate the outcomes under this assumption. If the conclusions are not changed, then the results are acceptable. If the conclusion changes, the credibility of the study is weakened. Attribution refers to the patients being analyzed in the group to which they had been randomized. The exclusion of noncompliant patients from analysis and exclusion of patients who do not receive the treatment to which they had been randomized are examples of this analytic error. The effect of these errors is to destroy the unbiased comparison provided by the randomization process. The three secondary guides dealing with the validity of the study results are listed in the table. These address blinding of the study personnel, similarity of treatment and control groups and co-intervention. If the investigators were blind to treatment allocation, there is less likelihood of bias. There is always a possibility that randomization will not provide balanced treatment groups. If imbalance is identified, the baseline differences can be adjusted in the statistical analysis. The third secondary guide deals with the possibility of imbalanced concurrent therapy or co-intervention might introduce additional bias.

The second major question is "What were the results?" There are 2 guides. These are: (1) How large was the treatment effect? and (2) How precise was the estimate of the treatment effect? [9]. The size of the treatment effect can be expressed in several different ways. These include the absolute risk reduction, the relative risk or the relative risk reduction. The perception of the size of the treatment effect is influenced considerably by these several methods of presenting the results of a study. The precision of the estimate of the treatment effect is best presented as the 95% confidence limits around the point estimate. Studies with larger sample sizes will have smaller 95% confidence limits and therefore have greater precision. The precision of the estimate must be interpreted with respect to clinical relevance.

The third major question is "Will the results help me in the care of my patients?" There are 3 guides. These are: (1) Can the results be applied to my patient care? (2) Were all the clinically important outcomes considered? and (3) Are the likely benefits worth the potential harms and costs? [9]. The first guide deals with the generalizability of the study results. Randomized clinical trials have inclusion and exclusion criteria. Rather than rigidly applying these criteria to one's own patient, the recommended approach is to ask if there is a compelling reason not to apply the study results to a particular patient. Subgroup analyses within a "negative" study must be interpreted with caution. Oxman and Guyatt [13] suggest that subgroup analyses are credible if the difference in the treat-

ment effect: (1) is large; (2) is very unlikely to occur by chance; (3) is from an analysis specified as a hypothesis before the study began; (4) was one of very few subgroup analyses performed and (5) is replicated in other studies. The second guide deals with the clinical outcomes selected in the study. Substitute outcomes (e.g. forced expiratory volume, correction of anemia) may not always be associated with improved survival. Another important outcome which may not be considered is quality of life. The third guide deals with the balance between the treatment benefits and the potential harm from the treatment.

The use of this approach for decision making for individual patient problems is intellectually attractive. It applies the principle of continuing medical education in the self-directed problem-based mode currently used in many medical schools and postgraduate programs. Graduates should have these skills but may not have sufficient time to apply them in a busy medical practice. An alternative is to consider the use of overviews and clinical practice guidelines.

SYSTEMATIC OVERVIEWS OF THE MEDICAL LITERATURE

A guide to understanding systematic overviews has been written by Oxman and colleagues [14]. They use the term overview for any summary of the medical literature and meta-analysis for reviews that use quantitative methods to summarize the results. They suggest that the clinician ask the same three questions as posed for evaluation of individual articles. These are: (1) Are the results valid?; (2) What are the results? and (3) Will they be helpful in my patient care?

The first question has 2 primary and 4 secondary guides (Table 1.5). The first primary guide is: "Did the overview address a focused clinical question?" If the question asked is broad or unclear, it is unlikely that the overview will provide an answer to a specific question. The second primary guide is: "Were the criteria used to select articles for inclusion appropriate?" The criteria should specify the patients, interventions and outcomes of interest. Moreover, the types of research design should be specified. Unless these criteria are explicitly defined, different overviews which

Table 1.5. Validity of overview results

Primary guides
1.   Did the overview address a focused clinical question?
2.   Were the criteria used to select articles for inclusion appropriate?

Secondary guides
1.   Have important relevant studies been missed?
2.   Was the validity of the included studies appraised?
3.   Were assessments of studies reproducible?
4.   Were the results similar from study to study?

appear to address the same question lead to different conclusions [15]. If the inclusion criteria are defined, the author's tendancy to cite studies which support their own opinions may be diminished. The four secondary guides are shown in Table 1.5. The completeness of the search for relevant articles is difficult to evaluate. The authors should provide a description of the search strategy used. Ideally, the validity of the articles included in the overview should be subjected to the scrutiny described earlier in this chapter. The process used by the authors of the overview should be explicitly stated. The decisions about which articles to include, their validity and the data extraction process are judgements made by the authors of the overview. If several different individuals do this independently, the conclusions reached will have greater credibility. The final secondary guide is related to the similarity of results among studies. Despite careful adherence to inclusion criteria, there may be differences in outcomes among studies. These differences may be due to chance or to differences among studies with respect to patients, interventions and outcomes. The statistical test to evaluate this is a "test of homogeneity". If it is significant, the differences are less likely due to chance alone and the validity of combining these studies is questionable.

The second question is: "What are the results?" There are 2 guides addressing this question. The first is: "What are the overall results of the overview?" If the overview simply adds up positive and negative studies, important information may be lost, especially in studies showing a clinically important but statistically non-significant effect. These studies contain potentially important information but have inadequate statistical power to detect a clinically important effect of an intervention. The quantitative techniques (meta-analyses) weight studies according to size and methodologic strength. The reader should be provided with a table showing the effect size for each study and the weighted average effect size for all studies combined. The second guide is: "How precise are the results?" This is addressed by providing the 95% confidence interval around the point estimate for each study and for the combined studies.

The third question is: "Will the results help me in caring for my patients?" The three guides are identical to those used for the evaluation of individual articles addressing interventions.

RANDOMIZED CLINICAL TRIALS VERSUS META-ANALYSIS

A large well designed and conducted clinical trial represents the strongest level of evidence for the evaluation of a particular intervention. Application of the users guides for validity and generalizability is an effective technique for evaluating the methodologic strength of the study. The studies which satisfy these criteria are few and they are often considered "landmark" publications. If such a study is not available, meta-analysis permits the combination of smaller studies, preferably randomized clinical trials, addressing the same question. The methodologic problems associated with meta-analysis have been described. Additionally, there is a bias toward the publication of positive rather than negative results. This means that the studies available for inclusion in a meta-analysis will tend to be positive. The situation in which a large randomized clinical trial reports a negative result and a meta-analysis reports a positive result should not be a surprise. In that situation, the randomized clinical result is more likely to be the correct result.

Several recent randomized clinical trials of interventions for patients with renal failure have not produced a result consistent with prior expectations [16, 17]. The use of subgroup analysis and meta-analysis [18, 19] provided evidence which differed from the main analysis but are subject to the biases discussed in the sections dealing with these methodologic issues.

CLINICAL PRACTICE GUIDELINES

The busy clinician may not have time to critically evaluate either the individual articles dealing with interventions or with systematic overviews. There has been increasing interest in the development of clinical practice guidelines. The Dialysis Outcome Quality Inititiative (DOQI) is a recent example of such a process.

The process of clinical practice guideline developement has been described by Browman and colleagues [20] and summarized in a succinct manner by Davis and Taylor-Vaisey [21]. They describe 7 steps in the process. These are: (1) a national body decides to develope guidelines in a clinical area in which there is a perceived need for such guidelines; (2) data are synthesized from research information and relevant practice patterns and weighing the strength of the evidence in a systematic manner; (3) a group of experts review these data and produce guidelines; (4) the data are endorsed by the sponsoring organization; (5) the clinical practice guidelines are disseminated; (6) implementation strategies are initiated; (7) guidelines are subjected to re-appraisal and re-evaluation.

In the DOQI process, the National Kidney Foundation initiated the process and was the sponsoring agency. The relevant literature was identified though systematic literature searches and relevant publications selected by a panel of experts. Each article was reviewed from a methodologic and from a content viewpoint. The expert panel then produced a series of guidelines. Some were based on evidence; others were based on opinion. This was followed by an extensive review process and the guidelines were modified. They have been disseminated [22, 23] in recent issues of the *American Journal of Kidney Disease*. The process of dissemination has commenced.

FUTURE DIRECTIONS

The clinical practice guideline process produces pragmatic recommendations based partly on evidence and partly on clinical experience. The idealistic expectation that all clinicians can apply the skills of evidence-based medicine to individual articles or overviews appears unrealistic. An alternative approach is the Cochrane Collaboration. This is an international effort to prepare, maintain and disseminate systematic reviews of the effects of health care [24]. This is organized by specialty with the Nephrology Cochrane group located in France. The systematic reporting of methodologically rigourous overviews is a potential solution for the busy physician who wishes to efficiently locate important high quality evidence for clinical decision making.

REFERENCES

1. Williamson JW, German PS, Weiss R, Skinner EA and Bowes F. Health science information management and continuing education of physicians: a survey of US primary dare physicians and their opinion leaders. Ann Intern Med 1989; 110:151–60
2. Antman EM, Lao J, Kupelnick B, Mosteller F and Chalmers TC. A comparison of results of meta-analyses of randomized control trials and recommendations of clinical experts; treatments for myocardial infarction. JAMA 1992; 268:240–8
3. Evidence-Based Medicine Working Group. Evidence-based medicine: a new approach to teaching the practice of medicine. JAMA 1992; 268:2420–5.
4. Kuhn TS. The structure of scientific revolutions. Chicago, Ill: University of Chicago Press; 1970.
5. Carruthers SG, Larochelle P, Haynes RB, Petrasovits A and Schiffrin EL. Report of the Canadian hypertension society concensus conference: 1. Introduction. Can Med Asoc J 1993; 149:289–93
6. Oxman AD, Sackett DL, Guyatt GH for the Evidence-Based Medicine Working Group.Users guides to the medical literature. 1. How to get started. JAMA 1993; 270:2093–5.
7. Haynes RB, McKibbon KA, Fitzgerald D, Guyatt GH, Walker CJ and Sackett DL. How to keep up with the medical literature, V access by personal computer to the medical literature. Ann Intern Med 1990; 112:78–84.
8. Guyatt GH, Sackett DL, Cook DJ for the Evidence-Based Medicine Working Group. Users guides to the medical literature. II How to use an article about therapy or prevention. A. Are the results of the study valid? JAMA 1993; 270: 2598–601.
9. Guyatt GH, Sackett DL, Cook DL for the Evidence-Based Medicine Working Group. Users guides to the medical literature. II How to use an article about therapy or prevention. B. What were the results and will they help me in caring for my patients? JAMA 1994; 271:59–63.
10. Chalmers TC, Celano P, Sacks HS and Smith H Jr. Bias in treatment assignments in controlled clinical trials. N Engl J Med 1983; 309:1358–61.
11. Colditz GA, Miller JN and Mosteller F. How study design affects outcomes in comparisons of therapy, I. Medical. Stat Med 1989; 8:441–54.

12. Haynes RB, Mukherjee J, Sackett DL, Taylor DW, Barnett HJM and Peerless SJ. Functional status changes following medical or surgical treatment for cerebral ischemia: results in the EC/IC Bypass Study. JAMA 1987; 257:2043–6.

13. Oxman AD and Guyatt GH. A consumer's guide to subgroup analysis. Ann Intern Med 1992; 116: 78–84.

14. Oxman AD, Cook DJ, Guyatt GH for the Evidence-Based Medicine Working Group. Users' guides to the medical literature. VI. How to use an overview. JAMA 1994; 272:1367–71.

15. Chalmers TC, Berrier J, Sacks HS et al: Meta-analysis of clinical trials as a scientific discipline, II: replicate variability and comparison of studies that agree and disagree. Stat Med 1987; 6: 733–44.

16. Klahr S, Levey AD, Beck GJ, Caggiula AW, Hunsicker L, Kusek JW, Striker G for the Modification of Diet in Renal Disease Study Group. The effects of dietary protein restriction and blood-pressure control on the progression of chronic renal disease. N Engl J Med 1994; 330: 877–44

17. Mehta R, McDonald B, Gabbi F, Pahl M, Farkas A, Pascual M, Fowler W for the ARF Collaborative Study Group. Continuous versus intermittent dialysis for acute renal failure in the ICU. J Am Soc Nephrol 1996; 7:1457 (abstract).

18. Levey AS, Adler S, Caggiula AW, England BK, Greene T, Hunsicker LG et al. Effects of dietary protein restriction on the progression of advanced renal disease in the Modification of Diet in Renal Disease Study. Am J Kidney Dis 1996; 27:652–63.

19. Pedrini MT, Levey AS, Lau J, Chalmers TC and Wang PH. The effect of dietary protein restriction on the progression of diabetic and non-diabetic renal diseases: a meta-analysis. Ann Intern Med 1996; 124:627–32.

20. Browman GP, Levine MN, Mohide EA, Hayward RS, Pritchard KI, Gafni A et al: The practice guidelines developement cycle: a conceptual tool for practice guidelines development and implementation. J Clin Oncol 1995; 13:502–12

21. Davis DA and Taylor-Vaisey A. Translating guidelines into practice: a systematic review of theoretic concepts, practical experience and research evidence in the adoption of clinical practice guidelines. Can Med Assoc J 1997; 157:408–16.

22. NFK-DOQI clinical practice guidelines for hemodialysis adequacy. National kidney foundation. Am J Kidney Dis 1997; 30:S15–66.

23. NKF-DOQI clinical practice guidelines for peritoneal dialysis adequacy. National kidney foundation. Am J Kidney Dis 1997; 30:S67–136.

24. The Cochrane Collaboration, Oxford, England UK. Cochrane Centre, National Health Service Research and Development Programme; 1994.

2. A continuous quality improvement paradigm for health care networks

EDMUND G. LOWRIE

"... it is necessary that a method should be found by which our beliefs may be determined by ... something upon which our thinking has no effect ... Such is the method of science.
'... there follows one corollary which itself deserves to be inscribed upon every wall of the city of philosophy: Do not block the way of inquiry."

(C.S. Peirce, 1887 & 1899) [1: pp 18 & 54]

The pragmatic method is primarily a method .... to interpret each notion by tracing its respective practical consequences. What difference would it practically make to anyone if this notion rather than that notion were true? If no practical difference whatever can be traced, then the alternatives mean practically the same thing, and all dispute is idle.

(William James, 1907) [2: p 377]

"Create a consistency of purpose ... Cease dependence on mass inspection ... Drive out fear ... Break down barriers between staff areas ... Eliminate slogans ... Eliminate numerical quotas ... Remove barriers that rob people of pride of workmanship ... The job of management is not supervision, but leadership ... Take action ... Improve consistently and forever."

(W. Edwards Deming, 1982) [3: Chapter 2]

Continuous Quality Improvement (CQI) is a matter of philosophy, not technique; hence, I offer those quotations. The paradigm is born of attitude more than discipline, particularly in distributed service networks like health care organizations. It applies practical, goal directed, clinical science to hierarchical human productivity systems. The goal is clear; define quality in some simple term(s) and pursue it with dispatch and vigor. Scientific inquiry is the method meaning that preconception, bias, and tradition for the sake of itself can play no role. Improvement is always possible, particularly in fields such as medicine where the knowledge base changes rapidly, so the inquiry is ongoing.

There is a purpose; the process has practical and urgent objectives. Therefore, bickering about minutia that have few practical consequences must be avoided just as preconception is purged from scientific thought. William James, a physician, understood. Debating inconsequence fritters time; matters should be kept as simple as possible.

The implementation strategy by which new knowledge is used to improve quality is perhaps the most important part of the paradigm. Quality can not be forced, or levered, into a health care system by algorithms, rules, or cook books delivered by those at the top. The many heads and hands closest to the action, the ones that provide the care, do not belong to mindless robots given to clinics simply to do piecemeal work on patients. Instead, most are professionals, many with advanced training, licensed to provide care. They are the ones with whom patients have the moral agency agreement[1] and therefore are directly accountable to the patient for the quality of care. Hence, the implementation strategy, its philosophy and structure, must consider carefully the nature of the human system in which quality is to be continuously improved.

The CQI process, while serious, should be fun; it should be a source of both pleasure and professional reward for active minded and involved clinicians who provide care in organized health care delivery systems. It is an ongoing process that is never finished because perfection is an ever receding goal. Practical information is used in practical ways to deliver better care. Information from many locations is pooled allowing the synthesis of new knowledge on a larger scale. However, both pooled knowledge and local information are used locally in deliberative ways to evaluate local performance and solve local problems using structured and quantitative tools. Command, control, and coercion from the top of the organization must yield to leadership, listening and support in such a system. Such things as records and charts,

L.W. Henderson and R.S. Thuma (eds.), Quality Assurance in Dialysis, 2nd Edition, 7–26.
© *1999 Kluwer Academic Publishers. Printed in Great Britain*

time trend, regression, and Pareto analysis (all illustrated later), and even technical or medical knowledge are only the tools of inquiry, responsiveness, and purpose.

I will first describe a health care network that could apply to clinical practice clusters, companies, or even governments. Next, will come conceptual development of the CQI paradigm discussing management of the human system before the technical process. I will then illustrate the paradigm, and some of the simple tools to support it, using "live" data accumulated over the years. Finally, I will close with mention of unanswered issues because the CQI paradigm must ask as well as answer questions.

CQI management is a matter of philosophy. All of the principles described herein, therefore, though drawn from others, are personal. Similarly, the data and anecdotes used as illustrations come from actual experiences during 15 years as administrative medical officer for a large network of hemodialysis providers.

THE HEALTH SERVICE NETWORK

Figure 2.1 illustrates schematically the configuration of a health services network showing the relationships that may exist between numerous remote facilities and a central organization. The central organization could be a company, a large hospital or practice organization, or a government. The facilities could be any set of activity nodes such as dialysis units or the operating subunits in any organization.

The facilities' staff include physician medical directors, and other affiliated physicians, who may or may not be directly employed by the facility or central organization. Even if directly employed, however, the control exercised over their discretionary actions on behalf of patients must be limited. Such control should be exercised only in circumstances indicating incompetence, malfeasance, or malpractice. Otherwise, control exercised by non-medical authority, or medical authority with no direct contact with individual patients, usurps the patients' rights to combine their physicians' judgments with their own to decide about appropriate treatment plans.

Indeed, the use of coercion to enforce desired

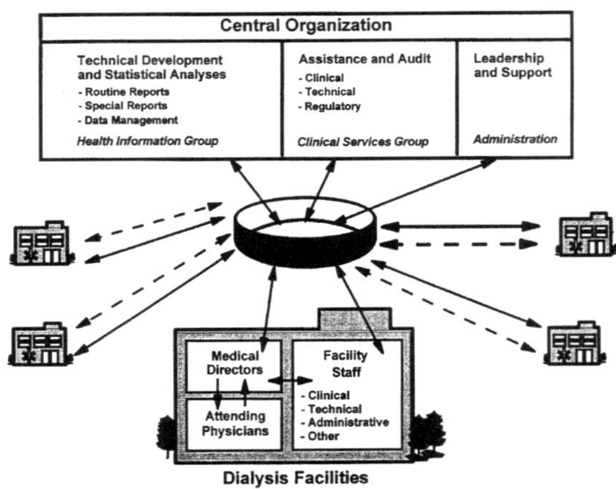

Fig. 2.1. Schematic illustration of a health service network with remote facilities connected through communication links to a central support organization.

practice patterns, or the setting of rigid practice rules by companies, governments, or other large organizations, have as their premise denial of the patient's right to participate fully in his or her own care. The right to complete disclosure, anticipating consent to treat, is effectively breached. The physician's choices are restricted and the patient can not possibly discuss individually his or her care plan with the company or government. Such blanket and possibly ill informed restrictions, for example, would not be tolerated by companies or governments if they were evoked by the clinical care teams to reduce work or enhance profit.

Physicians (and other licensed health care personnel) hold advanced degrees and have often received post-degree specialized education, neither often possessed by remote, administrative structures. They are licensed to provide service in the areas where they practice. The organizations are not licensed to prescribe; the physicians are. Finally, the administrative structures usually have no direct knowledge of the patient for whose benefit prescriptive actions are taken; the agency agreement granted by patients to providers is generally between the patient and individual humans – not facilities, corporations, or a government. Hence, we show dashed arrows between the care giving units in Figure 2.1 and the central organization to represent the nature of the clinical

↔ administrative relationship; they are bi-directional to show that communication is two-way.

The facility staff includes clinical, technical, and other administrative functions that usually do not prescribe treatment directly and are mostly employed by the facility or organization. It is appropriate that greater control be exercised over their daily activities so the bi-directional arrows are solid. Organizations, companies, or governments, however, must not interfere with the licensed practice of professional staff in the discharge of their daily duties with the exception of assuring the competence of staff to perform those duties.

Although the figure suggests a single organization exercising control over many facilities, a better paradigm would be illustrated by inversion of the figure so that the company, or government, is below the facilities showing that it supports them. The support includes the collection, digestion, analysis, and distribution of clinically related statistical material and assistance with clinical and technical process development. Clinical monitoring and audit are important functions. However, the central organization should not attempt to direct the behavior in facilities through command, control, coercion, or sanction.

Facility staffs, after all, are close to "where the rubber meets the road" and as such have detailed information about events and practices in the facilities. Only they can improve the quality of care provided in the unit because they are the ones who give the care. As such, their activities in the partnership with larger organizations will generally involve detailed on-site evaluation, planning, and clinical action. On the other hand, most facilities do not have the resources, information, capacities, or exposure to process, analyze, evaluate and distribute large volumes of data used to inform the CQI process. Larger organizations are more likely to have those capabilities.

The partnership between the support organization and the facility is illustrated by Figure 2.2. Support organizations evaluate outcomes and perform statistical analyses sharing them with the facilities. Facilities review both those reports and their own data as part of their CQI activities. As outcomes change, support organizations summarize, analyze and redistribute information to the facilities for use in their CQI processes. While support organizations might use powerful statistical instruments, like multi-variable analysis, relatively simple yet powerful analytical tools are available to both organizations. Those tools will be used later as part of a clinical illustration showing how the process works.

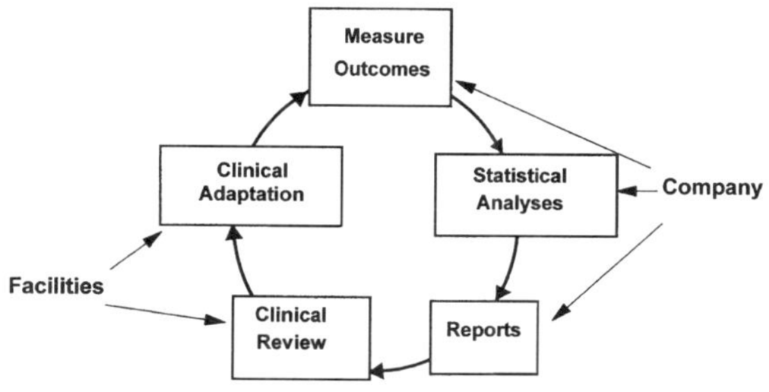

Fig. 2.2. Schematic illustration of the information flows and tasks roughly partitioned by responsibility in the facility-company partnership. The "company" could be any large, support organization including a government.

A STRATEGY FOR HUMAN SYSTEM STRUCTURES

W. Edwards Deming (1900–1993) earned a Ph.D. in Physics from Yale University in 1928. He had worked in manufacturing but after graduation began a career in government service with the US Department of Agriculture and later the Census Department. He encountered Walter Shewhart, a statistician with Bell Telephone Laboratories, early in his career. Shewhart was probably the father of statistical quality control (SQC) [4] and made major contributions to Deming's thought. Deming later commented that Shewhart's real genius lay in the fact that Shewhart knew when *not* to intervene in a manufacturing process.

Deming left government service in 1946 to establish a statistical consulting practice and to teach in the graduate school of business administration at New York University in which pursuits he remained until his death. He consulted with the Japanese government about the post-World War II census later becoming deeply involved with national movements to improve the quality of products manufactured in Japan. Those efforts assisted the transformation of Japanese industry so that the label, "Made in Japan", was associated with reliable product and was no longer used as a demeaning epithet to suggest poor quality. Indeed, in 1960 the Emperor awarded him the prestigious Second Order Medal of the Sacred Treasure. The Japanese Union of Scientists and Engineers instituted in 1950 an annual award(s) bearing his name for contributions by companies and persons to methods insuring the quality and dependability of products. In 1986, President Regan awarded him the National Medal of Technology for his forceful promotion of statistical methodology, contributions to sampling theory, and for his advocacy of philosophies that resulted in improved product quality for consumers and better efficiency for corporations.

Deming's greatest insights, however, applied not so much to statistical theory as to organizational and human resource management. By the 1950s, the statistical techniques advocated by Deming and his colleagues were being used less and less frequently in the United States. They were regarded as too difficult and time consuming. The technical people could be taught the methods, use them, and analyze the results but top management for the most part knew little about the process; without pressure from top management for quality nothing would happen in a company. Quality enhancement, Deming learned, is more a matter of organizational management than it is of technical process control. His insights, and the theories evolving from them, apply as much to service organizations as they do to the manufacturing environments for which they were originally intended.

The structure for Deming's understanding rests on four integrated, conceptual cornerstones [5] that are each as reinforcing to the others as are the corner posts of a well built home.

1. *Appreciation for a system.* A system, for our purpose, is an organized cluster, or network, of assets, processes, and people that function together to accomplish certain goals. The definition is thereby restricted to human enterprise systems. A system without a goal(s) is not a system; it is reduced to idle assets, unproductive processes, and confused people. The greater the interaction, or interdependence, between the system components required to achieve the goal(s), the greater will be the need for communication and cooperation between, and therefore management of, them.

The obligation of each human member of the system is to contribute to its efficient functioning in pursuit of the goal(s) and *not* to maximize his or her production, profit, or other "competitive" measure by which people are sometimes "judged". The obligation does not void the responsibility for encouraging necessary controversy; indeed, that is strengthened. To manage a system in that way, top management must understand how its components function together to achieve the goal(s) and must be very clear, in both word and deed, about what those goals are.

2. *Knowledge about variation.* If a person is above average with respect to a particular measure and another person is below average, is one better than the other? Of course not. If there is an average, some must be above and some below it. The issues are, by much and how often.

All measurements have distributions and the real question about measures that describe processes is, "Is the process stable and in control?" A process that is in statistical control has dependable capabilities; a random process does not. One must not aim, therefore, at discrete targets and then adjust processes repetitively to hit them after (near) misses. Such "tinkering" begets unstable processes. Rather, one should understand the distribution of outputs from a process and monitor the process, not whether target is hit exactly. The critical decision about particular measurements that depart from the goal is; 1) Is this (or are these) within the range of acceptable variation?, or 2) Is there some special cause that requires investigation or intervention.

There also exits substantial variation among the attributes of individuals even though each may have comparable potential to contribute to the efficiency and function of an organization. Understanding that principle is critical to efficient system management. The manager of people must understand the natural variation among them and how to extract potential from people converting it into contribution.

3. *Theory of knowledge.* Neither facts nor information are knowledge. Knowledge about a thing is little more than a belief system that informs and enables actions with respect to the thing. For example, "knowledge" that a red light at a traffic intersection means that oncoming automobiles must stop enables our decision to cross the street.

According to Pierce [1], beliefs are fixed in several ways. Many people, even most, simply submit to the *authority* of another – a parent, the church, a government, a professional organization. They may be decide by an *a priori* process such a pure reasoning absent empirical information or simple preference. Once formed, important beliefs are often held with great *tenacity* surrendered reluctantly despite evidence to the contrary. He rejected those methods in favor of careful observation followed by sound (logical) reasoning and called that method *science.*

James taught that the worth of beliefs should be judged by the results they produce because the practical function of beliefs is to enable actions [2]. The CQI paradigm focuses on practical and objective ways to improve quality; its cornerstone is endless inquiry. That is why quotations from those thinkers open this chapter. The principals are discussed more fully and in somewhat less abstract terms elsewhere focusing on the use of large, clinical data bases to support new dialysis related knowledge [7].

For our purpose, clinicians' knowledge usually derives from a combination of authority and experience. In so much as knowledge informs clinical action, new observations that contradict exiting beliefs create uncertainty – discomfort on the part of those who must act on behalf of patients. "How does one treat this symptom now anyway? I used to think…" or "Have I been doing it wrong?" or "How does everyone else do it now?" are not comfortable questions for the caring clinician. One must anticipate the discomfort, and therefore possible resistance, that new information causes in people if one is to take full advantage of clinicians' experience and understanding as new knowledge is introduced into the system.

Clinicians can rely comfortably on the authority of government or other large organizations such as professional organizations and companies to inform their "knowledge". That way they can minimize uncertainty, absolve themselves of responsibility, and avoid much of the discomfort associated with change – "Everyone else is doing it" or even "They made me do it" helps purge the stress. But then the system looses their specialized and highly valuable experience and understanding.

Relying on authority to evoke change in clinical belief systems is little more that a top down command to which clinicians are highly vulnerable these days. But what if the authority is wrong? The patients suffer on a large scale, not the clinicians or the authority.

4. *Psychology.* The manager of people must understand their differences and use them to achieve the goal(s) of the organization. This is not a performance ranking; it is understanding how human capability and motive can be used to support goal achievement. Different people have different motives; some (most) really are more intrinsically motivated to do a good job than extrinsically motivated to earn a large bonus. The job of a good hiring manager is to distinguish one from the other.

People learn in different ways and training systems should accommodate those differences. Some learn better from graphs and lectures; some do better with reading; others are hands on learners.

The manager of people should "manage" the people on their terms and not the manager's – which simply says that she or he should understand them as individuals and not as robot-like task renderers. Deming said it this way, "The most important act that a manager can take is to understand what it is that is important to an individual". He or she must also understand the goals of the system and how the system works else she or he can not assist the proper management of people to achieve the goal(s).

Finally, the manager of people must understand how to reduce human friction in the system. Promoting competition in the system with respect to quotas or other targets, for example, rather than cooperation may win a sales or production contest while sacrificing the larger goal(s) of the system as a whole. Creating systems of individual rewards creates systems of individual performers when it is cooperation among the parts that ensures an efficient system.

Deming illustrated his approach to organizational management with 14 key principles. I will list them and will comment about each briefly. As before, the principles are Deming's; the comments are mine; I refer the reader to Deming's books [3, 5] and also to a lucid explanation of his principles and practice [6].

1. *Create consistency of purpose for improvement of product and service.* We read the mission statements from large companies, "create shareholder value" they often say. Health care payer and provider companies have the same goal. The most pressing aim for the largest health care payer, government, is to control cost. Government must be considered an integral part of this health delivery system. It pays large fractions of the bills, writes regulatory standards, and inspects facilities to assure compliance with its standards. Its powers to inflict sanction are substantial no matter the right or wrong of a particular circumstance.

The mission statements of clinical service departments in the companies, on the other hand, usually start with words about giving high quality care. Which is the real first mission? If the answer is "both", which takes precedence when they are in conflict? Chief executives are responsible to their constituents, shareholders – large investment firms for the most part – not the ordinary citizens that consume health care. Clinical service departments respond to their constituents – patients and the people who care for them.

When conflict comes in American firms, the organization generally yields to the chief executive, not the clinician, because that is where the financial power resides. What is the nurse to say when she is told "quality" but is judged solely on her ability to beat a budget that is often not of her or his making? At the margin, then, greater weight will be given to the venture capitalist or fund manager than to the clinician unless the chief executive understands completely both the system for providing care and the principles of quality management; only then might she or he drive quality into the organization with the same (or more) fervor as he or she responds to large institutional shareholders in pursuit of greater shareholder value.

If government even threatens to withhold payment for beneficial therapies, or wrongfully pro-

motes a therapeutic guideline, quality enhancement suffers from practical reality – the fear of financial loss, administrative sanction, or charge of fraud. Quality yields to those realities. When government's motives conflict, as in companies, quality will suffer just as it does when companies are not clear about their real mission.

Unfortunately, there appears in our US systems of care these days substantial and evolving inconsistency of purpose among its actors. The party with the most to gain or lose, the patient, seems to have the least to say. Chief executives, government agencies, and other actors have the capacity to promote consistent quality oriented purpose but will do so only if they believe it is in their best long-term interest to do so. Patients seem to have little ability to demand it.

2. *Adopt a new philosophy.* Health service delivery systems are undergoing dramatic reorganization in the United States. Economic, not quality, matters are driving the change. Those who award health care contracts for large groups of patients – employees, unions, and beneficiaries – and who therefore pay the bills appear now more interested in price/cost than in quality. Patients have become little more than bartering chips in the negotiation.

If quality is to be established in the system, it must carry equal weight with price. Physicians, nurses, and executives with more than a financial mission and who understand their care systems can accomplish such a philosophical transformation if they focus on it and if they wish to do so.

3. *Cease dependence on mass inspection.* Systems that rely on "care rules", and inspection to insure compliance with them, can only improve quality much too late even if the rule is right. The "defect" has occurred by the time the inspector finds it; the paradigm has at its root the intent to manage defects.

The inspector does not trust the caregiver believing that the judgments of the inspector are superior to those of the caregiver. What if the rule is wrong? The paradigm then institutionalizes poor care and stifles constructive inquiry and therefore progress. It is better to get the care process right in the first place, leaving room for acceptance of new and better treatments, and eliminate mass inspection.

4. *End the practice of awarding business on the basis of price tag alone.* Price has little meaning without considering the quality of the service purchased unless the buyer is not concerned with quality. Patients are concerned with quality; purchasers who are not also the consumers of care may not be so concerned. If the primary concern is with short term cost or profit, then price tag becomes the controlling issue. That principle applies to governments as well as health service providers.

Health services are generally purchased on behalf of patients rather than directly by patients in the United States. Therefore, the price paid is determined by those with only indirect interest in the quality of service but direct interest in its price. Chief executives must realize and believe that it is in the long term interest of their firm, and government officials must believe that it is in the long term interest of the government, to promote quality systems for which they, as well as health service providers, are responsible. To properly implement such a belief, they, the executives and officials, must understand quality as well as they do prices and costs.

5. *Improve consistently and forever the system of production and service.* The idea is the heart of the CQI paradigm. But it really means that the paradigm, the philosophy, must be built into the health service system from the start. Quality must be designed into products and treatment delivery systems; the CQI paradigm is simply a matter of daily human behavior among all actors in the care delivery system. When asked why they do something in a particular way, the worker in a CQI driven organization would simply explain, "That is the right way and how things are done here".

6. *Institute training.* Training should be structured so that all levels of management and production understand the scope and nature of the services provided. Health regulators, and those setting payment, need to understand (receive training about) the services for which they set policy. That may include actually assisting in the operations of a facility or the delivering the care.

Deming observed that Japanese management had, by its nature, some important advantages over American management with respect to train-

ing. A person in management started his career with a long internship (4–10 years) "on the floor" and in other duties around the company. Those might include: purchasing, accounting, sales, distribution, manufacturing, or research and development. When assuming responsibility for general management then, the candidate was fully acquainted with all of the company's functions and its operating structures.

Too often, the emphasis in American organizations is placed on management more than understanding. Cost control, achievement of quotas, discipline and reward techniques, making budgets, and so forth often take precedence in the managers' pre-employment education and post-employment training with much less regard for the quality of service or product and how it is delivered or manufactured.

7. *Adopt and institute leadership.* Leaders must understand the work for which they are ultimately responsible but they do not direct the tasks by which it is accomplished. Supervision is not the same as leadership. Directorship is not the same as leadership. Commandership is not the same as leadership.

Leaders must know their work (both its cost [profit] and quality attributes) and be empowered to inform upper management about conditions that need correction. Subordinate leaders must not simply tell upper management what it is they think the boss wants to hear. Such persons should not be selected for promotion because they will one day want subordinates to tell them what they want to hear.

One attribute of leadership is responsiveness and upper management must evaluate and act on proposed corrections to the system. Another attribute of leadership is trust – two way trust between superiors and subordinates. Integrity, "plain talk", and honest motives are prerequisites for such mutual trust. From the subordinate: dedicated effort and honest opinion are appropriate, condescending agreement to tell the boss what he wants to hear is not. From the superior: guidance, direction and support are appropriate; punishment is not. Without such relationships, information cannot be reliably passed through the decision hierarchy of an organization from places where services are provided or product is made to higher levels where policy is determined and capital allocated.

8. *Drive out fear.* No one can perform well when they are afraid; fear evokes defensive, not cooperative behaviors; fear to an extreme is disabling. Fear of lost jobs, fear of government sanction, fear of reimbursement cuts for health service – all give birth to self-defensive, adaptive behaviors that often serve to defeat the best motives of those who instill the fear. The unintended result is often compromised quality.

When the US government cut the price for dialysis service, the industry responded making up the loss by capturing reimbursement for ancillary service revenue previously sent elsewhere. Government also changed the reimbursement method for an important new drug used to treat anemia (erythropoietin) from a fixed rate per administration, no matter the dose, to one that paid more money for larger doses. (Please see Figure 2.19 used elsewhere for illustrating another point.) Dialysis units responded by increasing the dose dramatically; blood counts increased by marginal amounts; the government paid millions more dollars; now government refuses to pay for any drug if the blood count is above a certain level that is still considered clinically anemic. Payment is proscribed even if physicians certify that the treatment is necessary for the patient's well-being.

In other words, fear of financial loss on the parts of both dialysis providers and the primary payer, government, drove (mal)adaptive behaviors on the part of both parties that resulted in government rationing effective care – denying it really – to its beneficiaries even though those providing the care believe it necessary for the patient's health. A federal overseer, or political leader, would not tolerate such a practice if the provider were denying the treatment in order make a profit. That denial by a provider would have been no different from the government's current denial in order to save money. They should have found a better, quality oriented, way to control expenditures.

Finally, many providers of dialysis care have agreed, for the time, to a method for describing dialysis dose, the urea reduction ratio (URR)[2] about which much more will be said later. There now exists a rough consensus about values associated with better clinical outcome. Government began inspecting facilities to see if those targets were met. Providers then began to adopt new methods for measuring the URR that yield higher numerical values of it but without changing the amount of therapy actually given the patient. The focus was now on the URR number, not on the outcome of treatment.

Thus, there occurred an "honest effort" to game the system caused by nothing but the fear of punishment. One might say that the books are cooked in pursuit of self-preservation. There was, for example, little, if any, pressure for a new URR measurement method during the 5 or more years that it was used as a clinical measure before the threat of potential sanction. Thus, instilling fear into the system by ill-informed policy served to compromise a potentially valuable quality measure.

9. *Break down barriers between staff areas.* We find in our health care system, a circumstance in which payers, frequently government, does not trust the motive of service providers and service providers trust even less the motive of payers, government pay setters, and regulators. I have already mentioned a few anecdotes. Wouldn't it be better if the barriers were broken down?

We see the same dynamic in organizations. In companies that both provide service and manufacture product, the product group often wants to sell more product at higher price to the service group; the service group wants to purchase less product at lower price. Success can only be achieved if the parts of a company, or system, work as a team – each understanding the strengths, weaknesses, problems, and frustrations of the others as well as their own. Only then can each part of the system optimize its own performance for the benefit of the whole. Self interested provincialism is a prescription for sub-optimal performance and ultimate mediocrity if not outright failure.

10. *Eliminate slogans, exhortations and targets for the work force.* Top management telling a work force that, "We tolerate zero defects" has no meaning. Neither do such slogans as, "Do it right the first time" or "Our goal is to increase productivity by 40%". They may work well as selling tools for upper management, management consultants, and perhaps institutional shareholders but they are effective only if those who do the work write the

slogan. How can a clinical staff reduce wasteful supply use if a purchasing department buys bad product in pursuit of low price? Slogans can not cure systematic problems; team work and planning can; relying on slogans can be destructive because they divert attention from the real tasks at hand.

11. *Eliminate numerical quotas for the work force and numerical goals for people in management.* Quotas are set of necessity at some statistical average for workers. Some can easily achieve or exceed the quota. About half should be able to do so statistically speaking. Once the quota is achieved, it's time for coffee. Peer pressure may hold down the achiever; where is the motive to excel? Others below average will struggle; the result is frustration, dissatisfaction, and turnover. Deming said, "A quota is a fortress against improvement of quality and productivity". I say that management quotas cannot solve systemic problems.

Management by numerical objective is little more than a quota. Relying on management by numerical objective can also be destructive. To manage and enterprise, one must lead its people. To lead, one must understand both the work and the workers. Management by numerical objective reflects an attempt to manage without understanding not knowing otherwise what to do.

12. *Remove barriers that rob people of pride of workmanship.* This principle is particularly true for health care companies the work forces of which are composed mainly of professionals with advanced education, many licensed by governments to practice their art. They know much more about the nature of the service provided than most managers at the top. How can those company or government managers set acceptable quality oriented work standards for physicians, nurses, dietitians, social workers, and others who provide care in today's health environment. The managers are frequently cost-driven – the number of patients seen per day, the number of hospital visits made per hour, the number and cost of tests ordered, and so forth. Who setting those quotas can assure the quality? How can one expect quality care from a physician or a nurse working in a system so managed when the manager cannot even tell them what quality is or how to achieve it?

13. *Encourage education and self improvement for everyone.* An organization needs good people that continuously improve themselves and are willing to return those personal improvements to the health care system in which they serve. The education includes not only matters of technical care but also the principles of quality management.

As noted earlier changing beliefs can be difficult. It creates uncertainty; orientation points for behavior are disturbed. Continuing inquiry is a critical cornerstone of the CQI paradigm as explained more fully later. As new knowledge is borne from inquiry, resistance is encountered. Participating in the development of new knowledge reduces resistance. Avoiding threat of punishment evolving from new knowledge reduces resistance. Strategies must be developed to overcome resistance gently so that the knowledge is introduced easily into the system without causing resistance or demoralizing care givers.

14. *Take action to accomplish the transformation.* Corporate executives and government policymakers should struggle with Deming's key principles and other beliefs. Refocusing from short term financial objectives to long term quality enhancement is not an easy matter. But if it is quality, or the quality/cost ratio, that is in the long term interest of a company or government, then Deming's prescription is a good one.

Much of the foregoing sounds insensitive of the needs of companies, profit or non-profit, to realize a surplus of revenues over costs – that is to say, make a profit. It sounds insensitive also to the needs of government to control its expenditures. Neither perception could be further from the truth.

I, as former operating officer in a large company, understand as well as any the need for companies to earn profits. Absent a return on invested capital there will be no capital to support the creation of service delivery systems. Arguing against the profit, therefore, is self-defeating if the aim is to deliver quality health care. However, the problem appears to be one of focus – on the short term financial expectation of some investors rather than on the long term health of a service delivery system. Unfortunately, that focus often serves to reduce revenue and increase cost.

As a taxpayer, I am sympathetic to the attempts of government to control its expenditures. But the efforts of government to control cost has often resulted in higher expenditures. As one physician said to me, "Every time they cut payment, we make more money". As one federal health executive said in a public forum, "Every time we pull something in, something else pops out". Of course, governments or health insurers could stop payments completely and save money. But then who in the long run would loose the most? Likely patients who could not find care; providers would simply do something else.

It seems to me that a government, and even companies, have a social obligation exceeding by a wide margin cost control; competent quality enhancement is one way to discharge that obligation. Even though controlling costs is important, even critical, service should not follow finance; finance should follow service. The faith must be kept among health service executives and government policy-makers that if quality and productivity are well attended to, then favorable finance will surely follow.

Deming's roots were in mathematics and physical science. He worked extensively with and taught the quantitative and statistical approach to process control and production management in pursuit of quality. Though firmly grounded in the hard sciences and quantitative methods, he came to realize through rich experience that the real key to quality enhancement is found in the creative management of the human system that produces the product or delivers the service.

THE CQI PROCESS

Figure 2.3 illustrates the three part process: assessment, action, and assurance. All three must function in both facilities and support organizations. "Assurance" is a large part of facility activities and involves record-keeping and evaluation of variances from the facility's standard practice that is adopted with the advice and consent of the parent. The job of support organizations is audit and information sharing. Facilities take "Action" to correct process variances and modify policy and procedure as new information becomes available. They evaluate both their own information and that

received from the support organization as a prerequisite for action.

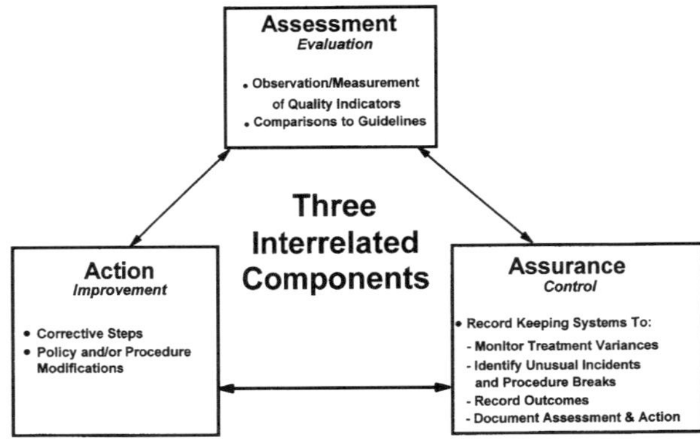

Fig. 2.3. The 3 interrelated components of a quality enhancement system.

Support organizations collect and evaluate information received from facilities before returning summaries of it for use by the facilities as suggested by Figure 2.2. Figure 2.4 illustrates a possible system to support that obligation. Laboratory and other clinical data are entered, screened for validity, and stored in a central location. Health information groups at the parent provide statistical reports to the facilities. Those reports are generally of two classes: 1) routine summaries of the facilities activities with benchmark data reflecting system wide performance, and 2) ad hoc reports intended to address matters of current interests. Both types of report will be illustrated later.

Quality Assurance

I will say little about quality Control at the facility level reserving most of my comments for Assessment and Action that are the hallmarks of the collaboration between central organizations and their affiliated facilities. Figure 2.5, however, illustrates a Quality Control process that is both cyclical and continuous. Information from internal audits and material, including the routine reports, information sharing flyers, and external audits performed by the company or government are reviewed; recommendations are made, proce-

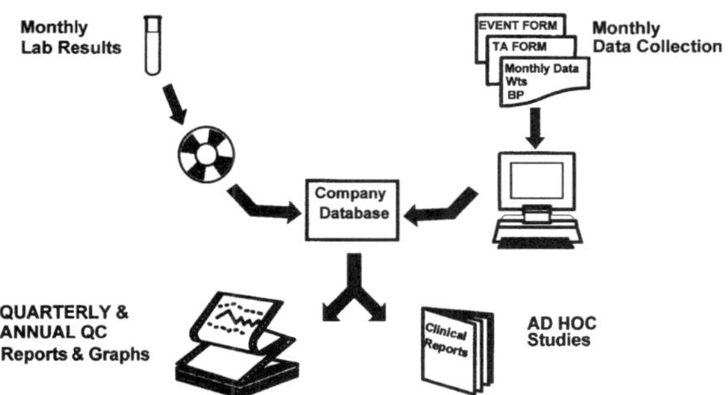

Fig. 2.4. Schematic illustration of a system architecture to support quality improvement activities. "Event" means admission (with baseline information) to the facility, discharge (and reason) from the facility, prescription change and so forth. "TA" means temporary absence for a variety of reasons including hospitalization (and reason).

dures are modified if necessary and documented. Logs, medical records, and other records are kept and reviewed as part of the facility's routine monitoring activities. The cycle starts once more when updated material is again reviewed, modifications to existing practice made, and so forth.

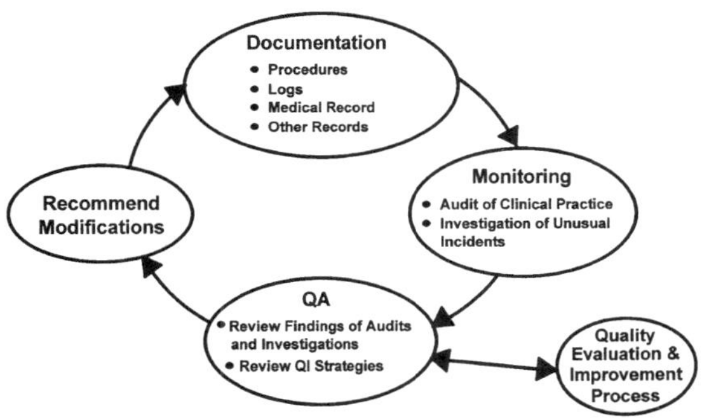

Fig. 2.5. Schematic illustration of the cyclical quality control process at the facility level and its interface with quality evaluation and improvement activities in both the facility and central support organization.

Quality Assessment and Improvement

Quality assessment is a focused, scientific process; it is neither abstract nor ill-defined. Outcome measures thought to reflect quality are identified unambiguously. A hierarchy of antecedent processes likely associated with the outcome, evalu-

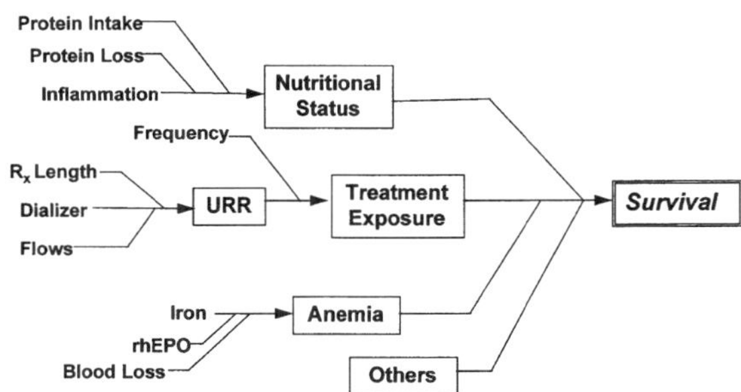

Fig. 2.6. Illustration of the relationship between outcomes and processes of care using a simplified cause and effect diagram. The designation of outcome or process is relative. The processes (designated at the left end of each line) can be the outcomes (shown in boxes) of other, antecedent, processes.

ated by measurement and themselves outcomes of other processes, are considered.

Figure 2.7 illustrates the idea. We choose survival for our illustrations because the purpose of dialysis is to preserve a life that would otherwise be lost. Many processes converge on the outcome of primary interests. But even those processes are outcomes of other processes. For example, Figure 2.6 suggests that treatment exposure influences survival. Treatment exposure, the dialysis process, here is measured by the URR and the number of treatments given during a week (say). However, the URR for a particular patient is the outcome of other processes such as the choice of dialyzer, the blood and dialysate flow rates at which it is operated, and the treatment time.

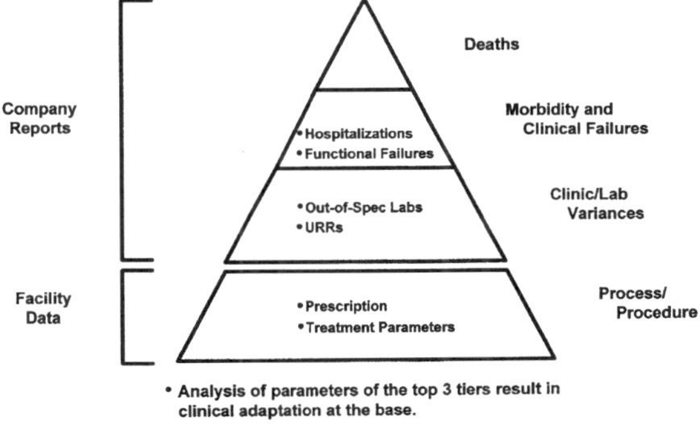

Fig. 2.7. The quality triangle. The hierarchy of failures and variances is illustrated according to the primary source of information used to summarize them.

The hierarchy of outcomes and processes can also be arranged as a quality triangle – Figure 2.7 – in which the outcome of primary interest is at the top. Hospitalization, subjective quality of life, or other such measurable quantities could well reside at the apex of this triangle. While hospitalization frequency could equally well be an outcome of primary interest, it can also be regarded as a subordinate associate of death. Similarly, the frequency with which laboratory values are found to be out of a specified reference range could be an outcome measure. However, such variances also can be considered antecedent to more serious failures. If they are not antecedent to more serious failure, why measure the tests? We use the URR here to reflect hemodialysis treatment exposure. It is only a specialized laboratory tests. All parameters can be monitored at the facility level but should be summarized across facilities for them by support organizations.

Understanding the chains of associations as they converge on outcomes is key to the CQI process. Only then can process be altered to improve outcome. The paradigm starts with a plan that leads to testing or perhaps changing techniques or process. The tests or effects of change are observed and the results studied. That process leads to another "plan, test or change, observe, evaluate" cycle; the cycle is repeated infinitely as suggested by Figure 2.8. It is called the Shewhart cycle after its author who first described the idea in 1939.

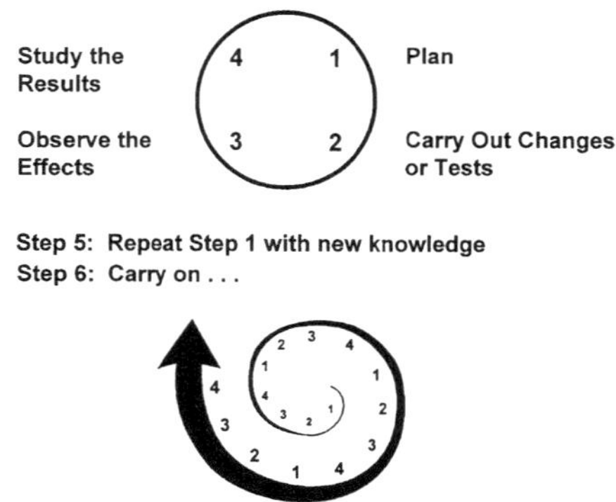

Fig. 2.8. Illustration of the Shewhart cycle in which sequential steps are carried out continuously in pursuit of improving quality.

Many of the analytic tools used by large support organization to support this paradigm will be sophisticated requiring specialized statistical knowledge. There are available, however, simple yet powerful tools easily used by persons with no statistical knowledge. Some are shown in Figure 2.9; the picture shows the tool; their use will be illustrated in following paragraphs.

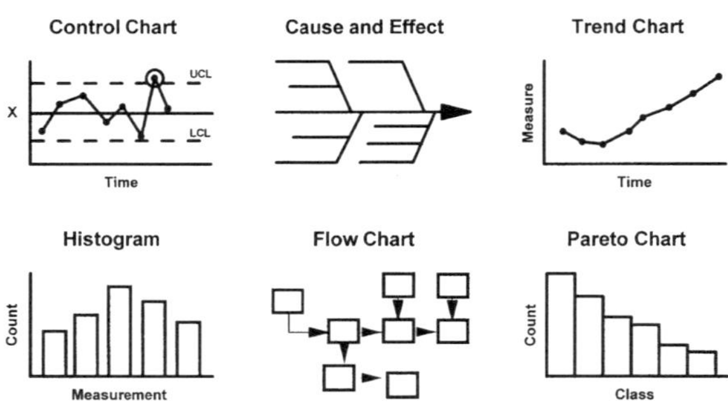

Fig. 2.9. Illustration of some simple yet powerful, quantitative tools that can be used to assist analysis as part of the quality improvement process.

Reports and their Use

Because the CQI paradigm is driven by information, I will review the nature and purpose of some important reports distributed by support organizations and illustrate the use of data to drive decisions.

Routine reports
Routine statistical reports summarizing the results of measuring key parameters for all facilities and for the individual facility are distributed frequently – say, every three months – for use in facility quality enhancement activities. Figures 2.10 show time trend charts of quarterly mortality ratios. Mortality is determined and adjusted statistically for age, sex, race, and the frequency of complicating conditions such as diabetes. The observed mortality rate (deaths per calendar quarter) is divided by the rate expected given system-wide experience and the mix of patients treated at the facility. Values of "one" suggests that mortality in the facility is similar to the system-wide average. A value under 1.0 suggests lower mortality; a value

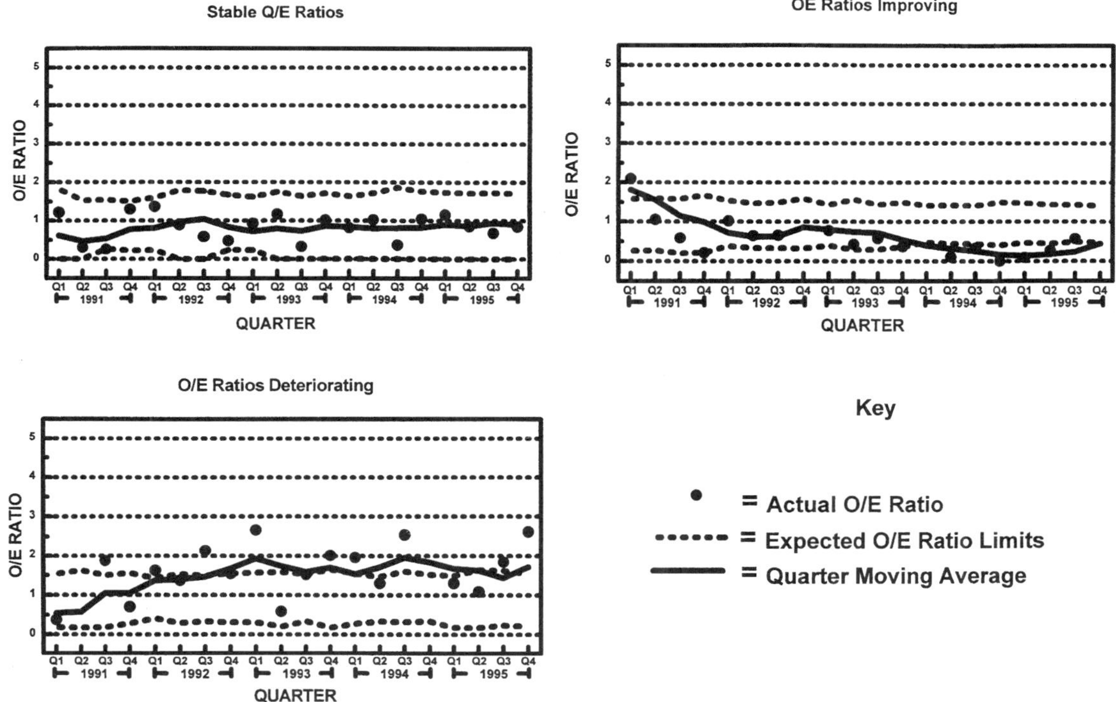

Fig. 2.10. Time trend charts of standardized mortality ratio (O/E ratio) from 3 dialysis units illustrating a stable trend (upper left), and improving trend (upper right), and a deteriorating but volatile trend (lower left). A moving average (solid line) as well as upper and lower control limits (dashed lines) are shown.

over 1 suggests higher mortality. But "lower or higher than average" does not necessarily deserve a complement or a call to action as explained earlier. The real question, remember, is, "How often and by how much?"

Ninety percent confidence limits are computed and bracket a moving average time trend. These are examples of the control charts illustrated in Figure 2.9; facility performance is plotted with tolerance ranges as a time trend.

The upper left panel of Figure 2.10 shows a facility with stable mortality over a 5 year time frame even though some mortality ratios exceeded 1.0 and a few were near the facility's upper control limit. The facility illustrated in the lower left suggests improving mortality. Quarter to quarter mortality is much more volatile in the facility illustrated in the lower left panel; the trend suggests deteriorating mortality early that remained high. While

occasional values were below or close to 1.0, the moving average suggests sustained ratios that were at or exceed the upper control limit.

Similar control charts can be constructed for other outcome measures such as the URR, nutrition-related measures, anemia, and so forth. Even absent such control charts, facilities should receive information frequently by which they can compare their own outcome and process measures to other facilities and evaluate changes in them over time.

Ad hoc reports

These describe the results of projects to: 1) set priorities, 2) evaluate the relationship(s) between outcomes and processes, 3) evaluate the result of system wide process change, and 4) evaluate statistical associations that may yield clues to disease processes. We chose survival as the outcome of primary interest and use it in these illustrations.

Figure 2.11 illustrates a *priority setting* exercise in which the strengths of association of patient attributes and medical process measures with odds of death were evaluated. The data suggested that of 24 variables analyzed 5 accounted for 80% of the explainable variance of death odds among those 16,000 or so patients [8–10]. Serum creatinine concentration and serum albumin concentration were strongly associated with death risk and are thought to reflect somatic protein mass and visceral protein mass respectively among dialysis patients. Anion gap, considered here at statistically comparable levels of all other variables, reflects acidosis. Age is an expected covariate of mortality. URR (the urea reduction ratio) reflects treatment intensity.

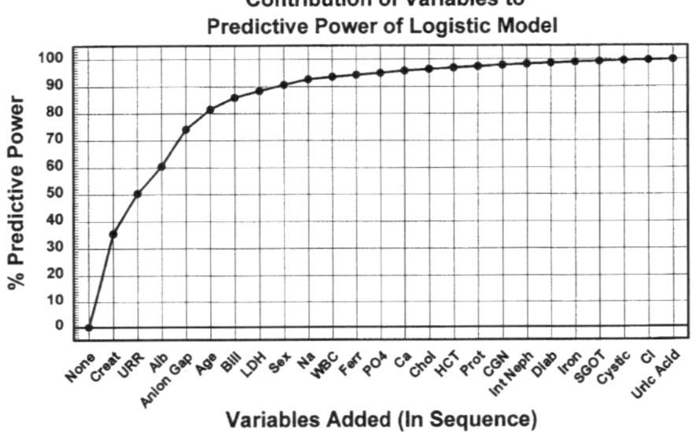

Fig. 2.11. Development of the predictive power of a logistic regression model as variables are added sequentially to it during a forward stepping analytical procedure. The tool can be used to develop priorities about which variables are most closely associated with an outcome of primary interest – in this case, odds of death. Number of patients = 16,163; Final model R^2 = 13.7%.

Reports such as these are sent to facilities and physicians providing the care [8]. Some are submitted in part as book chapters [9] or to journals for possible publication in the medical literature [10]. For example, reviewing the reference list at the end of this chapter, such as these references 8 through 10, will reveal frequent citation of internal memoranda, publicly available, followed by a literature citation. That format was chosen to illustrate this process.

I continue this example using the URR to illustrate the *relationship between an outcome and a process*. The URR is the fractional reduction of blood urea nitrogen concentration caused by a dialysis treatment. It is proportional to the urea clearance of the dialyzer times the length of the dialysis treatment divided by the patient's body water content. The left panel of Figure 2.12 is a bar chart comparing the odds of death among patients treated at various values of URR to those treated in a the reference range (here, URR = 65–70%). Statistical adjustments for patient attributes and those attributes plus a variety of laboratory values are made. It is clear that patients treated at low values of URR experienced higher mortal risk than those treated in the range over 60%. The right panel of Figure 2.12 shows the results of a curve splitting exercise suggesting that mortality tended to become worse at values less than about 60% but did not improve with values of URR increasing thereafter.

Armed with knowledge about the URR and information suggesting that low values of it are an important associates of death risk and also with information suggesting appropriate target values

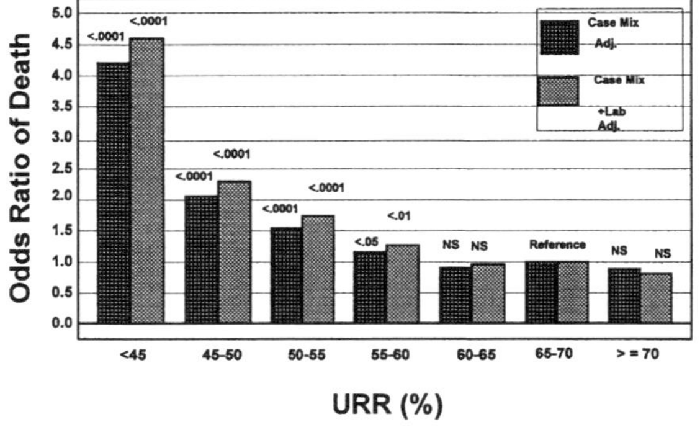

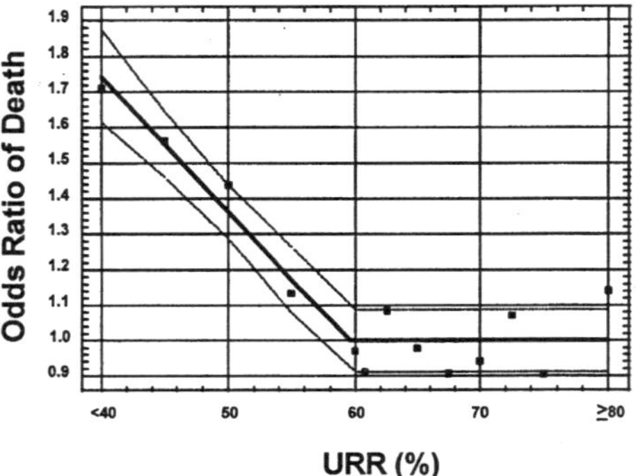

Fig. 2.12. Bar chart risk profile for the urea reduction ratio (left panel) and illustration of a curve splitting analysis to detect an approximate threshold for URR below which death risk becomes worse and above which it does not improve (right panel).

for URR [11–15], facilities were then able to develop quality enhancing strategies with respect to the URR.

THE USE OF INFORMATION TO ENHANCE QUALITY: AN ILLUSTRATION

The following figures illustrate hypothetical projects undertaken by a hypothetical dialysis unit to increase the level of dialysis exposure at which patients are treated. The clinical team uses information supplied by the support organization as well data gathered by them at their own facility.

Suppose the clinical staff understands facts such as those suggested by Figures 2.11 and 2.12. They also receive periodic reports describing the distribution of URR among patients treated in their facilities. Figure 2.13a illustrates such a distribution. The mean URR was 51.4% and only 12% of patients were treated at values exceeding 60%. The clinical team concluded that the distribution of URRs in the facility was much too low and plan to increase the values at which patients are treated.

Figure 2.13b illustrates their initial approach to the problem. They know, from prior understanding, that the value of the URR is determined principally by the dialyzer clearance and the length of the dialysis treatment. Fluid loss (UFR) and the amount of protein catabolism (PCR) during treatment also contribute but to a much lessor extent. They also know that the artificial kidney clearance is determined by the size of the dialyzer (KoA)

prescribed and the blood (Qb) and dialysate (Qd) flow rates at which it is used. They construct a cause and effect chart, otherwise called a "fish bone chart", as suggested by the figure. Understanding the processes that determines the value of URR, they can now proceed in an organized way to evaluate URR in their own facility. They check the adequacy of the dialysis prescriptions including the treatment time, dialyzer, and blood in dialysate flow rates increasing the values if they are low. They also evaluate the vascular access and whether patients are receiving their full measure of treatment time, again taking appropriate corrective action where warranted.

The distribution of URRs improved after those actions as suggested by Figure 2.14a. The mean is over 56% but still more than 60% of values are below URR = 60%. The clinical team concluded that their first project was worthwhile but the distribution of values is still too low. They plan to review the steps of the dialysis process to assure that the full measure of treatment is being delivered and begin with a process flow chart such as one shown in Figure 2.14b. The data suggest that some treatments are shorter than prescribed. Furthermore, patients' blood flow rates do not reach prescribed value early enough in the treatment and nurses and technicians are reducing those flows before the end of treatment. Therefore, the full measure of treatment was not delivered in the allotted time. They find less frequent treatment related problems and correct them as well.

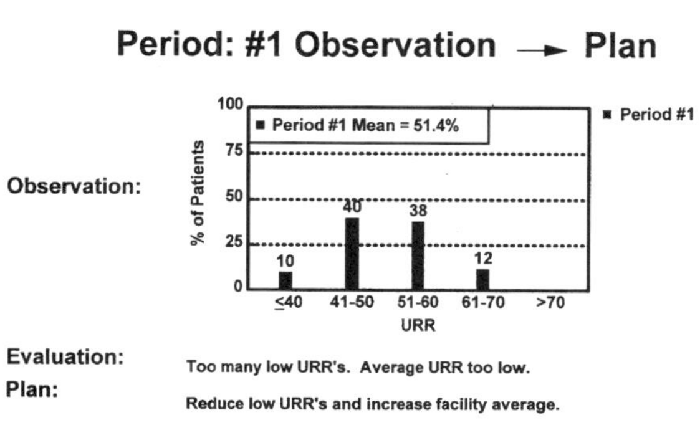

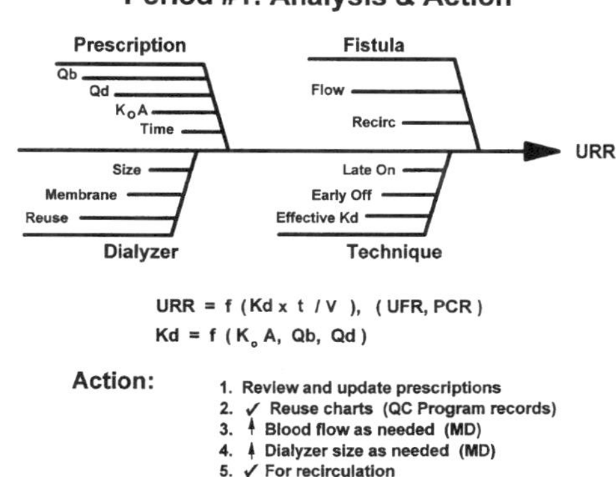

a

b

Fig. 2.13. (a) The observations of an initial (Period #1) distribution for URR and a plan evolving from it pursuant to a Shewhart cycle quality improvement project. (b) The analysis and actions resulting from observations shown in Figure 2.13a pursuant to a Shewhart cycle process.

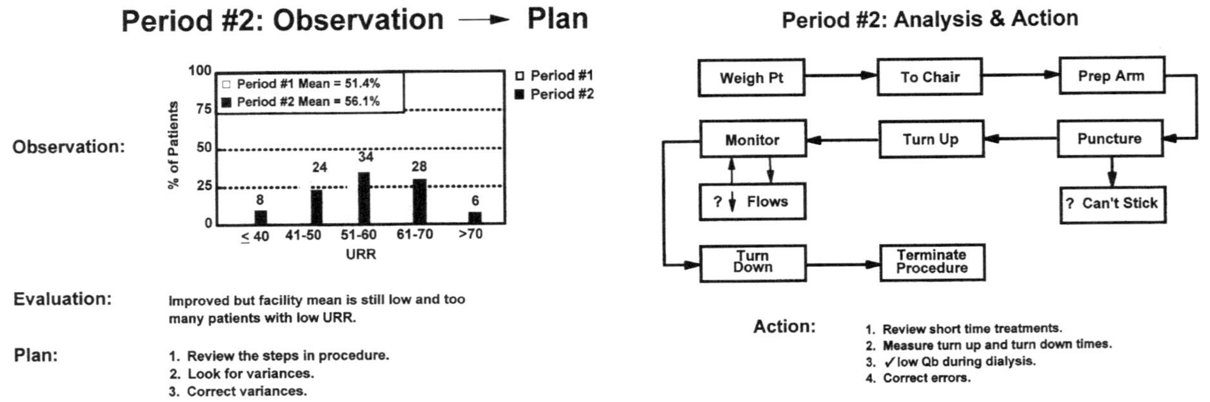

Fig. 2.14. (a) Evaluation of results achieved from Period 1 activities shown in Figures 2.13a and 2.13b and plans resulting from them. (b) The analysis and action resulting from observations shown in Figure 2.14a.

The third review of URR distributions shown in Figure 2.15a reveals an adequate average value. However, over 40% of values are still below 60% and nearly 20% are 50% or less. The clinical team concludes that more work is needed and decides to catalog treatment variances in a more formal way. They do so by ranking them in order of frequency using a Pareto chart such as that shown in Figure 2.15b. The data suggest that there remains a poor delivery of the dialysis prescription. Patients were also demanding shorter treatments and nurses and technicians often yielded to the demand. There-fore, the clinical leadership undertakes education programs for both staff and patients emphasizing the need to deliver the full measure of prescribed treatment and shares their recent findings with all of the facility staff.

Figure 2.16 shows the distribution of URR after those projects were completed. The facility mean now exceeds 64% and only 2% are treated in a danger zone less than 50%. Of course, some low URR measurements are expected. It is a diagnostic test, after all, and presumably low values lead to diagnostic and intervention actions by the clinical team on behalf of individual patients. Satisfied with progress, the clinical leadership, with their staff, now sets action thresholds for the purpose of making time trend process control charts (see Figures 2.9 and 2.10) as suggested in the figure.

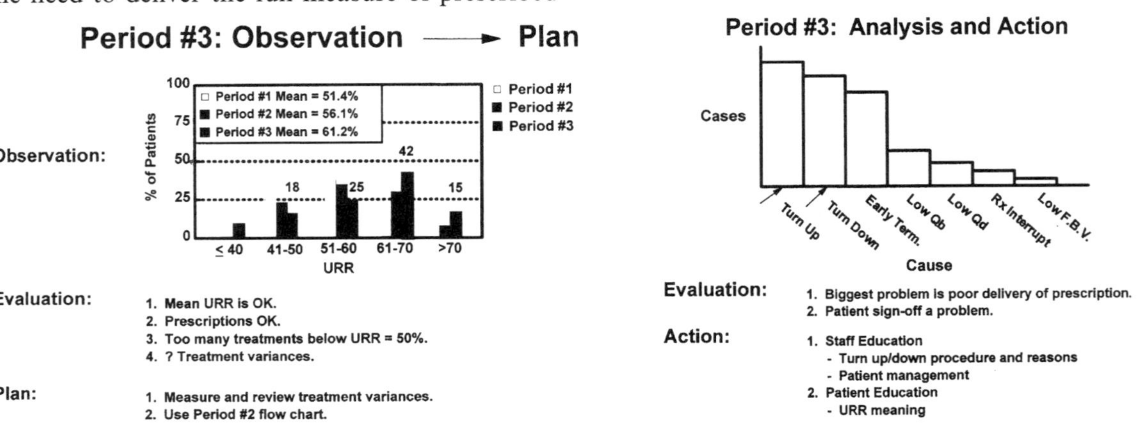

Fig. 2.15. (a) Evaluation of results from Period #2 activities shown in Figure 2.14a and 2.14b and the plan resulting from them. (b) Analysis and action resulting on the observations shown in Figure 2.15a.

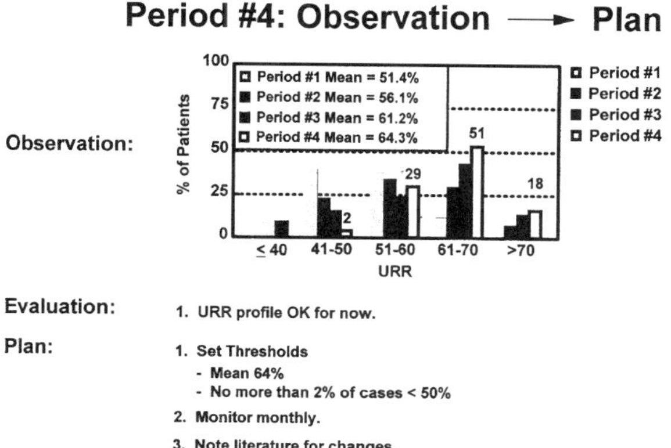

Fig. 2.16. Evaluation of Period #3 activities shown in Figures 2.15a and 2.15b. The distribution of URR has improved to acceptable levels and monitoring programs are established to assure continued acceptable levels of treatment.

EVALUATING SYSTEM-WIDE PROGRAMS

Figure 2.17 shows time trend charts illustrating URR distributions during 1991 through 1995. Between 30,000 and 45,000 individual tests are summarized each month from between 350 and 570 dialysis facilities. The median URR increased from approximately 58.5% to approximately 67%. Furthermore, the percentage of tests below an arbitrary warning threshold of 55% fell from over 37% to under 10% indicating that system-wide programs of information sharing, education, and assistance can achieve a desired result.

The real question, however, evolves not from the improvement of the test value itself but from the possible effect that such improvement might have on the real target of CQI activities – survival. The URR, after all, is only a test and improving the number associated with it is of little or no benefit if such improvement is not associated with a better outcome for patients.

Evaluating whether actions have their intended result may be a difficult task. Figure 2.11 shows that factors other than treatment exposure, the URR, are associated with survival likelihood. For example, the average age of patients increased from 57.7 years to 59.5 during the years covered by Figure 2.17 and the fraction of diabetic patients

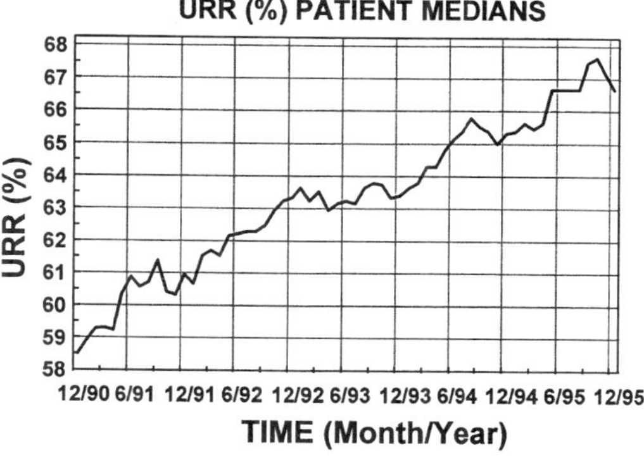

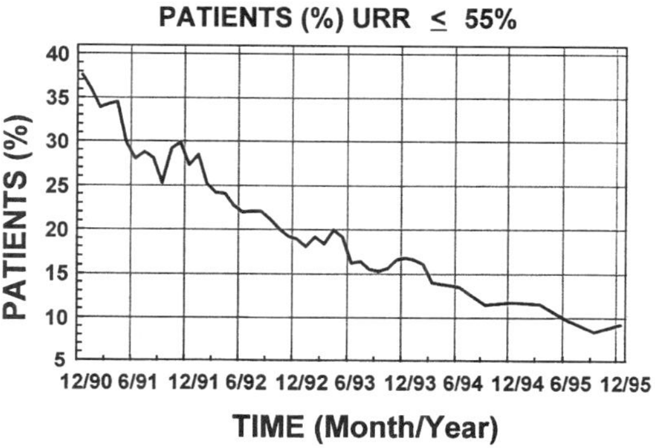

Fig. 2.17. Time trends of median URR (top panel) and the fraction of values less than 55% (bottom panel) monitored monthly in a large hemodialysis population.

increased from 34.5% to 41.6. Both advancing age and diabetes are associated unfavorably with survival thereby offsetting in part or in whole the possible benefits of improved URR.

How can one dissect the possible effect of improving a process/outcome from contemporaneous changes in other mortality associated dynamics? Such analyses are important prerequisites to evaluating the success of system-wide programs and evaluating the hypotheses that gave rise to them in the first place.

Figure 2.18 compares the evolving relative death risk importance associated with the URR to that associated with the concentrations of albumin, creatinine, and the anion gap all normalized to the importance for age [16].[3] The relative importance of URR fell as the distribution of values increased in this large population of patients suggesting that the majority of patients were being treated in the flat portion of the URR risk profile (Figures 2.12) at the end of this observation period. The importance of creatinine, albumin, and anion gap, on the other hand, remain relatively unchanged. A likely interpretation of the dual observations, decreasing importance with increasing values, suggests that programs to increase dialysis dose did achieve their ultimate goals to reduce death risk associated with low dialysis exposure.

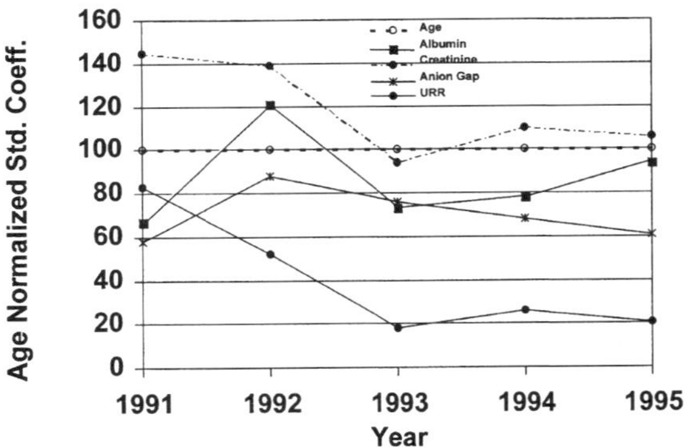

Fig. 2.18. Evaluating the association of changed URR distributions with improved mortality by associated cause of mortality. The associations of albumin, creatinine, and anion gap did not change in predictable ways during the period of observation. The association of URR, on the other hand, improved as prevalent values increased.

THE NEXT STEPS

I conclude with brief a description of an uncompleted group of projects because the essence of the medical CQI paradigm is endless goal directed inquiry to improve the outcome of clinical care for patients. It also illustrates the use of epidemiological data such as these to reveal clues about basic disease processes. Those clues can be used to develop diagnostic and treatment strategies that improve care quality. These are an important projects because they were undertaken to address the close association, repeatedly observed, of nutrition related measures with the odds of dying.

Figure 2.11 suggests that nutrition-related vari-

ables such as albumin and creatinine concentrations are associated in important ways with the odds of patient survival. Figure 2.18 suggests that the importance of those variables to survival has not improved. Other data, not shown here, show that the statistical distribution of nutrition related measures has not changed over time. Therefore, projects to evaluate causes contributing to, and possible treatments for, nutritional depletion among patients may result in improved survival for patients. There must be clues.

Figure 2.19 illustrates the time trend for certain hematological variables. The trend was constructed to evaluate changing erythropoietin dose which was a large cost/profit center of operation for most dialysis units. The real value of the chart, however, evolves not so much from better cost/ profit management but from the clues it provides

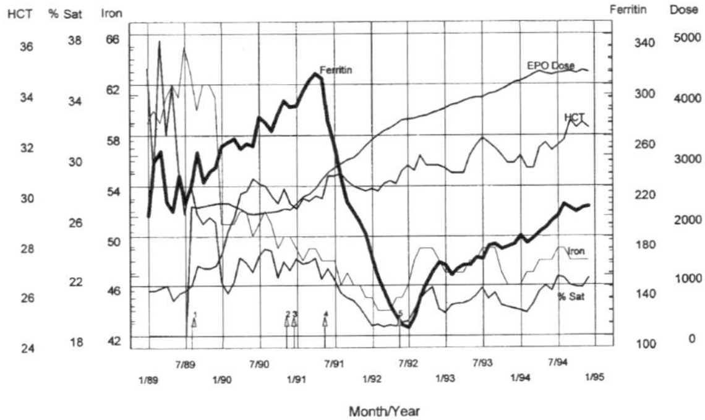

Fig. 2.19. Time trend chart showing the EPO dose per treatment and the median values for hematocrit, serum iron, % saturation of iron binding capacity, and serum ferritin concentration. The numbered arrows at the bottom of the chart indicate. 1) EPO becomes available, 2) reimbursement method changes from $ per administration to dose based, 3) Imferon importation stops, 4) Imferon inventory gone, and 5) Infed becomes available. HCT means hematocrit; % Sat means fractional saturation of iron binding capacity; Iron means serum iron concentration; Ferritin mean serum ferritin concentration; dose means the dose of erythropoetin (EPO) per administration.

about potential pathophysiologies contributing to malnutrition among patients.[4]

When erythropoietin became available, prevalent blood count values (hematocrit) increased among dialysis patients as expected. Iron is used biologically in the production of new red blood cells so prevalent values of serum iron and the fractional saturation of iron binding capacity decreased. Prevalent values reflecting stored iron (serum ferritin concentration), however, increased suggesting abnormalities of iron utilization among dialysis patients. Ferritin values fell when iron preparations were removed from the American market by the US Food and Drug Administration. When iron preparations were reintroduced, prevalent ferritin concentrations increased remarkably but the serum iron values increased by only small amounts. This, again, suggests poor use of available iron by dialysis patients.

Prevalent values for red blood cell and iron indices were similar to those commonly associated with the anemia of chronic disease (ACD) rather than iron deficiency [17–19]. ACD is also associated with impaired iron utilization and diseases associated with ACD frequently have malnutrition as part of their clinical syndromes. Could anemia and malnutrition, commonly prevalent among patients with kidney failure, be linked in some way?

Because ACD is commonly thought to be associated with sustained release of certain biochemical mediators, cytokines, we tested the hypothesis by measuring the serum concentration of a substance commonly associated with such cytokine release – the C-reactive protein. Figures 2.20 are scatter plots showing the association of both serum albumin concentration and blood hemoglo-bin concentration with the C-reactive protein. Both were highly correlated with it suggesting thereby that cytokine mediated processes are likely linked to both the malnutrition and anemia commonly prevalent among dialysis patients [20–22].

The tasks now seem to include efforts to confirm or refute the hypothesis that chronic inflammatory processes contribute in large measure to both the malnutrition and anemia associated with chronic kidney failure. Assuming confirmation, the tasks will include projects to reveal causes and efforts to develop interventions and treatments. Those efforts are not research abstractions, the products of idle inquiry. They should be highly focused, goal directed efforts performed as quickly, efficiently, and practically as possible in pursuit of improved care for patients.

Thus, quality driven inquiry has no end. I hope that I have succeeded, at least in some measure, illustrating the challenge of the CQI paradigm and showing its rewards for medical clinicians, researchers, and administrators. The only attribute that distinguishes it from other forms of inquiry is it goal directed focus. Deming once said that a project without a goal has no purpose. The only goal for the purpose at hand is improved care for patients and unless there is a clear connection, which transcends simple preference (please see the opening quotation from William James), between it and that goal no project is worth its undertaking.

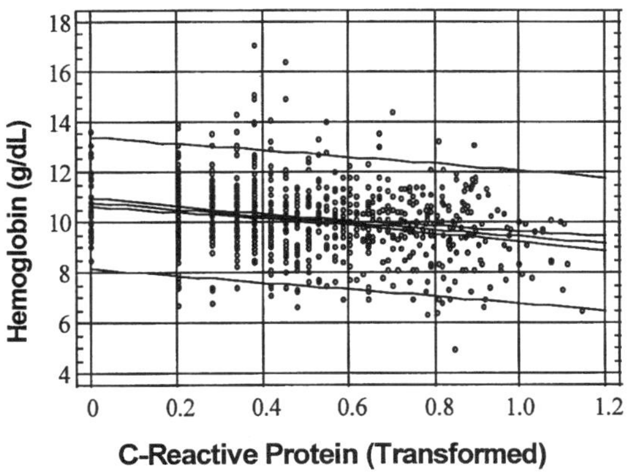
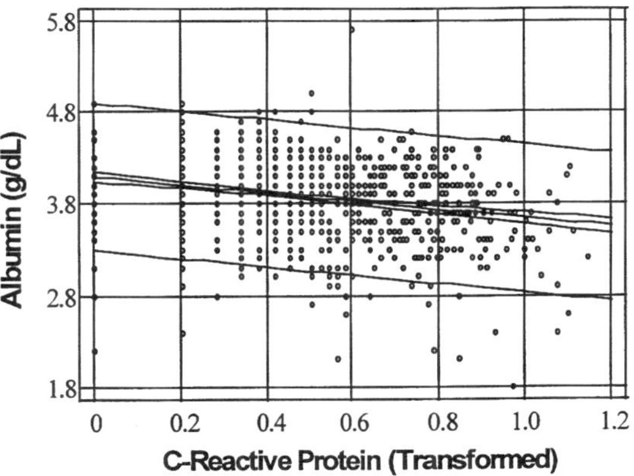

Fig. 2.20. The associations of blood hemoglobin concentration (left panel) and serum albumin concentration (right panel) with C-reactive protein concentration.

NOTES

[1] By "agency agreement" I mean the obligation of a professional to decide with a patient about health care matters just as the patient would on his or her own if the patient had all of the professional's medical knowledge.

[2] The URR is the fractional reduction of blood urea nitrogen concentration (BUN) caused by a dialysis treatment. Urea is a metabolic byproduct of protein metabolism and its concentration in the blood increases when the kidneys fail. URR = $100 \times$ (BUN before dialysis – BUN after dialysis) $\div$ BUN before dialysis.

[3] The absolute values of standardized logistic regression coefficients of the variables from routine annual analysis of mortality data were divided by the comparable coefficient for age and taken as a percentage value. The coefficients associated with age remarkably stable over time. The values are plotted as a time trend. Similar trends not expressed as ratios to age can also be used.

[4] By malnutrition I refer to body composition, particularly of proteins, and not food intake, per se. As such, malnutrition can result from causes other than simple starvation.

REFERENCES

1. Peirce CS. The fixation of belief. In Butler J, editor. Philosophical writings of Peirce.,New York, Dover Publications, 1955.
2. McDermott JJ. The writings of William James. Chicago, University of Chicago Press, 1977.
3. Deming WE. Out of the crisis. Cambridge, MA, MIT Centers for Advanced Engineering, 1986.
4. Shewhart WA. Economic control of quality of manufactured product. Van Strand, 1931. RPR Ed; American Society of Quality Control, 1980.
5. Deming WE. The new economics for industry, government, education, 2nd edition. Cambridge, MA, MIT Centers for Advanced Engineering, 1994.
6. Walton M. The Deming management method. New York, Putnam Publishing Group, 1986.
7. Lowrie EG. The United States renal data system, a public treasure – how best to use it? Semin Dialysis (In press).
8. Lowrie EG, Huang W, Lew NL, and Liu Y. Analysis of 1991 mortality data. Memorandum to DSD Medical Directors, February 26, 1993.
9. Lowrie EG, Huang WH, Lew NL and Liu Y. The relative contribution of measured variables to death risk among hemodialysis patients. In Friedman E, editor. Death on hemodialysis: preventable or inevitable? Hingham, Kluwer Academic Publishers, 1994; 121–41.
10. Lowrie EG. Chronic dialysis treatment: clinical outcome and related processes of care. Am J Kid Dis 1994; 24:255–66.
11. Lowrie EG. The measurement of urea reduction ratio (URR) and Kt/V: a laboratory enhancement for monitoring dialysis exposure. Memorandum to DSD Medical Directors, May 11, 1990.
12. Lowrie EG and Lew NL. Urea reduction ratios (URR): data to assist the interpretation of statistics for your dialysis unit. Memorandum to DSD Medical Directors, November 9, 1990.
13. Lowrie EG, Lew NL and Liu Y. The effect of differences in urea reduction ratio (URR) on death risk in hemodialysis patients: a preliminary analysis. Memorandum to DSD Medical Directors, November 5, 1991.
14. Lowrie EG and Lew NL. The urea reduction ratio (URR): A simple method for evaluating hemodialysis treatment. Contemp Dial Nephrol 1991; 11–20.
15. Owen WF Jr, Lew NL, Liu Y, Lowrie EG and Lazarus JM. The urea reduction ratio and serum albumin concentration as predictors of mortality in patients undergoing hemodialysis. New Engl J Med 1993; 329:1001–6.
16. Lowrie EG, Zhu X, Zhang H, Lew NL and Lazarus JM. Death risk profiles associated with the urea reduction ratio (URR) in review: 1991 through 1994. Memorandum to DSD Medical Directors, September 27, 1996.
17. Lowrie EG and Ma L. Time trends for EPO dose: Hematocrit, serum iron and other matters. Memorandum to DSD Medical Directors, May 30, 1995.
18. Lowrie EG, Ling L and Lew NL. The anemia of ESRD and related thoughts about iron and EPO therapy. Memorandum to DSD Medical Directors, August 10, 1995.
19. Madore F, Lowrie EG, Brugnara C, Lew NL, Lazarus JM, Bridges K and Owen WF: Anemia in hemodialysis patients: Variables affecting this outcome predictor. J Am Soc Nephrol 1997; 8:1921–9.
20. Lowrie EG, Ma L, Zhang J and Lew NL. Thoughts about anemia, iron, proteins, and a "chronic acute phase" state among hemodialysis patients. Memorandum to DSD Medical Directors, February 14, 1996.
21. Lowrie EG, Zhang J and Lew NL. Acute phase process among patients with kidney failure: extended observations and related thoughts. Memorandum to DSD Medical Directors, March 19, 1996.
22. Lowrie EG. Conceptual model for a core pathobiology of uremia with special reference to anemia, malnourishment, and mortality among dialysis patients. Semin Dialysis 1997; 10:115–29.

3. Process for initiating and maintaining continuous quality improvement in the ESRD setting

GREGORY HOHNER AND DIANE FENDER

BACKGROUND

A Proven Methodology Facilitates Change

For nearly two decades, organizations from all types of industries have attempted to implement an improvement process that could help them recognize a problem and formulate an effective and manageable solution. The healthcare movement towards quality improvement began formally when the Joint Commission of Accreditation of Hospitals. These early efforts increased the intensity of their requirements necessitating hospitals to develop quality indicators that could help ensure their ability to meet these requirements. They quickly discovered that by involving personnel at all levels of the organization, they could develop an effective and innovative approach to improvement, and cross-functional teams of employees including ancillary key individuals could make a detailed assessment of a situation, search for, and identify possible solutions.

Structured approaches to quality improvement have been based on the statistically-based work of Dr W. Edwards Deming and other quality scholars, such as Philip Crosby and J.M. Juran. Dr W.E. Deming, known as the father of quality management, laid to rest the idea that increasing quality leads to increased costs. He introduced quality control to Japan in the 1950s. He emphasized Statistical Process Control and believed that 85–90% of all problems were process (not people) problems. The publishing of Deming's 14 Points laid the foundation upon which quality improvement today has been based. The points blend leadership, management theory and statistical concepts which highlight management's responsibilities while enhancing the capacities of employees.

Phillip Crosby is a prominent expert in quality management and the founder of Phil Crosby Associates (PCA), a quality management consulting group. His approach is non-technical with emphasis on the belief that defect-free work is the responsibility of the line worker. Joseph Juran is one of the primary architects of the modern quality management discipline. His major contributions include development of a team-based, project-oriented method for making quality improvements. His emphasis has always been placed on distinguishing the "vital few" projects from the "trivial many" and planning for and managing results.

Research and methodologies of Deming, Crosby, Juran, and others have been instrumental in the design of continuous quality improvement tools for healthcare that have proven to attain desired results. Using quality assurance efforts as a starting point, hospitals and dialysis centers have been able to leverage data that has been historically available to them in new and innovative ways to achieve both clinical and operational quality.

Quality Assurance Programs

Quality assurance (QA) programs, patient records, clinical events, published studies and additional sources of dialysis center information provide good, solid data for successful Continuous Quality Improvement (CQI) process implementation. In fact, dialysis centers are implementing CQI to make consensus-building decisions by leveraging

L.W. Henderson and R.S. Thuma (eds.), Quality Assurance in Dialysis, 2nd Edition, 27–38.
© 1999 *Kluwer Academic Publishers. Printed in Great Britain*

their Quality Assurance systems as a valuable data source which is also assisting in the overall effort to more aggressively:

1. Identify improvement opportunities,

2. Position dialysis centers for a managed care environment,

3. Comply with heightened regulatory involvement, and

4. Compete in an increasingly competitive dialysis environment.

Best Demonstrated Practices (BDP) Program

In 1986, when the focus on quality assurance emerged in dialysis, the Renal Division of Baxter Healthcare Corporation launched a quality improvement support initiative for peritoneal dialysis, the Best Demonstrated Practices (BDP) program, to help dialysis centers analyze their PD performance by measuring individual center performance, and determining best practices from centers of excellence. The program enhanced activities related to PD patient retention by facilitating the analysis of treatment outcomes and modality transfer patterns. This program allowed professionals to more easily and quantitatively identify strengths, challenge weaknesses, and modify practices to affect outcomes.

Worldwide, BDP is the precursor to a cross-functional, team-based CQI approach. With hundreds of dialysis centers participating in data collection and analysis, and with many utilizing the practice guidelines that have evolved from this program, BDP continues to help dialysis centers evaluate and upgrade treatment practices.

Corporate Quality Leadership Process

At this same time, Baxter Healthcare Corporation began implementing a continuous quality improvement process, called the Quality Leadership Process (QLP), throughout its worldwide organization. As successes were realized internally, this process extended into customer partnership activities and then supplier excellence programs. Through QLP, Baxter created a workable quality improvement process and deployed tools and techniques to over seventy-five thousand employees. The process helps Baxter sustain management commitment, document measurements, and continually improve its own processes. As Baxter perfected this process internally, it was introduced and adapted to the healthcare community in materials management departments and eventually into clinical settings.

Baxter applied over sixteen years of research and development to the successful creation of continuous quality improvement (CQI) tools and techniques that, today, favorably improve patient care and organizational effectiveness in the dialysis community. Dialysis centers worldwide are actively implementing a CQI process that is resulting in sustainable clinical and financial improvements.

Overview of Baxter's CQI Process

CQI Process

A series of action steps and tools that have proven effective for successfully achieving results

Step one

Action:

Identify opportunity for improvement	*Tools:*
– Collect data	– Quality assurance data
– Form team	– Patient retention analysis
– Define problem/goal	(PRA)
	– Fishbone diagram

Step two

Action:

Review strengths and weaknesses	*Tools:*
– Brainstorm possible causes	– Root cause analysis
– Select cause(s) to investigate	– Potential cause summary
– Validate the issues through data analysis	– Data collection to investigate causes
	– Quality assurance data
	– Patient retention analysis (PRA)
	– Process flow diagramming

Step three

Action:

Select solution	*Tools:*
– Select one cause to impact	– Solution analysis
– Brainstorm possible solutions	– Cost effectiveness analysis
– Research potential improvements, practices guidelines, expert– opinions	– Solution analysis matrix
	– Action Plan
	– Practice checklists
– Select best solution	– Treatment recommendations

CQI Process (cont.)

Step four

Action:

Test solution

- Select one solution to test
- Design protocol
- Implement on pilot basis
- Collect and analyze data
- Evaluate outcomes: if positive, design standardized method

Tools:

- Data collection time lines
- POET model
- PD adequest/T.A.R.G.E.T.
- Simple APD model

Step five

Action:

Implement and track results

- Standardize process
- Measure to ensure success
- Perform post-assessment

Tools:

- Data collection time lines
- Quality assurance systems
- Clinical-based measurements and thresholds
- Advanced statistical methodologies

INTEGRATING CQI INTO A DIALYSIS CENTER

Impact of QA and CQI Integration

Effectively integrating a continuous quality improvement process into a dialysis center as a permanent part of a facility's clinical improvement effort is a significant challenge. Dialysis centers are, however, achieving successful results by integrating the CQI process and their QA efforts by applying the CQI process to their ongoing QA data collection activities. By combining and integrating the two approaches, the desired result that is being achieved is a methodology that allows for continued evaluation of clinical and operational areas. This integration improves quality proactively, is accepted and performed by everyone in the organization, provides a consistent process focused on outcomes, is internally driven for patients' benefits, and is systematic to help ensure desired results are continually attained.

Patient Retention

Increased patient retention yields psychological benefits to patients who may be able to continue home care rather than change lifestyle to accommodate in-center care. Increasing the average length of time a patient is treated at home leverages the dialysis center's orientation and training costs associated with establishing a home patient.

Rationale for CQI Process Implementation

The costs of providing patient care to an ESRD patient are almost 10 times the costs of an average Medicare patient. By the year 2000, it is expected that the ESRD program will be $24 billion if costs per patient are held to 0% annual growth. (Source: USRDS and Baxter Forecast)

An estimated 41% of the total ESRD costs are due to hospitalizations. Inpatient physician fees represent approximately 7% of the dialysis treatment cost. An estimated 1% of costs are in post-hospital services making 49% of the total ESRD therapy costs associated with hospital stays. (Source: Adapted from Burton, "Can A Global Payment System Work for the ESRD Program", Nephrology News and Issues, October 1993; 1994 Rand Study.) Reductions in hospitalizations represent the single most important way to reduce costs. Finally, it is rapidly becoming an accepted belief that the overall solution for controlling costs is managed care.

A managed care environment places emphasis on patient outcome at the lowest total cost as fixed revenue per patient becomes a reality. This shift from fee-for-service to global capitation requires an understanding of both therapy mix and improvement processes so that these results are achieved.

Emphasis on improving patient outcomes and reducing costs encourages dialysis centers worldwide to identify and evaluate these outcomes and objectives more closely than was necessary in past years. Oversight organizations, such as the Health Care Financing Administration (HCFA) in the U.S., has mandated that dialysis centers have a formal CQI process to manage quality and, therefore, work toward achieving these goals.

This health care regulatory change has motivated dialysis center management to focus more on improving patient outcomes, increasing patient satisfaction, increasing employee satisfaction and involvement, reducing costs, and enhancing patient care quality. These emerging trends panicked the competitive environment, as well. Implementing and sustaining a continuous quality improvement process helps to achieve these goals. Success in negotiating with managed care organizations is based on similar levels of performance including:

- Optimizing total annual cost per patient

- Reducing hospitalizations

- Increasing patient satisfaction

- Achieving and reducing standardized mortality rates

- Performing at key clinical measured outcomes

Elements for Successful Integration

To be effective, CQI must be integrated into the operations of the dialysis center as a continuous, supported activity, involving all staff members. Requirements for successful integration include: a quantitative baseline, trial, integration of key practices consistently across the dialysis center, and staff education and cooperation. People are empowered by working with the process.

At the onset of applying a continuous quality improvement process to routine dialysis center efforts, managers often ask these questions:

- How do we fit this additional activity into our daily workload?

- How do we get people involved?

- How long does it take and how do we know it's working?

- Where do we begin?

- Where do we go after the first project is completed?

Preplanning is needed to prepare an organization for successful integration of CQI. These early efforts ensure accurate and focused data collection, analytical tool selection, and sustainability of the process long-term. Following are ten elements necessary for successful integration of CQI into a dialysis center:

1. Transforming professional caregivers into an effective team requires each professional to have a clear perspective of the implementation issues, a problem-solving process, and the flexibility to handle change. Teams are formed to identify the cause of clinical obstacles and to eliminate them. Team-based decision-making, such as using multi-voting, involves many individuals in the dialysis center and helps to ensure total buy-in, good decisions, and successful implementation of the best ideas for improvement. Neither the work load nor the decision-making resides solely with one individual. A team leader coordinates the team, creates the agenda and facilitates the discussion. Decisions are made with input from a team consisting of key individuals who have been trained how to utilize a rigorous decision-making process.

2. CQI tools successfully applied to the dialysis center's area of study include brainstorming techniques, affinity diagramming, root cause analysis, process flow diagramming, force field analysis, short-and long-term goal identification, and the development of a workable action plan.

3. Successful implementation includes management involvement. The physician, or center manager, is responsible for ensuring that results are obtained. This begins by demonstrating commitment to the process, setting goals, and following through with action plans. A specially designed session to orient members to the responsibilities required to attain desired results is effective.

4. Identifying improvement opportunities and root cause of the problem focuses on the center's CQI effort. A well-selected project has potential clinical impact. Selected projects are based on an agreed-upon set of criteria that has been supported by a clinical and management group. Selected issues may be operational in nature, as long as a strong connection to the clinical area selected is substantiated. Improvement opportunities come from many areas such as quality assurance data, clinical outcomes data, protocol and practice reviews, and/or complaints and mistakes. An improvement opportunity needs to be measurable, achievable, and have a positive impact on a clinical outcome.

5. Initial data collection validates the issue by helping to better understand the magnitude of the situation and re-affirming the need for an improvement project. At the start of a CQI project, data collection validates or disproves an issue and helps establish the scope of a problem. Often, data collection is used to narrow the various causes of a clinical opportunity to its root cause. Insights from data help understand the situation prior to selecting the possible solution to the clinical issue. If possible, as the analytical skill set is identified, the use of advanced statistical methodologies may be appropriate.

Qualitative and/or quantitative data analysis in the CQI process will be employed at different points. Qualitative analysis positions data collection for attribute ranking which is especially effective in narrowing the scope of study, and multi-voting for solution selection. Quantitative analysis includes the use of statistical principles as well as multi-variant analysis. This type of analysis is effective for looking at trends and predictive equations.

Overusing data analysis at any time during a CQI project can misdirect the team by focusing team members on activity instead of results. The team leader and members must weigh the investment of time, effort, and change to the expected level of improvement. Managing the scope of data collection helps to set the parameters for analysis. Too little data collection and analysis is ineffective, and too much data collection and analysis is unproductive.

6. A formal approach to identifying possible solutions will help from focusing on a single solution too quickly. Analyzing possible solutions helps to better understand why a problem exists and identifies the best solutions that will prevent the problem from reoccurring. By testing these preliminary solutions, the process will identify which solution has the most profound impact on a single root cause.

7. Testing the solution indicates whether the solution works, whether there are hidden costs or problems and whether the solution is the best of the various solutions proposed. This test needs to be as "real world" as possible. A poorly designed test will yield unreliable results, and will prove devastating if the solution is chosen as the practice change for the whole facility. Testing the solution before full scale implementation ensures that what was hypothesized works. Measuring results is a critical component for testing the solution and requires a clear tracking system to measure results.

8. Implementation of the Action Plan focuses on installing the solution as a practice change. The scope of the plan should be clearly delineated, measurable, and achievable within a realistic time frame. The Action Plan may have required modification over time which may necessitate a second pass at the Action Plan. The Action Plan drives the success of a CQI project, represents unit-wide implementation and demonstrates measurable and achievable results within a realistic time frame.

9. Clinical and business outcomes are intertwined; in both, measurement determines the degree of success attained. The data chosen for measurement and the means used to measure are critical decisions in determining how the outcome is perceived as well as its success.

10. Evaluating an improvement opportunity involves reviewing both clinical and business implications of the results including what was learned from testing the solution and then full scale implementation.

Planning for Involvement

The physician, or center manager, is responsible for ensuring that clinical improvements are obtained. This begins by demonstrating commitment to the process, setting goals, and following through with action plans. A specially designed session to orient members to their level of responsibilities and involvement is effective. Once basic activities are defined and an inner structure of systems and techniques is positioned, planning for involvement can begin. Planning involves identifying key people, the subject/area requiring improvement action, and the proper structure – whether a small, two to three people working team, or a larger, ten to twelve people team needs to be established. Individuals responsible for making results happen must have the capability and authority to make decisions so that progress can be made.

Team Meetings and Structure

To be effective, team members meet regularly with everyone in attendance. A team leader calls a meeting of a quality working team every two to four weeks. It is management's responsibility to monitor and support meeting attendance. A meeting is always conducted with an agenda to keep everyone on track and to ensure that the team's activities, including topics discussed, remain focused. An agenda includes items for discussion as well as specific times allotted to each. The leader guides the discussion and ensures that every activity is assigned. Team members take responsibility, provide input and support for each other's efforts, and keep the process moving so that results are attained within a pre-defined time period. The scribe takes notes during the meeting, and distributes meeting minutes in a timely fashion after the meeting. This ensures that everyone knows the progress made and commitments assigned at the meeting. Facilitators ensure that the team understands how to work through the process, and has a required knowledge of the tools and techniques that will be applied for the process to be successful.

Baxter has a clinical support organization that assists dialysis centers in implementing CQI. Professionally trained and experienced CQI facilitators, located throughout the United States, help dialysis centers:

1. Establish a common vision and clinical improvement goal

2. Facilitate root cause identification and data collection

3. Review current and recommended practices

4. Identify possible solutions and implement practice changes

5. Monitor implementation progress

6. Create awareness and gain involvement from all staff members

7. Achieve and document results through tools and techniques

8. Understand and apply efficient methods for measurement

9. Initiate and manage a quality team

10. Prioritize project areas for improvement

IMPLEMENTING A QUALITY IMPROVEMENT PROCESS: FACILITY-BASED EXAMPLE

Introduction to Well-Designed Implementation

Most dialysis centers today have good, solid data and proven tools in place to facilitate successful CQI process implementation: quality assurance programs, patient records, clinical events, and published studies and standards. Successful efforts require that every dialysis center staff member be committed to:

- Implement a continuous quality improvement process,

- Have a common language regarding quality, and

- Possess a fundamentally sound understanding of quality improvement. Involvement of managers, supervisors and physicians, in conjunction with a competent and confident dialysis center staff, further ensures process implementation success.

ESTABLISHING AN OBJECTIVE FOR CQI

To describe objectives that have been effective in CQI process implementations, four examples from U.S. dialysis center studies are used.

Data collected every six months uncovered that 30% of a program's 188 PD patients failed to meet targeted adequacy parameters which affected patient well-being and nutrition. The center's CQI objective was defined as improving adequacy by increasing the program's total percent of patients achieving adequacy targets from 70% to 85%, and meeting targeted adequacy parameters of Kt/V of >1.7, and a creatinine clearance of >50 L/week normalized to 1.73 m^2 BSA. The dialysis center decided that additional data on patient compliance, residual renal function and adequacy would be collected and evaluated. Their CQI implementation plan included educating and training staff and physicians on prescription management and patient compliance to prescribed therapies. The CQI process identified ways to educate patients and bring about improved adequacy results, thus achieving their anticipated 85% target. (Note: This data represents results prior to the higher Kt/V standards now recommended by DOQI.)

A dialysis center identified their problem as 45% of their patient population not reaching the targeted hematocrit of 30% or greater. Mean hematocrit in the unit was 30.5%. Twenty percent of patients with hematocrits less than 30% were on non-reuse dialyzers which was significant because the center had experienced problems with occurrences of blood leaks and were unsure how much of a problem this represented. 8% of their patients were severely anemic. The agreed upon goal by all team members was that iron saturations would be greater that 25%, ferritin levels would be greater than 200 and hematocrits would be greater than 30 in this population within 3 months. The result of CQI was a significant improvement in the unit's hematocrit percentages greater than 30% along with an increase in the mean hematocrit. No appreciable difference in ferritin levels or percentage saturation levels were noted in the unit. One important factor that surfaced from their CQI efforts was an increased awareness among staff and patients regarding anemia.

Improving the unit's peritonitis rate from 1:21 months to 1:55 was one center's goal. They noted that 63% of their patients with peritonitis were using an Ultra-Bag of which 45% had been on peritoneal dialysis 9 months. Peritonitis was thought to be caused by inconsistent protocols and patient non-compliance. Through CQI implementation, the dialysis center decreased their peritonitis rate to 1:64 patient months within 6 months. By improving their protocol for training and retraining, the dialysis center decreased their incidence of peritonitis, and was able to realize an increase in comfort and convenience, with a decrease in cost to the patient. Cost savings came from decreased nursing time, medication costs, supplies and lab expenses. The dialysis center benefited from a better understanding of their patient population regarding percentage of patients with peritonitis on Ultra-Bag, percentage of patients with peritonitis on APD, and the percentage of peritonitis patients who had transfer sets changed every six months.

A dialysis center was concerned about hospitalization due to access failure. They felt that if they could minimize access failures, there would be a related drop in the number of hospitalizations. The decrease in hospitalizations would lead to an increase in patients' quality of life and decreased costs to the payer and patient. The center's efforts to minimize access failures, which would decrease hospitalizations, increased both patients' and staffs' morale. Patients expressed to the medical staff their appreciation and satisfaction with the clinic's efforts. Through education about their access, patients were able to identify problems with the access thrill and bruit and receive case-by-case consultations with their vascular surgeon on non-dialysis days. This prevented loss of revenue for the clinic which occurs when treatments aren't performed and the increased cost of managing vascular complications, consequently, increased the quality of life for patients as they deferred possible surgery.

EXAMPLE OF A CQI PROJECT

Pseudomonas Episodes Raise a Red Flag in Dialysis Center

A United States dialysis center, actively participating in CQI, attributes brainstorming sessions to the majority of their successful continuous quality improvements. During routine monitoring of peritonitis rates, which is performed on a monthly basis, by patient, by system, and by organism, three episodes of pseudomonas quickly prompted an investigation to find the cause. The individual responsible for monitoring peritonitis rates was selected as the group leader.

Data Collection

1. All of the patients, whether positive or not for pseudomonas, were on the same Ultra-bag system. Therefore, Ultra-bag was not felt to be a possible contributing factor for the peritonitis episodes.

2. The group affected were generally compliant patients who had been on peritoneal dialysis more than one year with no previous history of pseudomonas.

3. Most affected patients also had pseudomonas exit site infections prior to, or concurrent with, the peritonitis.

4. In reviewing technique and exit site care with patients, comments such as "the more I wash my exit site, the worse it gets" were frequently heard. The patients known to take the fewest number of showers had the best looking exit sites.

5. Given that pseudomonas is commonly found in soil and water, an environmental relationship was suspected. Upon researching the water source of all involved patients, it was discovered they all had wells. The entire patient population was surveyed to confirm well water as the possible root cause of the problem. Fifty percent of all patients with wells, either private or community, had pseudomonas. Zero percent of the patients with city water had pseudomonas. By the end of June, 1995, seven pseudomonas cultures had been confirmed in a patient population of approximately forty patients.

Data Analysis

Patients with confirmed pseudomonas cultures had used well water the previous year without a problem. The health department confirmed that wells were known to have higher counts of bacteria and pesticides than in previous years.

Solution Analysis

It was suggested that patients add bleach to their holding tanks since chlorine kills pseudomonas. Since the amount of chlorine could not be controlled, this was not a viable solution.

With physician input, an initial action plan was developed for aggressive exit site care. The goal was to prevent water from prolonged contact with the exit site where it might eventually make it's way down the catheter tunnel. Pseudomonas exit site infections were successfully eliminated with this plan, however, pseudomonas peritonitis still existed.

Driving forces: Issues

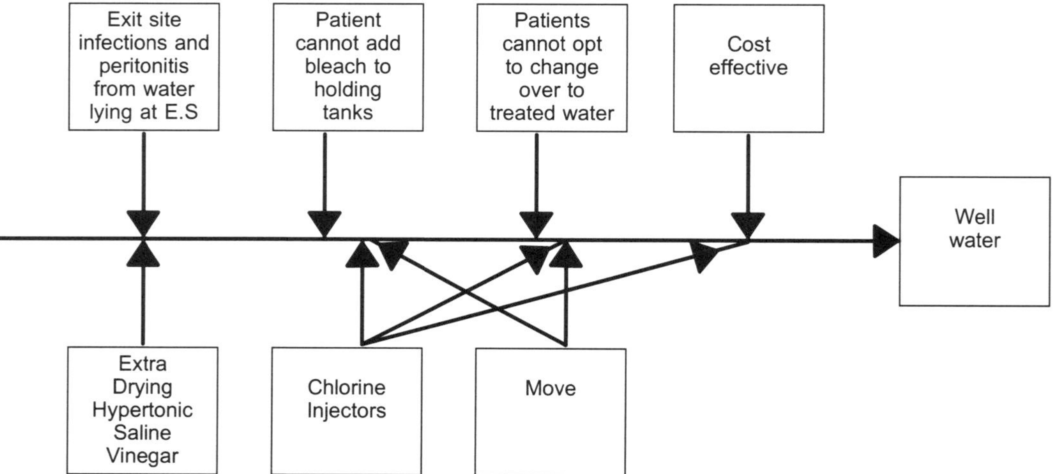

Restraining forces: Suggested solution for issues

Fig. 3.1

CQI Action Plan

I. Issue to address
Test the solution – installation of chlorine feeders and aggressive exit site care in patients with wells.

2. Desired outcome
Identify patients with contaminated well water. Prevent pseudomonas infection in patients with wells.

3. Action	*4. Staff responsibility*	*5. Start date*	*6. End date*	*7. Measurement/comments*
1. Culture remaining wells	Jennifer		11/30	One positive for pseudomonas
2. Reculture wells that have had chlorine feeders installed	Jennifer	10/15	10/30	All negative
3. Question each new patient regarding water source	Primary Nurse as poart of psych-social evaluation	Ongoing		
Teach aggressive exit site care to those with wells	Primary Nurse	Ongoing		
Culture new wells	Jennifer	Ongoing		
4. Monitor infection by patient, by system, by organism	Dolores	Monthly	11/30	Zero exit site or peritonitis by pseudomonas
5. Encourage downward directed exit sites	Physician	Ongoing		19 of 29 downward
6. Continue maintenance agreements on all treated wells	Water treatment company	Ongoing		
7. Aggressive exit site care in all patients with wells	Primary Nurse	Ongoing	11/30	Zero exit site infection rate by any organism

Prepared by: R.N.   Date: 2/29

Testing the Solution

There were three goals for the test:

1. Identify those patients with contaminated well water, therefore at high risk for pseudomonas infection, either exit site or peritonitis

2. Prevent pseudomonas exit site infections in patients with wells

3. Prevent pseudomonas peritonitis in patients with wells.

The County Health Department, responsible for developing a pseudomonas-specific testing procedure, assisted in culturing two wells in different areas. The samples which were obtained "midstream" after the water was on for five minutes, grew pseudomonas. The probable species was fluorescens. The health department bacteriologist indicated that the hospital laboratory, with less sophisticated equipment, would probably identify it as pseudomonas aeruginosa in patient cultures, and it did.

Test the Solution

Test objective: To determine if treating a patient's water, at either the source of the water or the source of entry into the patient can eliminate pseudomonas infections.

Test description: Chlorine feeders placed on wells: 1. Known to be contaminated and 2. Belonging to patients who have had pseudomonas infection. Aggressive exit site care for all patients with wells.

Test investigator(s): L.V.N., and R.N.
Time period of test: from 9/1 to 12/1
Sample size: 10 patients
Baseline period of measurement: Feb to May (7 cases of pseudomonas)

Data before solution test:
Seven cases of pseudomonas peritonitis over a four month period

Data after solution test:
Zero cases of pseudomonas peritonitis

50% of all patients with wells had pseudomonas infections. Cultured wells were positive for pseudomonas

Negative repeat well cultures

Other measurement before:
Pseudomonas exit site infections in three patients with wells

Other measurement after:
Zero exit site infections in this group by any organism

Comments:
The lack of any exit site infections in this group was surprising (will begin CQI project to investigate further)

Recorded by:
Head nurse 2/29

Communication Process

The physicians and administrator were kept informed at weekly intervals and findings were reported at the monthly CQI meetings. The Baxter representative and other Home Program Coordinators were informed of these findings to alert other units to potential problems

The Second Action Plan

There were two possible choices for the second action plan. The patients could move to city water, or their existing water could be chlorinated. A water treatment company suggested that a chlorine feeder be placed on the water line. The physicians and the administrator were supportive of the plan. Corporate managers expressed concern regarding liability if the feeders were not properly maintained by the patient. The dialysis center decided to lease the equipment with a monthly maintenance agreement. The unit administrator negotiated the contract and obtained corporate approval. The CQI team agreed that ethically the dialysis center had a strong responsibility to install the feeders and needed to provide the best, safest

care available to all patients, not just those financially able to have such basics as safe water.

Cost Effectiveness

The seriousness of the problem demanded that the dialysis center move as quickly as possible. Having implemented a completely successful action plan for exit site care, the cost of moving on to chlorine feeders was justified. The chlorine feeders were placed on two of the patients' wells. The water treatment company did all of the work, including some plumbing changes which each patient paid.

The unit paid for chlorine feeder installation, lease and maintenance agreements. The cost of pseudomonas peritonitis in patient suffering and risk cannot be measured, however, hospitalization costs were measurable. Over a six month period, 20 days of daily charges were lost while patients were hospitalized. One patient was on backup hemodialysis for 30 days. These 50 days cost the dialysis department revenue. Two patients' bags were medicated with Fortaz provided by the unit since there was no insurance coverage for medication. Treatment protocol calls for urokinase infusion when the bag clears, repeated seven days prior to completion of the medication.

Cost Summary
Related to Pseudomonas Episodes

Cost to treat pseudomonas	*Cost to proactively treat wells*
1. Nursing time to medicate bags 20 min/day × 28 days × \$21/hour × 3.5 episodes = \$686	1. Chlorine feeder installation – \$250/patient
2. Fortaz – \$874 (\$16.04 minus \$7.12 Medicare reimbursement = \$8.92/gm × 28 doses × 3.5 episodes	2. Lease agreement with maintenance – \$520/patient Total = \$670 per patient
3. Syringes and sterile water (not calculated)	
4. Nine cultures – \$675	
5. Urokinase infusions – medication – \$1160 – nursing time – \$672 – i.v. solution tubing and bags for dialysate for irrigation – \$307	
6. Medications at an outside pharmacy – \$720 (Fortaz, tobramycin, ciprofloxacin)	
7. Cost to Medicare, MediCal and private insurance included 20 hospital days and the cost of catheter replacement for one of the patients	
8. Lost patient work days (not calculated)	
9. **Total = \$5094+**	

The Future

The dialysis center realized that preventing further episodes of pseudomonas due to patients' well water required an ongoing commitment which included:

1. Culturing remaining wells at \$15.00 per well. Considering chlorine feeders on an individual basis.

2. Reculturing wells that had been treated to ensure effectiveness.

3. Questioning all new patients regarding water source.

4. Continuing to monitor infection rates.

5. More aggressively encouraging surgeons that all new catheters have a downward directed exit site to help prevent water from entering the tunnel.

6. Encouraging maintenance agreements to ensure adequacy and safety of the feeders.

7. Aggressively caring for the exit site on all patients known to have wells.

Impact on the Community

Community wells were discovered to be causing a unique problem. The city was contacted and reported that it did have very poor quality water and was trying to obtain grants for improvement. An article on the city's water problems reported that the filters had been changed for the first time in many years

Staff Involvement

The medical director assisted in the development of an exit site protocol and elicited support for the plan among the other nephrologists and dialysis units in the area. Each primary nurse reviewed exit site care, explained the project to patients and checked the source of water for all patients. The social worker, as part of her psycho-social assessment, also checks the source of water in all new patients.

LAUNCHING A MULTI-CENTER CQI INITIATIVE

Centers Adopt a Uniform Working Process

Today, with dialysis center mergers and acquisitions becoming more prevalent, the need for multi-center CQI initiatives is becoming a necessity and is demonstrating value. Dialysis centers are achieving results, as in the cases recently of regional launches. An organization selects an area of study and begins continuous quality improvement process implementation within a three-month period. Over a reasonable timeframe, the centers adopt a similar and uniform working process that helps the organization improve patient care, and streamline operational activities.

Efforts are focused on motivating management and clinicians to assume specific roles, moving key individuals onto a corporate leadership team, assigning those closest to the area of study onto individual dialysis center working teams, ensuring everyone is appropriately trained in tools, techniques, and the process, and that all meetings are facilitated uniformly.

The corporate team encourages and oversees the activities of each of the center teams, ensuring that results are communicated and measured. It is key that the corporate team commits to rewarding overall effort and success.

CONCLUSION

Implementation of a continuous quality improvement process helps dialysis center personnel focus on improving patient outcomes, increasing patient satisfaction, increasing employee satisfaction and involvement, reducing costs, and enhancing patient care quality. The dialysis center is consistently moving along the improvement continuum by collecting and analyzing data through CQI to benchmark against available best demonstrated practices and share successes. The result is a thriving dialysis center in a changing health care environment.

REFERENCES

1. Henderson LW and Thuma RS. Quality assurance in dialysis. The Netherlands, Kluwer Academic Publishers, 1994.
2. Fliehman DG and Auld DD, Customer retention through quality leadership – the Baxter approach. American Society of Quality Control, Milwaukee, Wisconsin, 1993.
3. Baxter CQI Educational Assistance Award Applications.
4. The team handbook, how to use teams to improve quality. Madison, Wisconsin, Joiner Associates, Inc., 1988.
5. Walton M. The Deming management method. New York, The Putnam Publishing Group, 1986.
6. Walton, M. Deming management at work. New York, G.P. Putnam's Sons, 1990.
7. Imai M. KAIZEN, the key to Japan's competitive success. New York, The KAIZEN Institute, Ltd, 1986.
8. Boyett J, Schwartz S, Osterwise L and Bauer R. The quality journey: how winning the Baldrige sparked the remaking of IBM. J.H. Boyett, S.B. Schwartz, L.L. Osterwise and R.A. Bauer. New York, Penguin Books USA Inc., 1993.
9. Stratton DA. An approach to quality improvement that works, 2nd edition. Milwaukee, Wisconsin, ASQC Quality Press, 1991.

4. Choice of statistical models for assessing the clinical outcomes of the efforts to provide high quality care for the ESRD patient

EDWARD F. VONESH

INTRODUCTION

The role of quality assurance (QA) and continuous quality improvement (CQI) in the managed care of ESRD patients is closely linked with the ideas of evidence- based clinical practice and outcomes research. With concerns over rising costs in the treatment of ESRD patients, evidence-based clinical practice provides a mechanism whereby clinicians can choose a cost effective treatment or therapy for a group or subgroup of patients while optimizing select patient outcomes (e.g. improved patient survival, better quality of life, reduced patient hospitalization, etc.). This chapter provides some basic statistical principles, methods and models which clinicians can use in pursuit of evidence based clinical practice, quality assurance, CQI and/or outcomes research. Specific attention will be paid to the use of proper statistical methods for collecting, analyzing and summarizing patient-specific outcomes as they relate to a set of explanatory variables (i.e. independent variables or covariates).

TYPES OF OUTCOMES (DEPENDENT VARIABLES)

Outcome variables, also known as dependent variables or endpoints, are those variables which are of primary interest to the investigator. Typically, the goal of the investigator is to relate the outcome variable(s) to a set of explanatory variables (also known as covariates or independent variables) using some type of statistical regression model. There are a number of different patient related outcome measures which clinicians routinely track. These outcome measures can be classified into two categories: discrete outcomes and continuous outcomes. Discrete outcomes correspond to measured endpoints having a countable and/or finite number of values. The outcomes are often categorical in nature. Examples of discrete outcomes include:

1. The number of infections a dialysis patient has over a given period of time (e.g. 0, 1, 2, 3, ... episodes of peritonitis in 1 year of follow-up).

2. The Karnofsky score (0 to 100 scale) describing patient functionality

3. The number of hospital admissions a patient experiences during a given time period (e.g. 0, 1, 2, ... admissions in 1 year of follow-up)

4. A subjective global assessment (SGA) of a patient's level of malnutrition (e.g. 0=none, 1=mild, 2=moderate, 3=severe)

5. Patient quality of life (QOL) which is based on tools like the KDQOL, a Kidney and Dialysis Quality of Life questionnaire.

In some cases, a discrete variable will be strictly categorical (e.g. the presence or absence of some condition or disease) while in other cases, the outcome will be ordinal in nature, that is, the levels of the outcome correspond to some natural ordering (e.g. the SGA score described previously is inherently ordered from $0 =$ none to $3 =$ severe).

Continuous outcome measures, on the other hand, correspond to measurements that can assume any value within a given line interval.

L.W. Henderson and R.S. Thuma (eds.), Quality Assurance in Dialysis, 2nd Edition, 39–54.
© *1999 Kluwer Academic Publishers. Printed in Great Britain*

Examples of continuous outcome measurements include

1. Serum chemistries (e.g. serum creatinine, blood urea nitrogen, serum glucose, calcium, etc.)

2. Patient anthropometric data (e.g. height, weight, body surface area)

3. Measures of dialysis adequacy (Urea Kt/V, Urea reduction ratio, weekly creatinine clearance, ultrafiltration)

4. Nutritional measures (dietary protein intake, serum albumin and total protein, nitrogen balance)

5. Time-related outcomes wherein the time to a certain event such as death (patient survival time) or transfer to another modality (technique survival time) are measured.

In some instances, continuous outcome variables may be classified into discrete outcomes. For example, a peritoneal dialysis patient undergoing a standard peritoneal equilibration test (PET) may be classified as a High, High Average, Low Average or Low transport patient depending on where the patient's measured dialysate to plasma (D/P) creatinine concentration ratio lies [1]. Here, the D/P ratio is a continuous variable which is used to form a discrete variable, namely the patient's PET classification. The PET classification, in turn, represents an ordered categorical variable which corresponds to the interval ordering of the actual D/P values.

As suggested by the above examples, there are numerous types of outcome variables used to track patient care. It would be nearly impossible to describe, in a single chapter, an appropriate statistical method and/or model for the various outcome measures used in routine clinical practice. For example, to compare a continuous outcome measure between two treatment groups, we might compare the sample means using a Student *t*-test provided the measurements are independent and normally distributed (i.e. when a histogram of the data is fairly symmetric and bell-shaped). However, if the distribution of measurements is skewed away from symmetry (i.e. one tail of the histogram is significantly longer than the other), then it would be more appropriate to compare the sample medians using a nonparametric test like the two-sample Wilcoxon rank sum test (equivalent to the Mann-Whitney test) [2–3]. Thus even in this simple scenario, there are choices to be made regarding an appropriate statistical method. Given the importance of tracking measures of adequacy and nutrition over time as well as tracking morbidity and mortality among ESRD patients, this chapter will focus primarily on methods for analyzing longitudinal data with particular emphasis placed on serial data (repeated measurements) and on time-related outcomes (e.g. patient and technique survival, infection rates, hospitalization rates).

TYPES OF COVARIATES (INDEPENDENT VARIABLES OR EXPLANATORY VARIABLES)

Covariates, also known as independent or explanatory variables, are those factors and/or variables which may be predictive of the outcome being measured. As with outcome variables, covariates may be continuous or discrete variables. Examples of explanatory covariates, both continuous and discrete, include:

1. Gender
2. Race
3. Age
4. Primary cause of ESRD
5. The presence or absence of comorbid conditions
6. A disease severity index like the Index of Coexisting Disease (ICED)
7. Treatment group or treatment modality

In some instances, covariates may be identified as key outcome variables. For example, baseline serum albumin may prove to be a useful explanatory variable in mortality studies in that, as a surrogate for baseline nutritional status, it may be predictive of patients with increased risk for death. Alternatively, serum albumin could serve as a key outcome variable in a nutritional study investigating the effect of a dietary supplement on the nutritional status of ESRD patients. Care must be shown, however, not to include certain outcome variables as covariates particularly when they have a cause and effect relation with the primary outcome variable.

STUDY DESIGN

In an effort to provide high quality care for patients, clinicians are often asked to choose from several different treatments. Ideally, such choices would be based on sound scientific evidence demonstrating the superiority of one treatment over another. The validity of such evidence depends, in large part, on the study design used. One can usually classify the study design by specifying each of three conditions: 1) Study Type – this describes the level of control the investigator has with respect to assigning patients to a particular treatment and/or exposure; 2) Data Type – this describes when and how observations are to be taken; and 3) Patient Type – this describes whether patients included in the study are current (prevalent), new (incident) or both. Table 4.1 gives a list of these conditions with each arranged in hierarchical order from best to least desirable. In designing a study, the investigator can choose from any combination of study type, data type and patient type; however, it is important to understand the advantages and disadvantages of each. The best design in Table 4.1 is the randomized prospective longitudinal study of new (incident) patients. By randomizing new patients to different treatment options, we minimize any chances there are for introducing bias into the study. The least desirable design, in terms of having the greatest potential for bias, is the observational cross-sectional study of current (prevalent) patients. Below, we briefly describe the benefits and drawbacks to each condition.

In terms of study type, experimental studies are those in which some sort of patient intervention is planned and the nature of that intervention is completely under the control of the investigator. The randomized prospective clinical trial comparing two treatments is the most commonly used experimental study, but there are examples of experimental studies where patient intervention occurs without randomization. By contrast, observational studies are strictly descriptive in nature.

Table 4.1. Key conditions for selecting a study design

Study type	Data type	Patient type
Experimental	Longitudinal	Incidence
– Randomized	– Prospective	
– Nonrandomized	– Retrospective	
Observational	Cross-sectional	Prevalent
	– Prospective	
	– Retrospective	

Unlike the experimental study, the investigator has no control over patient assignment to treatment (or exposure) in an observational study and there are no planned interventions. Here, the outcome variable is related to the treatment (or exposure) which the patient happens to be on. In experimental studies where intervention is possible, the investigator is in a position to formulate and test specific cause-and-effect hypotheses. In contrast, observational studies only allow the investigator to examine whether or not there is a significant association between treatment (or exposure) and outcome.

In measuring outcomes and/or covariates, the investigator can choose between collecting serial data over time on the same individuals (longitudinal data) or collecting a single measurement at a particular point in time across individuals (cross-sectional data). The advantage of collecting longitudinal data is that it enables us to distinguish changes over time within patients versus changes over time between patients. Cross-sectional studies allow us to evaluate changes between different cohorts of patients but they do not allow us to identify changes over time within patients. For example, in assessing the relationship between urea generation and age among a group of dialysis patients, a cross-sectional sample of baseline urea generation rates might reveal a trend like that shown in Figure 4.1. This trend shows that urea generation decreases with age, probably as a result of decreased protein intake. However, Figure 4.2 reveals that when follow-up data is included on each patient, there is actually an increase in urea generation during the first year or so of dialysis. In addition, the data in Figure 4.2 also reveals that older patients have a lower urea generation, at baseline, than younger patients. Although fictitious (the data were simulated), this example illustrates the advantages of longitudinal versus cross-sectional data. In particular, the analysis of the longitudinal data reveals the benefits of dialysis within cohorts of patients which the cross-sectional analysis fails to reveal. Finally, longitudinal studies also include those which track time-related outcomes like patient and technique survival, hospitalization rates, etc. Such studies are necessarily longitudinal in nature given that the measured outcome requires both a starting and ending date over which the event of interest is tracked.

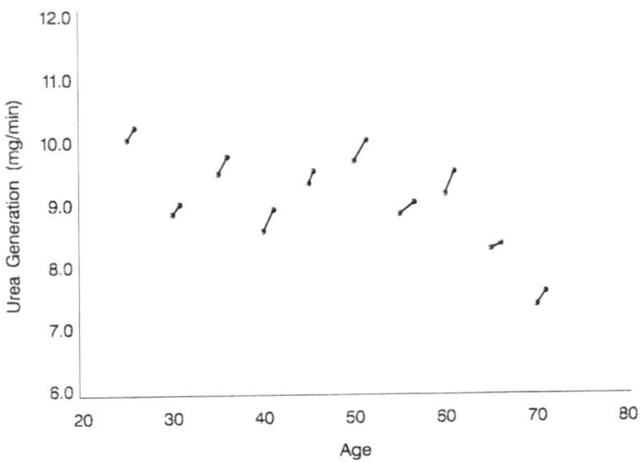

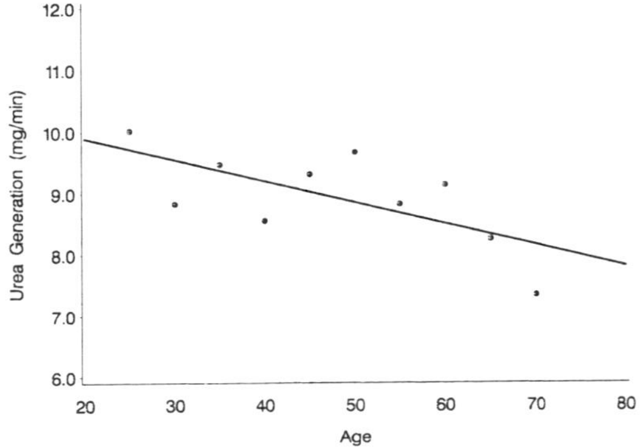

Fig. 4.1. Simulated data demonstrating cross-sectional trends between baseline urea generation rates and patient age at baseline. The regression line is given by:
Ug = 10.5921 − 0.0348 × age.

For both longitudinal and cross-sectional studies, the investigator may choose between 1) going back in time to acquire the necessary records (retrospective data); 2) collecting the data prospectively; or 3) doing both. The advantage of collecting data retrospectively is that it allows the investigator to summarize the information in a relatively short period of time. A disadvantage is that there are no guarantees regarding the quality and/or availability of the data being collected and special precautions should be taken in this regard. In a prospective study, the investigator has more direct control over the type and quality of data being collected, but this is done at the expense of time and cost. The investigator must weigh these considerations carefully when choosing between a retrospective versus prospective study.

Fig. 4.2. Simulated data demonstrating longitudinal trends between urea generation rates, time on dialysis, and age.

In terms of the type of ESRD patient studied, the investigator may choose to include 1) those patients new to dialysis (incident patients); 2) those patients currently on dialysis at a given date (point prevalent patients); or 3) those patients who are either new or current (period prevalent patients). Figure 4.3 presents a schematic illustrating prevalent and incident patients. In terms of statistical analysis, the ideal scenario would be to do a prospective longitudinal study of new (or incident) patients so that the relation between treatment (or exposure) and outcome may be determined from the very onset of treatment (exposure). This approach avoids any bias that might otherwise occur if one group of prevalent patients had been on dialysis longer than another. It would also require specifying a patient accrual period during which new dialysis patients are entered into the study. The chief drawback to a study of purely incident-based patients is that it usually takes an extended period of time to recruit the necessary number of patients. Consequently, many investigators include both new (incident) and current (prevalent) patients in their study population. If the study is a randomized prospective study, this will not be an issue since randomization will, in all likelihood, ensure the comparability of patients within each treatment group. If the study is not randomized, then additional precautions, usually in the form of statistical adjustments, are needed to help reduce bias in the group comparisons.

Prevalent (Current) versus Incident (New) Patients

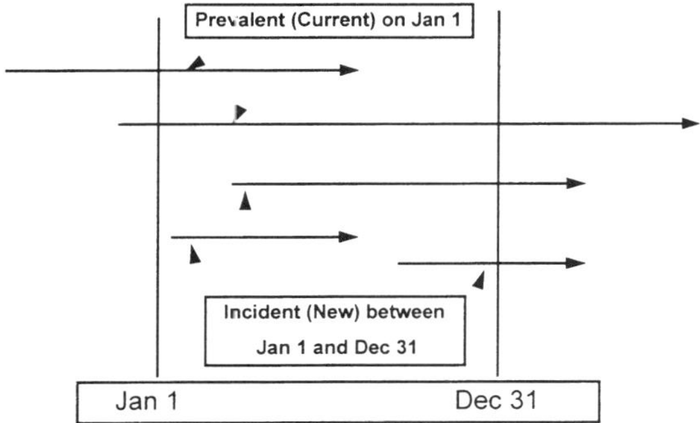

Fig. 4.3. Schematic of prevalent versus incident patients. Patients on dialysis January 1 are said to be point prevalent patients on that date. New patients who start dialysis between January 1 and December 31 of a given year are said to be incident patients for that cohort period. Period prevalent patients are all patients who received any form of dialysis during the cohort period (i.e. both point prevalent and incidence patients).

Finally, cross-sectional studies, by their very nature, are almost exclusively restricted to prevalent patients.

In summary, there are a number of study designs we can employ in pursuit of quality assurance, CQI and evidence based clinical practice. Despite the obvious advantages associated with randomized clinical trials, such trials are not always feasible. Consider, for example, a study designed to compare mortality rates between ESRD patients receiving maintenance hemodialysis (HD) versus peritoneal dialysis (PD). Significant differences in lifestyle between HD and PD make randomization all but impossible. Faced with this reality, the investigator must then choose an alternative design based on considerations like those just discussed. Since the focus of this chapter is primarily on methods for analyzing serial data and time-related outcomes (e.g. patient survival, technique failure, infection rates, hospitalization rates, etc.), the models and methods described in the following sections all assume the study is longitudinal in nature. Other study designs not discussed here include case-control studies, historical comparative studies, etc. all of which require additional considerations [4–6].

STATISTICAL MODELS FOR SERIAL DATA (REPEATED MEASUREMENTS)

Before addressing methods for analyzing time-related outcomes like patient survival, let us first consider methods for analyzing serial data like the urea generation rates shown in Figure 4.2. Serial or longitudinal data like this are referred to as repeated measurements reflecting the fact that each individual has repeat observations taken over time. There are special features associated with repeated measurements that we must take into consideration when performing an analysis. First and foremost is the recognition that individuals contribute more than one observation each to the data. Ignoring this aspect could seriously bias any inference we make. Suppose, for example, that we were to ignore this aspect of the urea generation rates (Ug) shown in Figure 4.2 and proceeded to fit the data using ordinary linear regression. The assumed linear regression model may be written as

$$Ug = \beta_0 + \beta_1 \times age + error$$

where β_0 is the intercept and β_1 the slope. Using any standard regression package, we would obtain the estimated linear regression equation:

$$Ug = 10.7129 - 0.0345 \times age$$

which, as depicted in Figure 4.4, is very similar to the cross-sectional results shown in Figure 4.1. Student *t*-tests based on the estimated intercept and its standard error (10.7129 ± 0.4662) and the estimated slope and its standard error (-0.0345 ± 0.0093) reveal that both the intercept and slope are significantly different from 0 ($p < 0.01$). These results indicate that urea generation decreases significantly with increasing age; a result similar to what we find for the purely cross-sectional data of Figure 4.1. This stands to reason even though the analysis incorrectly treats the data as though it were cross-sectional rather than longitudinal.

Suppose, instead, we were to take into account the repeated measures aspects of the data. To do so, we would first differentiate the effect of age at baseline from follow-up time on dialysis. Let time = the difference between the patient's age at follow-up minus his/her age at baseline. To relate

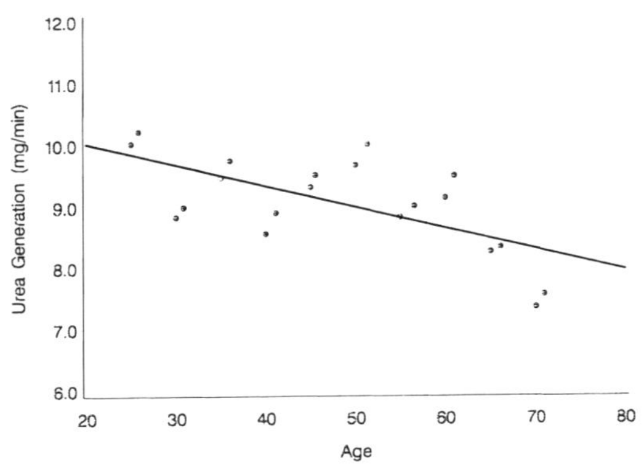

Fig. 4.4. Results obtained when one performs an ordinary linear regression on the serial urea generation rates data of Figure 4.2 as a function of age. Here the regression line is given by: Ug = 10.7129 − 0.0345 × age.

urea generation to time on dialysis and simultaneously account for differences in baseline age, statisticians would analyze this data using a two-stage random coefficient regression model (or, more generally, a linear mixed-effects model) [7–9]. Although mathematically complicated, two-stage random coefficient regression models are conceptually quite appealing. In the first stage, we specify a linear regression model for each individual. This within-subject regression is used to model the individual's repeated measurements as a function of time and/or other time-dependent covariates. Then, in the second stage, we specify a regression model across individuals (i.e. a between-subject regression model) which relates the patient-specific regression coefficients obtained from the first stage to a set of patient-specific covariates obtained at baseline. This second stage model accounts for between-subject variability while the first stage model accounts for within-subject variability.

In terms of our example on urea generation rates, we would specify a simple linear regression model for each patient which would relate the patient's urea generation rates to his/her time on dialysis. The resulting patient-specific intercepts and slopes would then be modeled as linear functions of baseline age. Assuming both the intercepts and slopes vary from patient to patient, the random coefficient regression model can be written in terms of the two-stage regression model:

Stage 1: $\mathrm{Ug} = \beta_{i0} + \beta_{i1} \times$ time+within-patient error
Stage 2: $\beta_{i0} = \beta_{01} + \beta_{02} \times$ baseline age+random intercept error
$\beta_{i1} = \beta_{11} + \beta_{12} \times$ baseline age+random slope error

where β_{i0} and β_{i1} are the ith patient's intercept and slope, respectively. Stage 1 represents a within-patient linear regression model relating urea generation to time on dialysis while stage 2 represents a between-patient linear regression model relating the individual patient intercepts and slopes to baseline age. Substituting the model from second stage into the first stage allows us to write one overall random coefficient regression model. For the simulated data shown in Figure 4.2, the urea generation rates were actually generated assuming only that the intercepts vary from patient to patient (i.e. the random slope error in the above model is set to 0). Thus, for our example, the overall random coefficient regression model is given by:

$\mathrm{Ug} = (\beta_{01} + \beta_{02} \times \mathrm{baseline\ age}) + (\beta_{11} + \beta_{12} \times \mathrm{baseline}$
$\mathrm{age}) \times$ time+within-patient error+random intercept error
$= \beta_{01} + \beta_{02} \times$ baseline age+$\beta_{11} \times$ time+$\beta_{12} \times$ baseline age$\times$
time+within-patient error+random intercept error

We fit the urea generation data of Figure 4.2 to this model using software specifically designed for random coefficient regression models [10]. The resulting regression equation is:

$\mathrm{Ug} = 10.5842 - 0.0345 \times \mathrm{baseline\ age} + 0.3399 \times \mathrm{time} - 0.0025 \times$
baseline age$\times$ time

The standard errors and *p*-values for testing whether these estimated regression coefficients are different from 0 are summarized in Table 4.2. The results show that urea generation rates increase significantly during the first year or so of dialysis (parameter β_{11} of Table 4.2) and that baseline urea generation rates are significantly lower in older patients (parameter β_{02} of Table 4.2). Also, there was no significant effect of baseline age on the rate of increase in urea generation following initiation of dialysis (parameter β_{12} of Table 4.2).

A second key feature of repeated measurements is that the observations within individuals tend to be positively correlated. More often than not, such correlation exists as a result of having both within- and between-patient variation. In our example above, between-patient variability is directly

Table 4.2. Parameter estimates, standard errors and *p*-values for the urea generation rate data taking into account both within- and between-patient variation

Effect	Parameter	Estimate $\pm$ SE	*p*-value
Intercept	β_{01}	10.5842 ± 0.6686	0.0001
Baseline age	β_{02}	-0.0345 ± 0.0135	0.0334
Time (on dialysis)	β_{11}	0.3399 ± 0.1191	0.0213
Age$\times$time	β_{12}	-0.0025 ± 0.0023	0.3103 (NS)

Table 4.3. Parameter estimates, standard errors and *p*-values for the urea generation rate data when within- and between-patient sources of variation are collapsed into one overall source of variation

Effect	Parameter	Estimate $\pm$ SE	*p*-value
Intercept	β_{01}	10.5770 ± 0.6626	0.0001
Baseline age	β_{02}	-0.0348 ± 0.0134	0.0334
Time (on dialysis)	β_{11}	0.3627 ± 1.0241	0.7279 (NS)
Age$\times$time	β_{12}	-0.0023 ± 0.0199	0.9104 (NS)

accounted for by allowing patient intercepts to vary randomly from patient to patient while within-patient variation is accounted for by modeling changes over time on dialysis. It is important to note that ignoring both sources of variation can result in overestimating or underestimating the standard errors associated with the regression coefficients. This, in turn, can produce misleading *p*-values. To illustrate, suppose we were to ignore the fact that there is within- and between-patient variation in the urea generation rates and, instead, collapsed both into one overall source of error. The resulting model would then be as follows:

$$Ug = \beta_{01} + \beta_{02} \times \text{baseline age} + \beta_{11} \times \text{time} + \beta_{12} \times \text{baseline age} \times \text{time} + \text{overall error}$$

We can easily fit the data to this model using almost any statistical software program that does multiple regression. Using the SAS procedure MIXED [10], we obtained the parameter estimates, standard errors and *p*-values listed in Table 4.3. Despite obtaining similar parameter estimates as in Table 4.2, here the standard error associated with Time (parameter β_{11}) has increased from 0.1191 to 1.0241. Consequently, the resulting *p*-value goes from 0.0213 to 0.7279 indicating, incorrectly, that urea generation does not significantly change with time on dialysis. The reason for the discrepancies between Tables 4.2 and 4.3 stems from having an inflated standard error of 1.0241 associated with β_{11}. This, in turn, is due to the failure of the incorrect model to differentiate the relative contribution of within and between-patient variation in the estimation of β_{11}. By correctly applying a random coefficient regression model to the urea generation data of Figure 4.2, we not only find the long-term trend of decreasing urea generation with increasing age, but we also identify the short-term trend of increasing urea generation within patients following initiation of dialysis. This is a key feature and a key advantage of longitudinal studies.

The methodology for analyzing random coefficient regression models and linear mixed-effects models has recently been extended to include non-linear regression models for both discrete and continuous data [7–9]. However, the methodology is very advanced and, in most cases, requires special software to implement [7–9]. While all this may seem quite intimidating, investigators really only need be concerned with some basic principles in order to avoid presenting a faulty analysis. First, investigators need to recognize when their data consists of repeated measurements. Secondly, any analysis they perform should take into account the correlation that exists in the repeated measurements. Thirdly, investigators should be careful when using routine statistical software programs since many of the programs either require special instructions for handling repeated measurements or they fail to account for the repeated measurements altogether. Armed with these principles, investigators will be in a much better position to judge when they can and should conduct their own analysis versus when they should consult a statistician.

STATISTICAL MODELS FOR TIME-RELATED OUTCOME VARIABLES

In analyzing morbid and mortal events, we can choose to analyze either the rate of occurrence or the "survival" time associated with the event. In analyzing the rate of occurrence, the response or outcome variable is the number of events that occur divided by the time at risk for the event. Analyses based on rates are more commonly employed when tracking multiple events within individuals (e.g. hospitalization rates, infection rates, etc.). For example, Poisson regression is often used to model peritonitis rates among peritoneal dialysis patients [11–13]. However, one can also model the time to first peritonitis or the times between successive episodes of peritonitis [14–15]. In analyzing survival time data, the response or outcome variable is the length of time until the event, or, in the case of multiple events, the lengths of time between successive events. Analyses based on survival times are most often used when tracking a single event like death or technique failure. The example most clinicians are familiar with is the analysis of patient survival times using a Cox proportional hazards regression model. However, by aggregating the number of events and corresponding exposure times over various subgroups of patients, one can analyze survival time data based on the rates of occurrence of the event [16–18]. In the following sections, we will present various statistical models and methods appropriate for analyzing event rates and survival time data. We begin by first discussing a key element present in both types of analyses; namely that of censored data.

Censored Data

A major issue in the analysis of time-related outcomes, particularly survival analysis, is the presence of censored data. In tracking events over time, censoring occurs whenever the elapsed time to an event or the time between two successive events is known only partially. For example, suppose we let the variable T denote the "survival" time to some event. Then T=(*event time – origin time*) where *event time* is the time the event of interest takes place (e.g. the date on which death occurs) and *origin time* is the time we first start following the individual (e.g. the date on which a patient first starts dialysis). If either the origin time or event time or both are unknown, then the "survival" time is said to be censored; otherwise it is said to be observed.

Figure 4.5 illustrates seven different cases of observed and censored survival times that one might encounter in a study of patient survival.

The solid portion of each line represents the fraction of the patient's survival time that is actually observed and the dashed portion is that fraction which is unobserved. Patients A and B are prevalent at the start of the study and both are depicted with unknown origin times. This would occur, for example, if there were no retrospective data available on their start dates. In the case of patient B, the event time is also unknown since the patient survives past the study end date. Thus both patients have recorded survival times (i.e. the solid portion of their lines) which are censored. Patients C, D, E, and F are incident (new) patients with known starting dates, but only patient D has a known event time. Patients C, E, and F therefore have censored survival times while patient D has a

Censored Survival Times

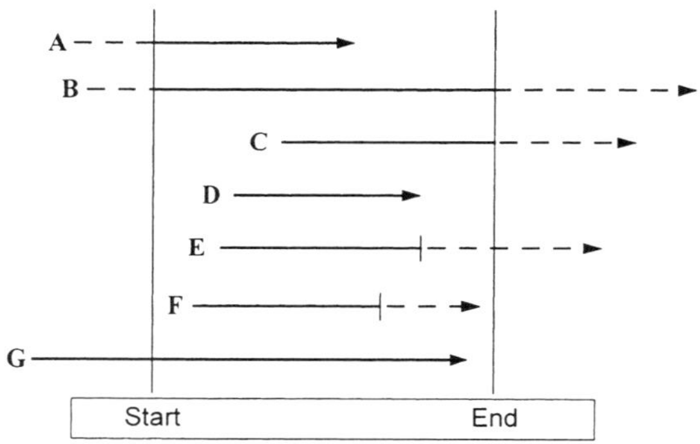

Fig. 4.5. Patient A is prevalent at the start of the study but has no known starting date (no retrospective data available). The patient dies during the study period resulting in a censored survival time (the origin time is unknown while the event time is known). Patient B is likewise prevalent at the start of the study with no known start date. This patient survives past the end of the study resulting in a censored survival time (both the origin time and event time are unknown). Patient C is an incident (new) patient who dies after the study end date resulting in a censored survival time (the origin date is known but the event date is unknown). Patient D is an incident patient who dies during the study period resulting in an observed survival time (both the origin time and event time are known). Patients E and F are incident patients who drop out before the study is complete and for whom the time of death is unknown resulting in a censored survival time (the origin times are known but the event times are unknown). Patient G is prevalent at the start of the study and has a recorded start date (retrospective data available). The patient dies during the study resulting in an observed survival time (both the origin time and event time are known).

completely observed survival time. Finally, patient G is a prevalent patient for whom retrospective data is available on the patient's start date. As this patient also dies during the study period, the patient's survival time is completely observed. Given the role of censoring, it is important to note that only patients D and G contribute fully in the estimation of expected survival while the remaining patients contribute only partial information.

Each of the statistical models which we will describe, can accommodate censored data. However, a key assumption of each model is that the censoring mechanism be unrelated to the event being tracked. For instance, the reason the survival time for patient C is censored is because the patient survived past the end of the study. In this case, the censoring mechanism is determined by the study start and end dates both of which are directly under the control of the investigator and both of which are independent of the event being tracked. Similarly, suppose patient E decides to move from the area for reasons unrelated to the study and, in the process, becomes lost-to-follow-up. If we let T_C denote this patient's censored survival time (i.e. the time up to when the patient is lost-to-folowup), then there is no reason to believe this patient will have any better or worse prognosis for survival beyond T_C than any other comparably based patient who survives to T_C. Consequently, there is nothing informative about this patient's censoring mechanism that would lead us to suspect an increased or decreased risk of death as a result of being censored. Hence, in both these examples, the censoring is said to be *uninformative* and we can proceed with our analysis assured that patients C and E will not introduce any bias into our results. On the other hand, suppose, patient F suffers a serious dialysis related complication and is transferred to another hospital where, unbeknownst to the investigator, the patient dies as a result of the complication. Here, the censoring mechanism is informative in that the prognosis for survival beyond the date of transfer is considerably worse in this patient than in other patients who have survived to the same point in time. In cases like this, the censoring is said to be *informative* and special precautions need to be taken to avoid introducing bias into the analysis. For example, when informative censoring is suspected, a sensitivity analysis can be employed to determine how robust the analysis is to those individuals with censored survival times.

Models and Methods for Analyzing Event Rates

There are numerous examples of studies involving ESRD patients where the primary outcome variable is an event rate. Examples include studies comparing mortality rates between HD and PD patients [19]; studies looking at hospitalization rates [20], and studies estimating and comparing infection rates (e.g. peritonitis rates, exit-site infections, access infections, etc.) [11–14]. In some cases, the rate is associated with a single outcome per patient (e.g. death) while in others it is associated with multiple events per patient (e.g. multiple episodes of peritonitis). In the former case, the rates are calculated by aggregating patients into subgroups according to their baseline characteristics (e.g. all Caucasian males between the ages of 20–24 for whom diabetes was their primary cause of ESRD). Once a subgroup is formed, we add up the number of events that occur within the subgroup as well as the number of years at risk contributed by each patient in the subgroup. The rate for that subgroup would then be the total number of events divided by the total number of patient years at risk. When there are multiple events per patient, we calculate a rate for each patient by simply adding up the number of events per patient and dividing by the number of days (or months or years) at risk per patient. Regardless of whether a rate reflects data from a subgroup of patients or an individual patient, we can write the rate symbolically as $R = X/t$ where R is the observed rate for the subgroup (or patient) while X and t are the corresponding number of events and time at risk. An estimate of the standard error (SE) of R is $S = \sqrt{R/t}$ so that inference about the true but unobserved rate can be made on the basis of the approximate 95% confidence interval, $R \pm 1.96 \times S$.

When comparing event rates across groups of patients, it is often necessary to adjust for differences in the demographic makeup of the groups. A failure to make such adjustments can result in misleading comparisons. For example, consider the annual death rates between the two groups of patients shown in Table 4.4. Ignoring age, the overall death rates (± 1 SE) are 27 ± 1.64 deaths per 100 patient years for Group A and 22.5 ± 1.5 deaths per 100 patient years for Group B. Based on these crude death rates and their standard errors, there appears to be a significantly higher risk of death among patients in Group A (risk ratio=1.20, p=0.043). However, when we examine the age-specific death rates, the data suggest the two groups have similar overall mortality. This apparent discrepancy is a result of having an older distribution of patients in Group A compared with Group B; a feature not accounted for in the comparison of the overall rates. Thus in this example, age is a *confounding factor or variable* which needs to be accountted for in the analysis. A confounding factor is any variable (continuous or discrete) which is predictive of the outcome being measured and which is unevenly distributed across the various groups being compared.

There are several ways to adjut estimated rates for the presence of one or more confounding factors. These include the methods of *direct* and *indirect standardization* [5, 21] and the use of Poisson regression [16–18]. Direct standardization entails calculating a weighted average of observed rates across the levels of the confounding factor(s). The weights correspond to a set of proportions from some reference population. The proportions, in turn, reflect the distribution of the reference population across the different levels of the confounding factor(s). In the example above, if we use as weights the overall proportion of patients aged 20–44 (30%), 45–64 (45%) and 65+ (25%), the standardized death rates for groups A and B would be:

Group A:
Standardized rate $= 0.30 \times 15 + 0.45 \times 25 + 0.25 \times 35 = 24.5$ deaths/100 pt. years
Group B:
Standardized rate $= 0.30 \times 17 + 0.45 \times 25 + 0.25 \times 32 = 24.35$ deaths/100 pt. years

With this direct standardization, we find there is no significant difference in the adjusted death rates (the adjusted death rate ratio is 1.006, p=NS). Indirect standardization uses a set of stable age-specific rates obtained from a reference population to calculate an adjusted rate (see Fleiss [21] for details). It is most useful in situations where we have sparse data within certain cells of the confounding factor [21]. The standardized mortality

ratio (SMR) is one form of indirect standardization.

Poisson regression is an alternative method for calculating and comparing adjusted rates. Regression techniques, in general, allow one to compare treatment groups after adjusting for the presence of other explanatory or confounding variables. Because the frequency distribution of count data often follows a Poisson distribution, we can model event rates or, equivalently, the number of events in a given time period, using Poisson regression [16–18]. To illustrate, suppose we are interested in comparing the event rates between two groups of patients (Group A versus Group B) adjusting for a set of p explanatory covariates, say $Z_1, Z_2, \ldots, Z_p$. Let Group be an indicator variable that takes a value of 1 for patients in Group A and 0 for patients in Group B. If the number of events per unit of time follows a Poisson distribution, then we can model the data using Poisson regression. The model, expressed in terms of the log of the expected rate, is given by

$$\log_e(\lambda) = \beta_0 + \beta_1 \times \text{group} + \beta_2 \times Z_1 + \ldots + \beta_p \times Z_p$$

where λ is the expected (as opposed to observed) rate associated with the set of explanatory variables. The intercept, β_0 is equal to the log of the reference baseline rate, i.e. $\beta_0 = \log_e(\lambda_0)$ where λ_0 is the expected rate for the reference group (i.e. the group of patients with values of 0 for Group, $Z_1, Z_2, \ldots, Z_p$. The remaining regression coefficients can be interpreted as adjusted log rate ratios. For example, β_1 is the log of the rate ratio between Group A and Group B adjusted for $Z_1, Z_2, \ldots, Z_p$. To see this, simply take the exponent of both sides of the model and substitute the appropriate values of Group into the resulting equation. Doing so, we end up with the expected rates for groups A and B as:

$$\lambda_A = \exp(\beta_0 + \beta_1 \times 1 + \beta_2 \times Z_1 + \ldots + \beta_p \times Z_p)$$
$$\lambda_B = \exp(\beta_0 + \beta_1 \times 0 + \beta_2 \times Z_1 + \ldots + \beta_p \times Z_p).$$

Upon simplification, the rate ratio (or relative risk), λ_A/λ_B, reduces to $\exp(\beta_1)$ which implies the log rate ratio (log relative risk) is simply $\log_e(\lambda_A/\lambda_B) = \beta_1$.

Applying a Poisson regression analysis to the death rate data of Table 4.4, we end up with the estimated regression equation:

$$\log_e(DR) = -1.0651 - 0.0025 \times \text{group} - 0.7460 \times \text{AGE20} - 0.3201 \times \text{AGE45}$$

where DR represents the expected death rate, AGE20 is an indicator variable taking a value of 1 if the age group is 20–44 and 0 otherwise, and AGE45 is an indicator variable taking a value of 1 if the age group is 45–64 and 0 otherwise. The regression coefficient for the variable Group is estimated to be -0.0025 ± 0.0977 ($p=0.979$) which yields an adjusted death rate ratio of exp(-0.0025)=0.9975; a result very similar to what we obtained using direct standardization.

Table 4.4. Observed deaths and years at risk for two groups of patients. Death rates are expressed as numbers of deaths per 100 patient years at risk

| | | Group | | | | | |
| | | A | | | B | | |
Age group	% of patients	Deaths	Years at risk	Death rate	Deaths	Years at risk	Death rate
20–44	30	30	200	15	68	400	17
45–64	45	100	400	25	125	500	25
65+	25	140	400	35	32	100	32
Total	100	270	1000	27	225	1000	22.5

In terms of variability, Poisson regression assumes the mean and variance of the counts are equal, and this feature needs to be taken into account when computing estimates of the regression coefficients and their standard errors. There are times, however, when count data (or rates) exhibit greater variation than can be explained by standard Poisson regression [22]. In this case, a further adjustment is needed to estimate the standard errors of the regression coefficients [22]. Examples of this occur frequently in the analysis of peritonitis rates among PD patients [11–12]. The excessive variation in the number of episodes of peritonitis across patients can be accounted for in the Poisson model by allowing the patient-specific rates to vary randomly from patient to patient. This type of Poisson regression is known as gamma-Poisson regression and the model is a gamma-Poisson model (also known as a negative binomial model or a mixed-effects Poisson model)

[11–12]. It is important to note that failure to account for excess Poisson variation can produce misleading results.

Models and Methods for Analyzing Survival Time Data

In contrast to methods for analyzing event rates, the analysis of survival time data necessarily requires having the survival times for each patient. This feature leads to more efficient inference when compared to methods based on aggregated data and summary rates [22]. This is particularly true when dealing with outcome variables which represent one and only one event (e.g. death). However, when the data entail multiple events over time per patient (e.g. number of hospital visits per year), an analysis based strictly on the time to the first event will be less efficient than an analysis on the individual patient rates [14].

Rather than working with rates or the numbers of events in time, the analysis of survival time data focuses on the individual's actual survival time, say T. Also fundamental to the analysis of survival time data are the concepts of the *survivor function* and the *hazard function*. The survivor function, denoted by S(t), describes the individual's probability of "surviving" beyond some time point, t. Specifically, $S(t) = Pr[T>t]$ where $Pr[T>t]$ stands for the probability that an individual's "survival" time, T, exceeds t. Here, use of the term "survival" stems from the many applications where death is the primary event of interest. In our more general setting, the survival time, T, simply refers to the time to an event and S(t) is simply the probability that an individual remains free of the event beyond t. The hazard function or hazard rate, denoted by h(t), is a potentially complicated mathematical function which describes the individual's instantaneous risk of an event occurring at time t. It is not a probability, per se, but rather a rate which may or may not change with time. The hazard function has much the same interpretation as an event rate in that it is a dimensional quantity having the same form, namely the number of events per interval of time [23]. In fact, the observed event rate, as defined in the previous section (i.e. $R = X/t$), may be viewed as an estimate of the hazard rate provided the hazard rate is nearly constant over the interval of follow-up on which X and t are observed. However, a key feature of the hazard function is that it is not necessarily constant over time. For example, we know the risk of dying will eventually start increasing as a person ages making the hazard rate, at that point, an increasing function of time. Figure 4.6 contains examples of various hazard functions or rates. When the hazard rate is constant, i.e. $h(t) = h$, the distribution of survival times follows what is known as an exponential distribution and the survivor function is simply $S(t) = \exp(-h \times t)$.

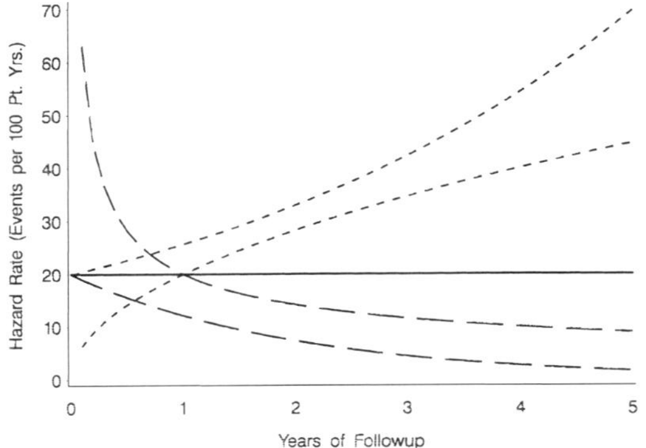

Fig. 4.6. Examples of increasing, decreasing and constant hazard rates expressed as events for 100 patient years.

Methods for analyzing survival time data are divided into two areas: descriptive and predictive. Descriptive methods include estimating unadjusted survival curves using either the Kaplan–Meier method (also known as the product-limit method) or the lifetable (actuarial) method, and comparing these unadjusted survival curves using a log-rank test [23, 24]. Predictive methods utilize regression techniques like the Cox proportional hazards regression model to estimate and compare adjusted survival curves with adjustment made for other explanatory or confounding variables [23, 25].

The Kaplan–Meier method produces a non-parametric estimate of the survivor function $S(t)$ and, as such, requires no information about the underlying hazard function $h(t)$. It is best used when one has precisely measured survival times (e.g. the event dates are known exactly). The lifetable or actuarial method also produces a non-

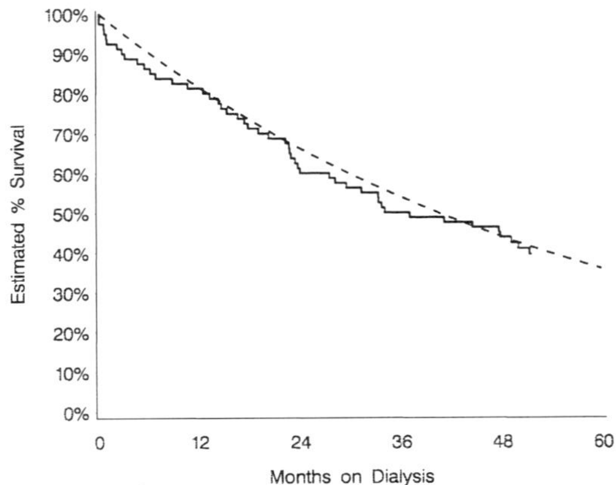

Fig. 4.7. Example of a Kaplan–Meier estimated survival curve (solid line) where the true hazard rate is constant over time versus an estimated survival curve obtained assuming a constant hazard rate (dashed line).

parametric estimate of the survivor function, but it is better suited when survival times are less precisely known (e.g. the month an event occurs is known but not the exact date). In the rare instance when the time to the event is known exactly for everyone, the Kaplan–Meier estimate of survival at time t is readily computed as the fraction of patients with event times greater than t. However, more often than not the event times will be subject to censoring and one will need the assistance of a computer program to calculate the Kaplan–Meier estimate. Alternatively, if we know what form the hazard rate takes, we can plot the survival curve using a parametric estimate of $S(t)$ such as the exponential survivor function, $S(t) = \exp(-h \times t)$. For example, the patient survival data shown in Figure 4.7 were simulated assuming a constant death rate of 20 deaths per 100 patient years (i.e. the hazard rate is assumed constant at $h = 0.20$ deaths per year). As we would expect, the estimated exponential survival curve (dashed line) provides a good fit to the "observed" Kaplan–Meier survival curve (solid line). In contrast, the survival data shown in Figure 4.8 were generated assuming a decreasing hazard rate. Here, the estimated exponential survival curve overestimates the "observed" Kaplan–Meier survival curve everywhere but at the very beginning and end. This example highlights a key benefit of the Kaplan–

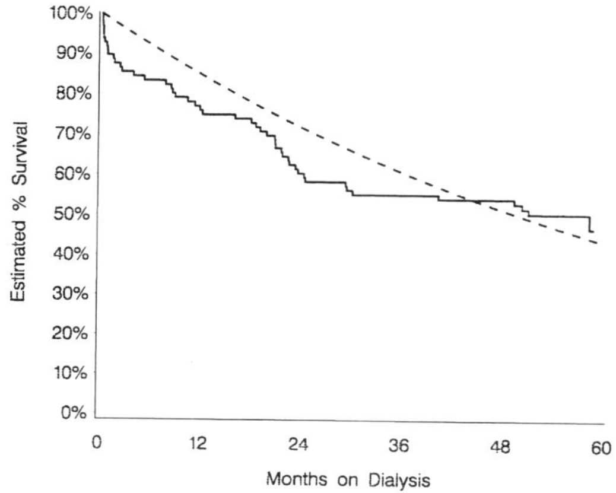

Fig. 4.8. Example of a Kaplan–Meier estimated survival curve (solid line) where the true hazard rate is a decreasing function of time versus an estimated survival curve obtained assuming a constant hazard rate (dashed line).

$$\log_e(h(t)) = \log_e(h_0(t)) + \beta_1 \times \text{Group} + \beta_2 \times Z_1 + \ldots + \beta_p \times Z_p$$

where Group is the indicator variable defining what treatment group patients belong (e.g. Group=1 if patients are in Group A; Group=0 if patients are in Group B).

In contrast to Poisson regression where we directly model the observed event rates (i.e. $R = X/t$), the hazard rate, $h(t)$, is neither observed nor estimated under the Cox model and regression is carried out on the basis of the ranks of the observed survival times. Specifically, Cox regression is based on a technique known as partial likelihood to estimate the regression coefficients [26]. It is, in part, due to this technique that the Cox regression model has achieved such wide spread appeal. Because it is semi-nonparametric, partial likelihood estimation is similar to Kaplan–Meier estimation in that it does not require knowledge of the baseline hazard rate, $h_0(t)$. Indeed estimation and inference are carried out solely on the basis of the ranks of the event times.

Finally, the term proportional hazards simply refers to the fact that under the Cox model, the ratio of hazard rates for any two patients will always be constant regardless of the shape of underlying hazard rates. Consequently, the hazard rates for two patients will always be proportional to one another. To see this, consider the hazard rate for a patient in Group A and a patient in Group B, both of whom have the same set of values for the explanatory variables, $Z_1, Z_2, \ldots, Z_p$. According to the model, we have

$$
\begin{aligned}
h_A(t) &= \exp\{\log_e(h_0(t)) + \beta_1 \times 1 + \beta_2 \times Z_1 + \ldots + \beta_p \times Z_p\} \\
&= h_0(t) \times \exp\{\beta_1 \times 1 + \beta_2 \times Z_1 + \ldots + \beta_p \times Z_p\} \\
h_B(t) &= \exp\{\log_e(h_0(t)) + \beta_1 \times 0 + \beta_2 \times Z_1 + \ldots + \beta_p \times Z_p\} \\
&= h_0(t) \times \exp\{\beta_1 \times 0 + \beta_2 \times Z_1 + \ldots + \beta_p \times Z_p\}
\end{aligned}
$$

Taking the ratio of $h_A(t)/h_B(t)$ and simplifying, the unobserved and unknown baseline hazard rate, $h_0(t)$, cancels and we are left with the constant rate ratio or relative risk (RR):

$$h_A(t)/h_B(t) = \exp(\beta_1) = \text{adjusted rate ratio for Group A}$$
relative to Group B.

Thus, the term $\exp(\beta_1)$ is the relative risk of death for patients in Group A compared with patients in Group B adjusted for the covariates, $Z_1, Z_2, \ldots, Z_p$.

Meier estimate, namely its ability to estimate patient survival without requiring the investigator to know anything about the underlying hazard rate.

If the primary focus of a study is to compare "survival" between two randomized groups of patients, then the estimated Kaplan–Meier survival curve and log-rank test are appropriate tools. However, for an observational study, these methods will be somewhat limited by virtue of their inability to adjust for other explanatory variables that may be present in the data. In a landmark paper, the British statistician, Sir David R. Cox, extended the standard lifetable approach to survival analysis by introducing regression-type arguments into what is now called the Cox proportional hazards model [24]. In its most basic form, this model is not much different from the Poisson regression model of the previous section except that the expected Poisson rate, λ, is replaced by the unspecified and possibly time-dependent hazard rate, $h(t)$, and the intercept, $\beta_0 = \log_e(\lambda_0)$, is replaced by the log of the baseline hazard rate, $\log_e(h_0(t))$. Thus, for our set of baseline explanatory variables, $Z_1, Z_2, \ldots, Z_p$ the Cox regression model can be written in terms of the unknown hazard rate as:

Note that the rate ratio we get from the Cox model is similar to what we get using Poisson regression. This stands to reason since the Poisson model is also a proportional hazards model; the only difference is that it assumes the hazard rate is constant, an assumption which is not unreasonable for studies with relatively short periods of follow-up. In fact, by partitioning patient follow-up periods into smaller segments, we can use Poisson regression to fit survival time data to what is known as a piecewise exponential survival model [23]. This highly flexible model provides an alternative to the Cox model; its chief advantage lies in its ability to estimate the shape of the underlying hazard rate.

The Cox model is a widely used regression technique for tracking morbidity and mortality among ESRD patients. It has been used in a number of studies comparing patient and technique survival [19, 20, 27–30], and time to infection [14, 15]. By allowing one to simultaneously assess the effects of various explanatory variables, the Cox model gives us an ideal tool for comparing different treatment groups while controlling for case-mix differences. There are, however, some precautionary notes regarding the use of such a powerful tool. First, it is important to verify the primary assumption of the model, namely that the hazard rates are proportional over time. This can be accomplished in a variety of ways which we won't go into but which are described in most texts on survival analysis [23, 26]. Violation of this assumption, although not always serious, can lead to bias inference. For example, in a study reported by Mairorca et al. [27], diabetes would not have been found to be a significant risk factor for death when included in the Cox model. However, the factor diabetes was found to violate the proportional hazards assumption. When re-evaluated using a stratified lifetable analysis, diabetes was found to be a significant predictor of mortality.

Second, we need to be careful with the types of explanatory variables we include in the model. For example, we should not include, at baseline, any covariate that is measured after the patient's start date. This would be like predicting the future from the future which, of course, defeats the whole purpose of including baseline covariates as predictors of patient outcome. An excellent example of this and other potential pitfalls associated with the Cox model can be found in a paper by Wolfe and Strawderman [33]. Third, in some cases, two factors will interact with one another to produce an effect which is not evident by looking at each factor independently. For example, age has been shown to significantly interact with treatment therapy in studies comparing PD and HD [27, 29, 30]. It is important, therefore, to try and identify such interactions since ignoring their presence could also lead to bias inference. These are just a few issues we must grapple with when applying the Cox model. In the following section, some additional issues are presented which we need be aware of when applying many of the statistical techniques presented here.

ADDITIONAL TOPICS

A number of statistical models and methods have been presented for the analysis of longitudinal data as it pertains to improving the care of ESRD patients. Despite the great flexibility many of these models and methods exhibit, there are three other issues related to their use which we need to address. First, we need to recognize what limitations these models have in the presence of substantial dropout. Specifically, any time we analyze data from a longitudinal study of ESRD patients, particularly those on dialysis, we encounter the problem of patient dropout. If patient dropout is related to the outcome being measured, there is potential for introducing bias into the analysis as was seen in our discussion of informative censoring. Methods for handling informative censoring are extremely complicated and are best left in the hands of a professional statistician. Nonetheless, one concept investigators can appeal to when dealing with dropouts is the idea of performing an *Intent-To-Treat* analysis.

In randomized clinical trials, investigators often conduct what we call an *Intent-To-Treat* (ITT) analysis. Under such an analysis, all comparisons are made on the basis of the groups to which patients are originally randomized. The idea is to preserve the benefits of randomization in the actual comparisons. Specifically, the principles of randomization assure us that, on average, patients randomized to different treatment groups will be comparable to one another in terms of both measured and unmeasured factors. Consequently, any differences between groups following randomization can safely be ascribed to differences in the *intended* treatments even if some patients dropout, change treatment, or fail to comply with their treatment. In the area of ESRD, the ITT approach is advocated for use when comparing mortality between HD and PD [32–34].

Opponents of the ITT approach argue that noncompliant patients, and patients who switch treatments should be excluded from the analysis as these patients no longer receive the benefits of the actual treatment under investigation. Instead, they suggest performing an *As-Treated* analysis whereby the measured outcome is ascribed to the actual treatment the patient is on at that time. In most cases, this will force us to drop patients from the analysis which may lead to a bias comparison. For example, suppose we are comparing an active treatment to a placebo control and there is a higher rate of dropout and noncompliance in the group receiving the active treatment. If we restrict our analysis to those patients who complete the study and who are compliant, we may find the active treatment does better than the control. However, we can no longer be sure that these differences are due to the treatment or whether they are do due unforeseen factors related to compliance and dropout. The simple fact is, the two "As-Treated" groups will be different from the groups we started with since we have selected out patients from the analysis. Hence, we can not be sure that the benefits observed in the treatment group are truly due to the active treatment or whether they are do to the selection process.

There are numerous arguments both for and against the ITT and As-Treated approaches [35]. It is probably in the best interest of the investigator to do both types of analysis. However, when reporting the results, the investigator should emphasize the question each approach addresses. For example, in a study comparing mortality between HD and PD, an ITT analysis addresses the question of whether the initial treatment modality has any effect on subsequent mortality regardless of what path the patient takes following the initial choice of treatment. An As-Treated analysis, on the other hand, addresses the question of whether or not the current modality has any effect on mortality.

A second issue pertains to the use of relative risks and *p*-values. In summarizing results from studies examining patient survival, for example, we often find results reported in terms of relative risks. The problem with relative risks and *p*-values is that, when reported alone, they fail to give an accurate portrayal of what the actual risks are [35]. To illustrate, suppose there are two groups of patients, say groups A and B, with patients in group A having a 20% higher mortality rate than patients in group B (i.e. relative risk = 1.20). Suppose, also, these results are based on a study with over 200,000 patient years at risk and over 50,000 deaths. The *p*-value associated with this 20% increase in mortality is 0.001 indicating patients in group A have a *statistically* significant higher risk of death than patients in group B. What are we to conclude? Well, it is possible to achieve these results in any number of ways some of which may not bear any clinical relevance. For example, the death rate in group B might be 32 deaths per 100 patient years. This yields a one year survival of 73% (= 100% × exp(−.32)). The death rate in group A would be 1.20 × 32 = 38.4 deaths per 100 patient years with a corresponding one year survival of 68%(= 100% × exp(−.384)). The resulting 5% difference in absolute survival stands out as being clinically relevant and perhaps consistent with what we may have thought initially when told only that the relative risk is 1.20 and the *p*-value is 0.001. Suppose, however, the death rate is only 12 deaths per 100 patient years for group B. The corresponding one year survival would then be 89%. The death rate for group A would be 1.20 × 12 = 14.4 deaths per 100 patient years and the corresponding one year survival would be 87%. Do these results have the same clinical impact as the previous results? Are we swayed into thinking this difference in absolute survival of 2% has the same clinical impact simply because the risk ratio is 1.20 and the *p*-value is 0.001?

Hopefully, this example illustrates why we need to evaluate both relative and absolute risks. Moreover, we should never confuse statistical significance with clinical significance. By carefully choosing the sample size to be large enough, we can always "prove" that one group is statistically different from another even though the difference may be clinically meaningless. Likewise, we can always select a small enough sample size so as to conclude the two groups do not differ statistically even though the difference may have a profound clinical impact.

Finally and most importantly, we should never view the use of statistical tools like the Cox regression model as substitutes for performing well-controlled prospective randomized clinical trials. No matter how many covariates we include in a regression model, we can never be sure that all the relevant confounding factors have been accounted for. It is only by randomizing patients that we can ever be assured of an unbiased comparison between groups.

REFERENCES

1. Twardowski ZJ, Nolph KD, Khanna R et al. Peritoneal equilibration test. Perit Dial Bull 1987; 7(3):138–47.
2. Conover WJ. Practical nonparametric statistics, 2nd ed. New York: John Wiley & Sons, 1980.
3. Lehmann EL. Nonparametrics: statistical methods based on ranks. San Francisco: Holden-Day, 1975.
4. Friedman GD. Primer of epidemiology. New York: McGraw-Hill, 1974.
5. Monson RR. Occupational epidemiology. Boca Raton: CRC Press, 1980.
6. Breslow NE and Day NE. Statistical methods in cancer research, volume 1: the analysis of case–control studies. Lyon: IARC Scientific Publications No. 32, 1980.
7. Diggle PJ, Liang K-Y and Zeger SL. Analysis of longitudinal data. Oxford: Clarendon Press, 1994.
8. Davidian M and Giltinan DM. Nonlinear models for repeated measurement data, 1st edition. New York: Chapman and Hall, 1995.
9. Vonesh EF and Chinchilli VM. Linear and nonlinear models for the analysis of repeated measurements 1st edition. New York: Marcel Dekker, 1997.
10. SAS Institute Inc. Master Index to SAS System Documentation, Version 6, 3rd edition. Cary: SAS Institute Inc., 1991.
11. Vonesh EF. Estimating rates of recurrent peritonitis for patients on CAPD. Perit Dial Bull 1985; 5:59–65.
12. Vonesh EF. Modeling peritonitis rates and associated risk factors for individuals on continuous ambulatory peritoneal dialysis. Stat Med 1990; 9:263–71.
13. Luzar MA, Coles GA, Faller B et al. Staphylococcus aureus nasal carriage and infection in patients on continuous ambulatory peritoneal dialysis. N Engl J Med 1990; 322:505–9.
14. Tranaeus A, Heimburger O and Lindholm B. Peritonitis during continuous ambulatory peritoneal dialysis (CAPD): risk factors, clinical severity, and pathogenetic aspects. Perit Dial Int 1988; 8:253–63.
15. Vonesh EF. Which statistical method to use when analyzing the incidence of peritoneal dialysis related infections? Perit Dial Int 1991; 11:301–4.
16. Holford TR. The analysis of rates and of survivorship using log-linear models. Biometrics 1980; 36:299–305.
17. Berry G. The analysis of mortality by the subject-years method. Biometrics 1983; 39:173–80.
18. Frome EL. The analysis of rates using Poisson regression models. Biometrics 1983; 39:665–74.
19. Fenton SSA. Schaubel DE, Desmeules M et al. Hemodialysis versus peritoneal dialysis: a comparison of adjusted mortality rates. Am J Kidney Disease 1997; 30:334-42.
20. Canada-USA (CANUSA) Peritoneal Dialysis Study Group. Adequacy of dialysis and nutrition in continuous peritoneal dialysis: Association with clinical outcomes. J Am Soc Nephrol 1996; 7:198–207.
21. Fleiss JL. Statistical methods for rates and proportions, 2nd edition. New York: John Wiley & Sons, 1981; 237–55.
22. Dean CB and Balshaw R. Efficiency lost by analyzing counts rather than event times in Poisson and overdispersed Poisson regression models. J Am Stat Assoc 1997; 92:1387–98.
23. Allison PD. Survival analysis using the SAS system: a practical guide. Cary, NC: SAS Institute Inc., 1995.
24. Kaplan EL and Meier P. Nonparametric estimation from incomplete observations. J Am Stat Assoc 1958; 53:457–81.
25. Cox DR. Regression models and life tables (with discussion). J Royal Stat Society 1972; B34:187–220.
26. Kalbfleisch JD and Prentice RL. The statistical analysis of failure time data. New York: John Wiley & Sons, Inc., 1980.
27. Maiorca R, Vonesh E, Cancarini CG et al. A six year comparison of patient and technique survivals in CAPD and HD. Kidney Int 1988; 34:518–24.
28. Serkes KD, Blagg CR, Nolph KD, Vonesh EF and Shapiro F. Comparison of patient and technique survival in continuous ambulatory peritoneal dialysis (CAPD) and hemodialysis: a multicenter study. Perit Dial Int 1989; 10:15–19.
29. Maiorca R, Vonesh EF, Cavilli P et al. A multicenter selection-adjusted comparison of patient and technique survivals on CAPD and hemodialysis. Perit Dial Int 1991; 11:118–17.
30. Held PJ, Port FK, Turenne MN, Gaylin DS, Hamburger RJ and Wolfe RA. Continuous ambulatory peritoneal dialysis and hemodialysis: comparison of patient mortality with adjustment for comorbid conditions. Kidney Int 1994; 45:1163–9.
31. Wolfe RA and Strawderman RL. Logical and statistical fallacies in the use of Cox regression models. Am J Kidney Dis 1996; 27:124–9.
32. Nelson CB, Port FK, Wolfe RA and Guire KE. Comparison of continuous ambulatory peritoneal dialysis and hemodialysis patient survival with evaluation of trends during the 1980s. J Am Soc Nephrol 1992; 3:1147–55.
33. Nelson CB, Port FK, Wolfe RA and Guire KE. Dialysis patient survival: evaluation of CAPD versus HD using 3 techniques [Abstract]. Perit Dial Int 1992: 12:144.
34. Fisher LD, Dixon DO, Herson J et al. Intention to treat in clinical trials. In Peace KE, editor. Statistical issues in drug research and development. New York: Marcel Dekker, 1990.
35. Vonesh EF. Relative risks can be risky. Perit Dial Int 1993; 13:5–9.

5. Assigning severity indices to outcomes

NASEEM S. AMIN

INTRODUCTION

In other disease states the influence of both the severity of the primary disease and unrelated other comorbid diseases on the course of patients has been studied [1, 2]. However the majority of observational studies examining the End Stage Renal Disease (ESRD) population are hampered in the conclusions they arrive at, because they have not quantified the severity of patient indices at baseline and related these to patient outcomes.

In the quest to improve the analysis of outcomes, researchers have developed instruments, that measure the severity of indices such as comorbidity, functional status and the quality of life of patients. These instruments have been developed because of the realization that adjusting just for the presence or absence of comorbid conditions does not accurately describe the risk profile of a patient population. These instruments that adjust for severity, used either in the research or clinical arena, offer an opportunity for clinicians and researchers to better compare outcomes in differing dialysis patient populations.

The other challenge is that in the ESRD patient population, depending on whom you ask that are involved in the delivery of patient care, different outcomes are given relatively different importance. From a patients perspective, the impact of dialysis care on their physical functioning, and quality of life, as well as how satisfied they are with the delivery of care, maybe most important. However, from a care givers perspective, the impact on mortality and morbidity outcomes may be the most important. From a payers perspective the cost effectiveness of the care their members are receiving, may be the most important outcome.

A number of instruments have been developed or adapted for use in ESRD patients to assess these different outcomes. These instruments are being used to both, better case mix adjust at baseline, and to track the impact of the delivery of care, on patient outcomes through repeat measurements.

The presence of comorbidity and measurement of other indices such as functional status and quality of life have predicted early mortality and hospitalizations among patients entering treatment for ESRD.

Measuring comorbidity in end stage renal disease (ESRD) studies is important not only for case-mix adjustment but also because the incidence of a comorbid condition is a clinical outcome [3–6]. However there are a limited number of instruments that adjust for severity of comorbid conditions, and even fewer have been tested in the ESRD population. It has recently been shown that scoring systems which adjust for the severity of coexisting diseases can refine survival predictions. Among patients beginning dialysis, the presence of diabetes mellitus, congestive heart failure, coronary artery disease, peripheral vascular disease and hypertension have each been shown independently to increase the risk of death in ESRD [7]. Mortality rates have been compared for patients receiving dialysis or transplants, using a method that categorizes patients into different risk groups based upon the number of coexisting diseases [8]. Much of the higher mortality in dialysis patients was attributable to the presence of a greater number of coexisting diseases in dialysis patients. However, this classification did not take into account the severity of the coexisting diseases.

Tabulation of the number of coexisting diseases affecting dialysis patients shows that patients beginning dialysis now have more coexisting diseases than in the past. Elderly diabetic patients

L.W. Henderson and R.S. Thuma (eds.), Quality Assurance in Dialysis, 2nd Edition, 55–60.
© 1999 *Kluwer Academic Publishers. Printed in Great Britain*

have been observed to have a greater number of coexisting diseases and to have higher mortality. The inference has been made that the higher mortality was due to the greater number of coexisting diseases [9–11].

Low functional status (as measured by the Karnofsky Index) and quality of life (as measured by the Spitzer Quality of Life Scale) have also been shown to be associated with higher dialysis mortality [12]. The same study also showed increased mortality when patients with a coexisting disease were compared to patients lacking that coexisting disease. However, neither the interaction between coexisting disease and functional impairment nor the impact of more than one coexisting disease was explored. Subsequent multivariant analysis showed angina, congestive heart failure, nutritional impairment and low Karnofsky scores to be independent risk factors for dialysis mortality [13].

Analysis of United States Renal Data System (USRDS) has allowed estimation of the relative mortality risk associated with each of 25 coexisting conditions among 3,399 incident dialysis patient [14]. Peritoneal dialysis patients had fewer comorbid conditions than hemodialysis patients [15].

In the USRDS 1997 Annual Data Report, comorbid conditions account for the majority of causes of death in the ESRD population. Comorbid conditions also account for the majority of reasons for hospital admissions.

From some large registry databases we learn that survival is comparable for PD and HD [16–18], however the USRDS reported, lower survival on PD than HD for the >65 year old diabetics, and higher for younger diabetic patients [19]. The Canadian Organ Replacement Register shows better survival across all cohorts for PD [20]. Some multi-center clinical studies show patient survival on PD and HD being similar [21–26]. Other studies have shown better results on HD [27–29].

A number of studies have compared Quality of Life (QOL) for patients on HD or PD [30–34]. Home HD patients appeared to have the best quality of life, PD patients appear to have a better QOL compared to in center HD patients. However few longitudinal QOL studies are available that take into account severity of comorbid conditions and impact on QOL.

All these comparative studies examining outcomes for dialysis modalities, have been retrospective and non-randomized studies. These studies have been hampered by having a differing case-mix by modality. Differences in the severity of preexisting comorbidity have either not been, or only partially corrected for by statistical analysis. These conflicting results highlight that major pitfalls exist in physicians making conclusions based on results obtained without adequate risk adjustment of patient populations.

The development of a method to measure and classify by severity, comorbidity, faces several difficulties. Pathogenic connections can muddy the distinction between coexisting disease and complications of a primary disease. For example, a disease causing ESRD could also act as a comorbid disease (e.g. diabetes mellitus), and conditions resulting from ESRD could also act as independent comorbid conditions (e.g. secondary hyperparathyroidism). In order to avoid confusion, the following definition of a comorbid condition is a useful way to view comorbid conditions. A comorbid condition is any distinct additional clinical entity that has existed or that may occur during, the clinical course of a patient who has end-stage renal disease [35].

Classification of diseases and their severity is a technically difficult task, especially if the data for the recording and classification of each condition are extracted from patient records. Probably for this reason, most comorbidity studies in ESRD have ignored variability in the severity of comorbid conditions. In previous studies of comorbidity in ESRD, comorbid conditions reducing long-term survival were emphasized, it is important that comorbid conditions which do not lead to death be included in the comorbidity assessment, since these can play a major role, in other patient outcomes besides mortality.

A chart-based comorbidity index, the Index of Coexisting Disease (ICED), was introduced to control for the influence of coexisting diseases on cancer management [36]. This tool was developed by estimating the relative risk of death for each coexisting condition and then these are used to calculate a weighted index of comorbidity. A three grade severity system combined with a four grade scoring system predicted one year survival in a population of 685 women with breast cancer [37].

This scheme relied on physician interpretation of clinical data. Several studies have been published using this ICED instrument [38–40].

The ICED is a composite comorbidity index that has two components, the individual disease severity (IDS), which grades the severity of each condition from 0 to 4, and individual physical impairment (IPI) from each condition, graded from 0 to 2. This instrument allows categorization of both comorbid conditions and physical impairment into different levels of severity. It takes into account the severity of each condition and the impact of the condition on patient functional status. In order to use the ICED for ESRD, the modifications involved lengthening the list of conditions which commonly occur as comorbidity in ESRD. Scoring of the severity of functional impairment has been adjusted to reflect the level of impairment commonly found in dialysis charts.

This modified instrument has been validated in the ESRD population and is currently being used in several large dialysis studies. The NIH sponsored, Hemo study and the CHOICE study. It has been shown to predict mortality in a cohort of ESRD patients. The study was retrospective. It showed ICED score to be an independent risk factor of death in ESRD patients. A Cox proportional hazard model incorporated data from a retrospective review of 255 patients dialyzed at one Italian center during a 15 year period and the ICED score, predicted mortality independently of patient age, sex, the presence of diabetes or other systemic disease causing renal failure, or treatment modality [40]. In another study a single reviewer using the dialysis chart, examined ICED scores as a predictor of patient outcomes in peritoneal dialysis patients. An ICED score was assigned to all 69 patients who began chronic PD at one center over 12 years. Mean follow up was 7 years. ICED level correlated with hospitalizations ($r=0.28$, $p=0.019$) and cumulative ensuing hospital days ($r=0.28$, $p=0.02$). A multivariate model using age, diabetes and ICED level gave an good prediction of survival (area under the receiver operating characteristic ROC curve 86%) [41].

Since the ICED is derived from data abstracted from patient records, for practical reasons, the occurrence of comorbid conditions is best assessed by trained physicians or nurses most involved in patient care at the clinical center.

The Comorbidity Assessment Form includes 19 individual disease categories, each of which has three levels, and allows for IDS classification. The general guidelines which describe the individual disease severity classifications are explained below:

IDS O. Absence of coexistent disease in that category.

IDS 1. A comorbid condition which is asymptomatic or mildly symptomatic, where there is little or no morbidity. There are no complications and there is no indication for hospitalization. There is no limitation in activities of daily living.

IDS 2. A mild to moderate condition that is generally symptomatic and requires medical intervention. This also includes past conditions, presently benign, that still present a moderate risk of morbidity. There is need of medications: chronic administration from chronic conditions and short course administration for acute conditions (infections, etc.). Hospitalization, surgery or other invasive procedures may be indicated. Complications may occur, but are not life threatening in the near future. There may be mild limitations in the activities of daily living.

IDS 3. An uncontrolled condition which causes moderate to severe disease manifestations during medical care. These conditions are usually acute or subactive and require medical intervention. Symptoms persist despite medical or surgical or other invasive treatment. Frequent hospitalizations may be necessary. Life threatening complications may occur. There is a high degree of morbidity and a moderate risk of mortality. There may be severe limitations in the activities of daily living.

Coexisting diseases are often not considered consequential in an episode of care or hospitalization when they are medically well-controlled. Such diseases may actually have an impact on outcomes, but even a careful chart review may not identify and classify a given disease because little information is in the medical record. The concept underlying the assessment of physical impairment is that some not diagnosed but relevant diseases may have an impact on the function of the patient.

The second component of the ICED, the IPI

includes 11 categories, each of which has two levels. The IPI, rates the patient in eleven areas or dimensions of physical function impairment using a three level scale, 0, 1 or 2.

Level 0: No significant impairment, normal function,

Level 1: Mild/moderate impairment, symptomatic, may need assistance with activities of daily life.

Level 2: Serious/severe impairment, symptomatic.

The Karnofsky Index was developed to quantify the overall functional ability of the patient. It has been used in several cross-sectional and longitudinal ESRD studies, and was used in the USRDS special study on Erythropoietin and Quality of Life [42]. The instrument is easily administered, requires minimal interviewer training, and can be completed within ten minutes. Limitations include interobserver variability and limited scope [43]. The Karnofsky Index (KI) like the IPI form should be completed by dialysis unit staff person who is most familiar with the patient's functional ability, usually the unit social worker or a dialysis nurse. The frequency of assessment has been at baseline and annually so each assessment covers a one year period.

Many instruments intended to measure quality of life or general health status assessment have been used in individual studies in ESRD. Only a few have been used in more than one or two studies. Instruments for Quality of life status assessment should provide information about physical functioning, mental health, social functioning and other domains which are related to health. These include pain, fatigue, and the patient's overall perception of his or her well-being. The Short Form 36 Health Survey (SF-36) was developed on the basis of experience in the Medical Outcomes Study. It assesses physical function, role limitations attributable to physical problems, pain, mental health, role limitations attributable to emotional problems, social function and vitality. The SF-36 is available in a computer-scored format and can be completed in less than ten minutes. Minimal instruction is needed to administer the instrument. The SF-36 has been used extensively in ESRD and appears to be reliable and valid in this population [44–46].

The KDQOL-SF version 2.1 was recently developed at the RAND Corporation. It intersperses SF-36 questions among other questions from the Medical Outcomes Study long form questionnaire and ESRD-specific questions. Results of validation among 165 hemo and peritoneal dialysis patients have been published [47].

It should be noted that although in presenting their instruments and findings, the authors of ESRD-specific instruments assert the necessity of supplementing generic health surveys, the value of the additional information in characterizing ESRD, in comparing treatment strategies or in improving care has not been demonstrated.

In summary these new instruments that allow us to better quantify the severity of patients comorbid diseases, their physical functioning and QOL, are not yet widely used in either research studies or in the clinical arena. If ongoing large population based studies, show that use of these instruments do provide better predictive powers than existing methods, then these instruments will make there way into routine clinical practice, especially in an environment where payers are increasingly demanding that providers document outcomes.

REFERENCES

1. Feinstein A. The pre-therapeutic classification of comorbidity in chronic disease. J Chron Dis 1970; 23:455–68.
2. Kaplan M andFeinstein A. The importance of classifying comorbidity in evaluating the outcome of diabetes mellitus. J Chron Dis 1974; 27:387–404.
3. Greenfield S, Blanco D, Elashoff R et al. Development and testing of a new index of comorbidity. Clin Res 1987; 35:346A.
4. Greenfield S, Blanco D, Elashoff R et al. Patterns of care related to age of breast cancer patients. JAMA 1987; 257:2766–70.
5. Greenfield S and Nelson E. Recent developments and future issues in the use of health status assessment measures in clinical settings. Med Care 1992; 30:23–41.
6. Greenfield S, Apolone G, McNeil B et al. The importance of co-existent disease in the occurrence of postoperative complications and one-year recovery in patients undergoing total hip replacement. Med Care 1993; 31:141–54.
7. Hutchinson T, Thomas D and MacGibbon B. Predicting survival in adults with end-stage renal disease: An age equivalence index. Ann Intern Med 1982; 96:417–23.
8. Hutchinson T, Thomas D, Lemieux J et al. Prognostically controlled comparison of dialysis and renal transplantation. Kidney Int 1984; 26:44–51.

9. Collins A, Hanson G, Umen A, Kjellstrand C and Keshaviah P. Changing risk factor demographics in end-stage renal disease patients entering dialysis and the impact on long-term mortality. Am J Kidney Dis 1990; 15:422–32.

10. Collins AJ, Ma JZ, Umen A and Keshaviah P. Urea index and other predictors of renal outcomes study dialysis patient survival. Am J Kidney Dis 1994; 23:272–82.

11. Kjellstrand C, Hylander B and Collins A. Mortality on dialysis – on the influence of early start, patient characteristics, and transplantation and acceptance rates. Am J Kidney Dis 1990; 15:483–90.

12. McClellan W, Anson C, Birkeli K et al. Functional status and quality of life: predictor of early mortality among patients entering treatment for end-stage renal disease. J Clin Epidemiol 1991; 44:83–9.

13. McClellan W, Flanders W and Gutman R. Variable mortality rates among dialysis treatment centers. Ann Intern Med 1992; 117:332–6.

14. USRDS. Comorbid conditions and correlations with mortality risk among, 3,399 incident dialysis patients. Am J Kidney Dis 1992; 20:32–8.

15. USRDS. Patient selection to peritoneal dialysis versus hemodialysis according to comorbid conditions. Am J Kidney Dis 1992; 20:20–6.

16. European Dialysis and Transplantation Association: European Renal Association (EDTA-ERA). Report on management of renal failure in Europe, XXIII, 1992. Nephrol Dial Transplant 1992; 9:1–48..

17. United States Renal Data System: USRDS 1993 Annual Data Report. Betheseda MD, The National Institute of Health, National Institute of Diabetes and Digestive and Kidney Disease, February 1993.

18. Registration Committee of Japanese Society for Dialysis Therapy: An overview of regular dialysis treatment in Japan. Japanese Society for Dialysis Therapy, 1993.

19. United States Renal Data System: USRDS 1992 Annual Data Report. Betheseda MD, The National Institute of Health, National Institute of Diabetes and Digestive and Kidney Disease, 1992.

20. Fenton SA, Schaubel DE et al. Hemodialysis versus peritoneal dialysis: a comparison of adjusted mortality rates. Am. J Kid Dis 1997; 3:334–42.

21. Maiorca R. Vonesh EF. Cavalli PL et al. A multicenter selection-adjusted comparison of patient and technique survivals on PD and hemodialysis. Perit Dial Int 1991; 11:118–27.

22. Mion C, Mourad G, Canaud B et al. Maintenance dialysis: a survey of 17 years experience in Languedoc-Rousillon with a comparison of methods in a standard population. ASAIO J 1983; 6:205–13.

23. Kurtz SB and Johnson WJ. A four-year comparison of continuous ambulatory peritoneal dialysis and home hemodialysis: a preliminary report. Mayo Clin Proc 1991; 59:659–62.

24. Charytan C, Spinowitz BS and Galler M. A comparative study of continuous ambulatory peritoneal dialysis and center hemodialysis. Arch Intern Med 1986; 146:1138–43.

25. Maiorca R, Vonesh E, Cancarini GC et al. A six year comparison of patient and technique survivals in PD and HD. Kidney Int 1988; 34:518–24.

26. Lupo A, Cancarini G, Catizone L et al. Comparison of survival in PD and hemodialysis: a multicenter study. Adv Perit Dial 1992: 8:136–40.

27. Gokal R, Jakubowski C, King J et al. Outcome in patients on continuous ambulatory peritoneal dialysis and haemodialysis: 4-year analysis of a prospective multicentre study. Lancet 1987; ii:1105–9.

28. Gentil MA, Cariazzo A, Pavon Ml et al. Comparison of survival in continuous ambulatory peritoneal dialysis: a multicenter study. Nephrol Dial Transplant 1991; 6:444–51.

29. Capelli JP, Camiscioli TC and Vallorani RD. Comparative analysis of survival on home dialysis, in-center hemodialysis and chronic peritoneal dialysis (PD-IPD) therapies. Dial Transplant 1985; 14:38–52.

30. Evans RW, Manninen DL, Garrison LP et al. The quality of life of patients with end stage renal disease. N Eng J Med 1985; 312:553–9.

31. Morris PLP and Jones B. Transplantation versus dialysis: A study of quality of life. Transpl Proc 1988; 20:23–6.

32. Simmons RG, Anderson CR and Abress LK. Quality of life and rehabilitation differences among four ESRD therapy groups. Scand J Urol Nephrol 1990; 131:7–22.

33. Wolcott DL and Nissenson AR. Quality of life in chronic dialysis patients: a critical comparison of PD and HD. Am J Kidney Dis. 1988; 11:402–12.

34. Tucker CM, Ziller RC et al. Quality of life of patients on incenter HD versus PD. Perit Dial Int 1991; 11:341–6.

35. Feinstein A. The pre-therapeutic classification of comorbidity in chronic disease. J Chron Dis 1970; 23:455–68.

36. Greenfield S, Blanco D, Elashoff R et al. Patterns of care related to age of breast cancer patients. JAMA 1987; 257:2766–70.

37. Greenfield S, Blanco D, Elashoff R et al. Development and testing of a new index of comorbidity. Clin Res 1987; 35:346A.

38. Greenfield S, Apolone G, McNeil B et al. The Importance of co-existent disease in the occurrence of postoperative complications and one-year recovery in patients undergoing total hip replacement. Med Care 1993; 31:141–54.

39. Bennett C, Greenfield S, Aronow H et al. Patterns of care related to age of men with prostate cancer. Cancer 1991; 67:2633–41.

40. Nicolucci A, Cubasso D, Labbrozzi D et al. Effect of coexistent diseases on survival of patients undergoing dialysis. Trans Am Soc Artif Intern Org 1992; 291–5.

41. Athienites NV, Sullivan L, Fernandez G et al. Pretreatment comorbidity and patient outcomes in peritoneal dialysis (PD). J Am Soc Neph 1994; 5:432.

42. USRDS 1993 Annual Data Report. Appendix B. EPO and Quality of Life Study.

43. Hutchinson T, Boyd N, Feinstein A et al. Scientific problems in clinical scales, as demonstrated in the Karnofsky Index of Performance Status. J Chron Dis 1979; 32:661–6.

44. Meyer KB, Espindle DM, DeGiacomo J et al. Monitoring dialysis patients' health status. Am J Kidney Dis 1994; 24:267–79

45. Kurtin P, Davis A, Meyer K et al. Patient-based health status measures in outpatient dialysis: early experiences in developing an outcomes assessment program. Med Care 1992; 30:136–49.

46. Meyer K, Kurtin P, DeOreo P et al. Health-related quality of life and clinical variables in dialysis patients. J Am Soc Neph 1992; 3:379.

47. Hays, RD, Kallich JD, Mapes DL, Coons SJ and Carter WB. Development of the kidney disease quality of life (KDQOL) instrument. Qual Life Res. 1994; 3:239–338.

6.   The role of quality assurance in preventing legal actions

JAMES T. O'NEILL

INTRODUCTION

As is true of any other health care providers, dialysis caregivers are potentially subject to being sued for malpractice in connection with real or perceived injury to a patient. This chapter discusses the ways in which quality assurance can reduce the risk of lawsuit, and improve the caregiver's chances in court in the event a lawsuit is filed.

TEXT

Every patient-treatment decision made by a health care provider brings with it the risk of a lawsuit for malpractice. Any time a caregiver makes a choice to act, to refrain from acting, or to act in a certain way in treating a patient, the potential exists for that choice later to be attacked in a lawsuit filed by the patient or the patient's family. This is as true in the context of dialysis as it is in any other field of medical practice.

The risk of lawsuit cannot be eliminated entirely, both because a patient does not need to have a winning case in order to sue and because patients can have a plethora of different motivations for filing lawsuits. But the risk can be reduced, and quality assurance is one of the most powerful means available to achieve that reduction. As this chapter will explain, quality assurance can reduce the risks of legal actions in at least three ways.

First, quality assurance, to the extent it can result in better outcomes, can help avoid the very conditions – the injuries – that lead to lawsuits.

Second, quality assurance can enhance the quality of care that patients *perceive*. Many if not most malpractice lawsuits stem more from patient perceptions than from objective evidence of negligence.

Third, if a patient ultimately does file a lawsuit, quality assurance programs can help to improve the caregiver's chances of a favorable result in court.

This chapter shortly will address these three lawsuit-related benefits of quality assurance programs. Before doing that, however, the chapter will (1) provide some general background on malpractice lawsuits, including the requirement that physicians meet the applicable "standard of care", and then (2) examine some of the kinds of malpractice claims raised in lawsuits involving dialysis.

Because the author practices in the United States, and because the U.S. appears to be a far more litigious society that most, this chapter addresses legal principles under U.S. law. It is the author's hope that the general concepts discussed in this chapter also will be of use to persons whose practices are governed by the laws of other nations.

BACKGROUND: CLAIMS AND LAWSUITS FOR MALPRACTICE

Malpractice Claims and Lawsuits in General

The vast majority of claims for medical malpractice never see the inside of a jury room. In the first place, some of these claims are not filed as lawsuits (at least initially), but instead are raised by patients

L.W. Henderson and R.S. Thuma (eds.), Quality Assurance in Dialysis, 2nd Edition, 61–72.
© 1999 *Kluwer Academic Publishers. Printed in Great Britain*

or their lawyers with hospital or clinic management. In some cases a patient may reach a settlement with a hospital's risk management staff, or
may decide for other reasons not to pursue the
matter further, and no lawsuit ever will be filed.

Where a patient or patient's family does file a
lawsuit, the odds are that the suit will be resolved
before trial [1–4]. In many cases the parties reach a
financial settlement short of trial. In other cases
the patient decides not to pursue the case, or loses
on preliminary motions, and the case is dismissed
[3].

If a malpractice lawsuit goes to trial, some data
(such as they are) suggest that the physician generally is likely to win [2, 3]. For example, a series of
published reports examining data in various jurisdictions found that patients won between 13.5%
and 53% of malpractice cases, with a median win
rate of 29.2% and a mean win rate of 29.6% –
suggesting that physicians won roughly 7 out of 10
malpractice cases [2]. These data should be taken
with a grain of salt because they are, for lack of
any centralized information source, drawn from
scattered jurisdictions and incomplete [1, 2]. In
any event, even a "70% win rate" for physicians in
general might have little meaning in the context of
a specific case, since that 70% figure is an average
across a number of divergent jurisdictions, and
also covers a wide variety of medical disciplines
and factual circumstances.

If a jury finds that a health care provider's
malpractice caused injury to a patient, the jury
may award the patient "compensatory damages"
as compensation for the patient's injuries. Compensatory damages may include such relatively
objective measures of damage as medical bills and
lost earnings, as well as more subjective items such
as an award for pain and suffering. If the jury finds
the malpractice to have been particularly egre-
gious, it may (depending upon the particular
state's laws) award the patient punitive damages
designed to punish the treater and to deter a
repetition of the malpractice.

Malpractice Standards in General

Whether they are filed in a state or a federal court,
malpractice cases generally are decided under
state law. Depending upon the state, some of the
applicable malpractice principles may be drawn

from laws enacted by the state legislature (sta-
tutes), while others may be drawn from judge-
made law (often called "common law"). There are
some broad common standards running though
the malpractice laws of the various states; these
commonalities will allow this chapter to discuss
some of the general terms of "malpractice law".

At the same time, however, there are a variety of
differences (some subtle, some not so subtle)
between various states' malpractice laws. This
means that any given case might be decided under
different standards if it were filed in one state as
opposed to another state, depending on the facts of
the case and the exact legal principles involved.
The author recommends that any person interested in the legal principles applicable to his or
her jurisdiction consult legal counsel, and indeed
that all readers view this chapter as general
commentary (that in some respects sacrifices precision for the sake of brevity) rather than specific
legal advice.

In general, in order to win a malpractice case,
the person bringing a lawsuit (called the "plaintiff") must show the following: (1) the standard of
care that the physician being sued (the "defendant") owed to the plaintiff; (2) that the physician
deviated from that standard of care; and (3) that
the physician's deviation from that standard of
care was the "proximate" (i.e. legal) cause of the
plaintiff's alleged injury [1, 5].

The question of whether the health care provider met his or her "standard of care" may be asked
in a slightly different way: Did the provider supply
care *of sufficient quality* to meet his or her legal
duties? [3] One often-quoted state court decision
explained it this way:

> "Medical malpractice is legal fault by a physician or
> surgeon. It arises from the failure of a physician to provide
> the *quality of care* required by law"[6].

The precise formulation of the applicable "standard of care" can vary from state to state [7–10].[1]
However, one illustrative formulation by a state
court is that a physician must exercise "that degree
of care, skill, and proficiency exercised by reasonably careful, skillful, and prudent practitioners in
the same class to which he belongs, acting under
the same or similar circumstances" [10].

This chapter will return to a more detailed discussion of the "standard of care" when it discusses how quality assurance can help caregivers win malpractice lawsuits. For now, and with the foregoing background of malpractice principles in mind, this chapter will offer some background on malpractice cases in the specific context of dialysis.

Lawsuits and Dialysis

For a variety of reasons, it is difficult to determine with any precision how frequently providers of dialysis care are sued for malpractice. Certain legal databases and jury verdict reporters contain information about cases that actually have gone to trial, but even then their coverage is spotty. More importantly, the great majority of medical malpractice cases are settled out of court, and public reporting of settlements is limited; indeed, settling defendants often insist on confidentiality of the settlement amount (to the extent the applicable law allows it) as a condition of the settlement agreement.

For purposes of this chapter, the author did not undertake a systematic study of malpractice lawsuits in the dialysis context. Instead, he conducted a number of searches through some of the available computer databases containing state judicial decisions, federal judicial decisions, and jury verdict reporting publications [13]. The objective was less to determine the number of lawsuits brought against dialysis providers than to ascertain the types of allegations made by the patients who brought suit.

Fortunately or unfortunately (depending upon one's perspective), the author's searches did not locate very many reports of lawsuits against dialysis providers. Leaving aside several civil rights lawsuits (in which people in jail or prison sued claiming a right to receive dialysis), the author could find at most a few dozen reports of malpractice suits involving dialysis. (This small number may be *consistent with* a low rate of malpractice lawsuits against dialysis providers, but the data located by the author are best viewed as inconclusive on this point.)

The small number of reports located by the author makes it difficult to draw any generalizable conclusions about the types of malpractice claims typically brought against dialysis providers. Nevertheless, even this limited number of reports contains some small "clusters" of cases addressing similar issues, suggesting the identification of at least a few areas of possible malpractice risk.

For example, the following general types of allegations[2] appear to have arisen in two or more malpractice lawsuits against dialysis providers:

- *Disconnection of hemodialysis needles with resulting blood loss.* In at least two cases, the next of kin of the patients alleged that during hemodialysis treatment the patients were left unattended and the needles connecting them to the dialysis machines became disconnected, causing them to die from complications of blood loss. For one of these cases, the court's decision on a preliminary motion has been published, but this author does not know the ultimate outcome [14]. For the second case, a jury found $361,000 in damages, although this may have been reduced by 40% based on negligence by the patient [15].

- *Puncturing the vena cava while inserting a catheter.* In at least two cases that went to trial, the plaintiff alleged that a catheter inserted into the patient's chest punctured the patient's superior vena cava, ultimately causing the patient to die. In a case tried in Georgia, the plaintiff received a jury verdict of $585,000 against a nephrologist and his nephrology partnership ($500,000 compensatory and $85,000 punitive damages), in addition to undisclosed settlements with a medical center and its radiology group [16]. In a case tried in California, a jury returned a verdict in favor of the defendant surgeon, although the surgeon who had punctured the vena cava was not a defendant; the plaintiff sought to blame the defendant internist for the other doctor's actions [17].

- *Failure to remove a catheter in response to infection.* In one case, the plaintiff contended that the defendant general surgeon was negligent in removing a PD catheter using traction rather than surgery, with the result that a portion of the catheter remained and became infected. The jury awarded the plaintiff $40,000 [18]. In a second case, the next of kin of a patient contended that the defendant vascular surgeon negligently had failed to remove a patient's shunt, resulting in a lung infection that caused several months of pain and suffering. (The patient had died from multiple myeloma, and apparently his next of kin did not claim that his death had anything to do with the shunt.) The jury found in favor of the defendant [19]. In a third case, the plaintiff claimed that the defendants hematologist and nephrologist had failed to remove a shunt placed in the patient's leg, despite signs of infection at the shunt site, contributing to a longstanding infection. (The plaintiff also contended that the defendants had administered two contraindicated drugs, Ancobon for a systemic fungal infection and Oxymetheleone for anemia.) The jury found negligence in failure to remove the shunt earlier and in continuing to administer Ancobon after a certain point, and awarded a total of $125,000 for pain and suffering [20].

- *Placement of hemodialysis shunts.* One plaintiff contended that the defendant surgeon was negligent in regard to three surgeries performed on the plaintiff's right arm for purposes of creating an access-site for dialysis. The patient developed severe complications to his arm which led to gangrene, requiring partial amputation of the hand. The jury returned a verdict in the amount of $273,125 [21]. A second patient alleged that the defendant surgeon had negligently implanted a dialysis shunt and failed to revise the shunt, resulting in compromised blood flow and ischemia. The plaintiff asserted that the shunt was drawing too much blood from the plaintiff's hand and had caused ischemia, a claw hand, hypersensitivity of the non-dominant left hand and arm, and neurological damage. Plaintiff also claimed that the shunt implanted was too large. The defendant contended that the plaintiff only had four viable shunt sites due to small vessel disease of his hands, and that two of these sites already had been used, meaning that it was appropriate not to move the shunt as long as it could be tolerated. Defendant also contended that the plaintiff's condition was a well known risk of shunt use, and that the plaintiff, although instructed to return for treatment if needed, had failed to return. The jury awarded $100,000 against the surgeon, which

was reduced to $50,000 because the jury found that the patient was 50% negligent. The nephrology associates and four associated physicians who treated the plaintiff settled before trial for an undisclosed amount [22].

With these examples in mind as illustrative of some of the types of malpractice claims that patients may bring against dialysis providers, this chapter now will consider how quality assurance can help prevent lawsuits.

QUALITY ASSURANCE AS A MEANS TO REDUCE LAWSUIT RISKS

While nobody is immune from lawsuit, prudent health care providers can, and do, take measured steps to reduce their risks of being sued. They also seek to reduce the chances that, if they are sued, they will be required to pay a judgment. The remaining sections of this chapter will examine some of the ways in which quality assurance can reduce lawsuit risks.

Quality assurance can operate on at least three levels to reduce the risk of legal actions. First, quality assurance can facilitate positive patient outcomes, and minimize negative patient outcomes. Put another way, quality assurance is good for human health, and people who do not suffer what they would consider to be "harm" are less likely to sue. Nowhere is the value of quality assurance clearer than in regard to routine procedures that, if not performed properly, pose serious potential health risks.

Second, quality assurance can help reduce patient and family motivations to bring lawsuits. Patients and their loved ones generally understand that ESRD is a very serious medical condition, and realize that the dialysis patient may suffer setbacks or even die. If the patients and their loved ones *perceive* that the care provided is of high quality, they may be less likely to view a negative event as the "fault" of the health care provider, and correspondingly less likely to bring a legal action.

Some research suggests that patient perceptions of the quality of care depend largely upon patient reactions to the attitudes and the communication behavior of caregivers. Perceptions thus become double-edged: While a patient who views his or her treaters' attitudes and communications favorably may give the treaters *at least* as much credit for quality as they are due, a patient who reacts negatively to caregiver attitudes and communications may subjectively underrate treatment quality. Although there are no absolutes in this regard, some research suggests that the perceived quality of caregiver communication and attitude matters even more to patients that the objective "correctness" of the care administered.

Third and finally, quality counts in court. It counts in the eyes of the law, and it counts in the eyes of juries. A dialysis provider who has a strong quality assurance program in place ought to be, at least in general, in a better position to defeat a malpractice lawsuit (or, at a minimum, avoid a large damages award) than a provider without such a program.

Quality Can Reduce the Risk of Lawsuits By Improving Patient Outcomes

The better people feel, the less reason they have to sue. Hence, the ideal defense – but unfortunately one that is unattainable in the real world – is to ensure that all patients recover completely from their ailments and suffer no pain.

The reality in dialysis is that discomfort and mortality among patients are tragic facts of life. The health care provider can prolong life, improve life, and in many cases – by helping to build a "bridge" to eventual transplantation – effectively give life back to the ESRD patient. But ideal outcomes will be the exception more than the rule, meaning that the risk of lawsuit will always be present to some degree, even with the best quality of care [23].

The risk of negative outcomes, however, is one that *declines* as quality increases, because quality reduces negative outcomes. Of course, quality *alone* may not determine outcomes, at least in any given case. But viewed from the standpoint of a series of patients and a series of outcomes, quality should make a difference.

The author is generally aware that certain questions surrounding dialysis "outcomes" are the subject of current medical debate. As an attorney and not a physician, the author cannot pretend to offer judgments about how quality systems will affect one specific measure of outcome or another.

Based upon his research, however, the author can state with confidence that a large percentage of malpractice lawsuits – including lawsuits against dialysis providers – allege problems that can be avoided or reduced though the application of quality systems.

Some malpractice lawsuits result from subtle second-guessing of sophisticated medical judgment exercised in emergency situations with little time for reflection. With regard to this type of lawsuit, the author suspects, but does not know, that quality assurance systems may improve outcomes incrementally. But a huge proportion of lawsuits (as well as claims that are resolved short of a lawsuit) result from what is claimed to be simple carelessness, sloppiness, or neglect on the part of a medical professional or organization in performing routine, day-to-day functions [23].

For example, a claimed breakdown in medical "fundamentals" might be alleged in a lawsuit on the grounds of:

- Ignoring repeated alarms from a dialysis machine;

- Failing to ask a patient some simple, and critical, questions about medical history;

- Failing to note that a patient has a known allergy to an antibiotic; or

- Missing or ignoring critical information recorded on a patient's chart.

This kind of error in routine, "fundamental" procedures can lead directly to a negative outcome, and then to a lawsuit. Moreover, a failure in performance of medical "fundamentals" creates obvious risks in a courtroom. While jurors often are sympathetic to the difficult judgment calls doctors must make, this sympathy will be of little help where the case concerns a simple, precise requirement that a health care practitioner simply failed to meet. The issues will be relatively straightforward and accessible to the jurors' everyday experiences – and a decision against the health care provider will be relatively easy to render.

Breakdowns in medical fundamentals can lead to negative outcomes and lawsuits specific to the dialysis context. The following examples of allegedly flawed dialysis procedures, which are drawn from reports of medical malpractice lawsuits as well as other legal proceedings, are illustrative:

- *Mistaking a PD catheter for a feeding tube.* In a criminal case, a physician was convicted of "reckless endangerment" after the death of a patient. The doctor had mistaken the patient's Tenchkoff catheter, which had been placed for PD, for a gastrointestinal feeding tube, and ordered that the patient be given Isocal (a feeding solution) via that tube. Even after discovering the error, the doctor did not attempt to remove all of the Isocal from the patient's peritoneum, and did not begin antibiotic coverage in an effort to prevent or arrest the onset of bacterial peritonitis [24].

- *Lack of communication of blood chemistry results.* A patient in a hospital for cardiac evaluation developed acute renal failure, and was placed on hemodialysis. After her condition stabilized, the patient's doctor had her transferred to a skilled nursing facility. The patient's orders at the nursing facility called for daily blood chemical studies. However, the blood chemistry results – which indicated rising levels of blood impurities – were recorded in the patient's charts by the facility's nurses *but not reported to any physician.* The patient did not receive any dialysis at the nursing facility, and she coded three days after being transferred to the nursing facility, and died (her DNR orders precluded efforts to resuscitate her). The jury awarded $10,000 to each of the patient's five children, but the appeals court increased this amount to $25,000 per child, or a total of $125,000 [25].

- *Inadequate treatment and monitoring of water for dialysis.* A hospital did not perform periodic chemical testing of the water used in its renal dialysis unit. The local tap water had an extremely high aluminum content. One morning, five of the eight patients receiving dialysis at the hospital began having sleep disturbances, seizures, and difficulty walking – symptoms of dialysis encephalopathy or dialysis dementia. After the dialysis unit was closed and the patients transferred to another dialysis facility, personnel of the U.S. Centers for Disease Control (CDC) discovered that the hospital's main-

tenance personnel had not examined the reverse osmosis unit of the hospital's water purification system in a year and a half, and that the purification system was nonfunctional or broken in many respects. A CDC doctor testified that the patients were poisoned with aluminum. The state settled with the patients for undisclosed amounts, then brought a lawsuit against an accrediting body and two insurance companies to try and recover the settlement amounts [26].

- *Cross-contamination of access needles with HIV.* In August, 1993, one dialysis center in Columbia, South America reported that 13 of its dialysis patients were HIV positive. A cohort study of patients at the center found (among other things) that the center had reprocessed access needles by soaking 4 pairs of needles at a time in a common container with benzalkonium chloride, a low-level disinfectant (which the center reused for 7 days), creating the potential for cross-contamination or use of a patient's needles on another patient. The study's researchers concluded that improperly-processed patient-care equipment, and most likely the access needles, was the probable mechanism of HIV transmission from HIV-seropositive patients to previously uninfected patients [27].

Because a patient undergoing dialysis well may suffer from medical conditions besides renal failure, malpractice claims against dialysis providers also can arise from negative outcomes related to these other conditions. Hence, quality assurance can improve outcomes by ensuring that dialysis patients, while in a dialysis unit, continue to receive necessary monitoring or treatment for their other conditions. The following example is illustrative of the kind of malpractice allegations a patient or patient's family may make regarding non-renal care in a dialysis unit:

- *Inadequate cardiac monitoring in dialysis unit of patient transferred from another unit of a hospital.* A patient suffered from non-sustained ventricular tachycardia and atrial fibrillation, as well as chronic kidney failure. His cardiologist, concerned that the patient's arrhythmia problems posed a risk of fatal ventricular fibrillation, referred the patient to a hospital with an electro-physiology service. The patient was placed in the hospital's telemetry unit, meaning that he was connected automatically to a cardiac monitor under continuous observation. When doctors in the telemetry unit were satisfied that it was safe for the patient to undergo dialysis, he was taken to the dialysis unit. He was disconnected from the monitor in the telemetry unit and not monitored during his transport to the dialysis unit, although his chart contained no order for the discontinuation of monitoring. Although the patient's full chart accompanied him to dialysis, *the practice in the dialysis unit was for the dialysis nurse to concern herself only with the nephrologist's dialysis order.* The original attending nurse in the dialysis unit was not even aware that the patient had come from the telemetry unit. She noted that the patient had an irregular heartbeat, *but did not report this finding to a physician.* The dialysis order did not mention monitoring, and the patient was not connected to a monitor in the dialysis unit, even though that unit did have a monitor. While the patient underwent dialysis, nurses periodically checked his vital signs. When a nurse checked his vital signs 25 minutes after the previous check, she found him unresponsive with no blood pressure. While the patient eventually was resuscitated, he had sustained irreversible brain damage as a result of loss of oxygen, and remained in a coma for a month before he died. The jury found the hospital liable in the amount of $150,000 (which was reduced to $10,000 under a state law limiting hospital liability), and found the doctors and nurses not liable. However, because of certain errors in jury instructions and other rulings by the trial court, the appeals court ordered a new trial of the claims against one doctor and one nurse [28].

As suggested by the above examples of lawsuits, a dialysis provider can reduce liability risks by focusing on day-to-day "fundamentals" and executing them methodically and consistently. Errors in "fundamentals" such as routine procedures seem particularly well-suited to being addressed by systematic quality assurance programs: These procedures will arise frequently and relatively predictably, and can to a large degree be reduced to a "checklist" form that (unlike at least some procedures or treatments) is relatively mechanical and uncontroversial.

Quality Assurance Can Reduce Lawsuit Risks By Improving Patient Perceptions of the Health Care Provider

To a large degree, malpractice lawsuits are about perceptions. In a sense, the quality of care that the patient *believes* he or she has received it at least as important as the objective quality of the care.

Quality assurance programs, to the extent they result in quality that a patient can see – in the form of systems that clearly are operating smoothly, and the competence of well-trained professionals – can reduce the likelihood that the patient will want to bring a lawsuit even if he or she suffers a negative outcome. At the same time, however, quality that appears to manifest itself in a mechanical, unfeeling fashion may, while improving patient outcomes, paradoxically increase patient alienation – and with it the likelihood of a lawsuit.

A number of commentators have suggested that physician *attitude* and physician *communication* are key factors in patient decisions to sue [29–33]. For example, a 1991 survey of attorneys by the American Trial Lawyers Association found that perhaps 75% of decisions to sue result from physician attitude and communication [23]. There probably are a number of reasons for the importance to patients of caregiver attitude and communication, perhaps including the following:

- A patient may not have the technical knowledge needed fully to assess the quality of the care received, and general impressions of competence and caring may serve the patient as surrogate measures of quality [34].

- A patient who is dissatisfied as a result of a caregiver's apparent attitude or lack of concern may be predisposed to anticipate injury or to perceive outcomes negatively [31].

- A patient who is ill may perceive himself or herself as highly vulnerable and highly dependent upon the treater (powerless), meaning that the perceived quality of the interaction will be felt deeply and personally by the patient [35]. If the patient experiences a negative outcome and also has negative perceptions of the treater, the patient may seek to "retaliate" by resorting to a lawsuit [30, 32]. A lawsuit will force the treater to respond and put the treater at risk – and thereby give the patient *power* over the treater.

Regardless of the precise motivations behind lawsuits, it is apparent that patient perceptions play a key role in the decision to sue. The appearance of sloppiness or carelessness – i.e. the opposite of quality – may increase the likelihood that a patient will view as negative event as a reason to sue. Conversely, the appearance of careful, well-constructed procedures may reduce lawsuit risks.

Patients' assessment of treatment quality also depend heavily upon patient perceptions of caregiver attitudes and communication. The *manner* in which quality care is delivered, therefore, may have a significant impact upon the probability that a given patient will choose to sue. Efforts to develop rapport with patients, to answer their questions without condescension, and to show care may improve patient satisfaction while simultaneously reducing liability risks. This suggests that dialysis providers should consider including, as elements of quality assurance or risk management programs, (1) mechanisms to assess and improve interpersonal behavior and (2) measures of patient satisfaction.

Quality Assurance Can Reduce the Risk That a Caregiver Who is Sued Will Lose a Lawsuit or Be Required to Pay Large Damages

From the perspective of the health care provider, the best lawsuit is one that never is filed. Ideally, patients and their families alike are satisfied with the care the patient received, and do not wish to sue even if the patient suffers a severe medical setback – because they do not blame the health care provider.

Unfortunately, even under the best of conditions every health care provider – regardless of how strong his or her commitment to quality – faces a risk of being sued. Whether it because a patient or her loved one assumes that "someone must be responsible", or because a personal injury lawyer's television advertisement catches a family member's attention, even the most careful physician, nurse, clinic, or hospital ultimately may become a defendant in a lawsuit.

Fortunately, however, quality counts in lawsuits. It counts as a technical legal matter, and (at least as importantly) it counts in the eyes of jurors. This means that in the event a patient or patient's family does decide to bring a lawsuit, and the lawsuit goes to trial, quality assurance can reduce both the risk that the caregiver will be held liable and the risk that the jury will award large damages.

The law recognizes quality as a major factor in deciding a personal injury lawsuit: The legal requirement that caregivers meet the "standard of care" looks to the quality of the care provided [3, 6]. At a theoretical level, if the health care provider's quality assurance systems implement well-accepted care standards (assuming there are any), then the defendant health care provider should (assuming the standards were followed in a given case) be less likely to be found negligent.

The technical legal meaning of the "standard of care", however, may be less important that a jury's own views of what constitutes acceptable patient treatment [37]. Jurors are human beings who – especially because they generally are laypersons and not experts – tend to apply their own subjective views and visceral impressions to their decisions in court [36, 37]. In addition, when judges instruct jurors on the "standards of care" that the jurors are to apply to a case, the judges generally speak in broad terms that offer few concrete guidelines [9–11].[3] Thus, the task of deciding what standard of care applies in a given case ultimately rests with the jury, with relatively sparse guidance from the court – and relatively broad latitude to decide based upon their own views.

While jury instructions about standards of care can be quite general, the parties on both sides of a lawsuit usually seek to offer more detail through their witnesses: A jury in a malpractice case can expect to hear expert witnesses, often presenting diametrically opposite views of the applicable standard of care [7]. Courts in fact generally *require* expert testimony about *both* (1) what the applicable duty of care was and (2) whether that duty was breached by the defendant [6, 7].

In their testimony, the experts on both sides in a malpractice suit generally have broad latitude in selecting the sources to which they look for standards of care. For example, where practice guidelines exist (formulated by, for example, medical societies) those guidelines can be one source of evidence to which the parties' experts ask juries to look. A jury well may hear the two sides' experts advocating entirely different standards from entirely different sources.

The jury's role in a malpractice case therefore includes evaluating the persuasiveness of each side's medical experts on "standard of care" issues, including the various different "standards of care" that the experts advocate [7]. While juries often display admirable abilities to absorb complex principles, they generally lack the depth of training to make fine judgments about medical standards. Both because of this and because of natural human tendencies, juries appear to make decisions in malpractice cases based largely upon whether they think the physician acted *reasonably* or whether they would trust the physician to treat their loved ones [29, 36].

As a formal legal matter, then, one of the battle-grounds in a malpractice case will be the "standard of care" and the physician's compliance with that standard. In practice, however, success in that battle will depend largely upon convincing a jury that the caregiver's actions were *reasonable*. Quality assurance programs can help with this task.

Quality assurance programs can simultaneously provide (1) a structure of quality for the jury to see and (2) a reasoned rationale for the treatment choices at issue. For example, where a lawsuit calls into question a physician's choice of a procedure or a treatment parameter, the presence of institutional guidelines supporting that choice may prove quite powerful as evidence. If the jury sees that the institution or the particular physician explicitly decided on certain guidelines in advance – and had good reasons for the choices made – the jury may be more likely to see the caregiver's actions as reasonable, and in accordance with the standard of care.

This suggests that quality assurance programs should include more than the "what" of the steps and procedures to be followed. Quality assurance programs also should include the "why" of the reasoning behind those steps and procedures. For example, if a hospital or clinic selects a particular set of measures for what it will consider to be "adequate" hemodialysis, it should base that selection on an overt consideration of the available literature and data bearing on that choice.

Consideration of procedures to be followed also should include a careful assessment of any available practice standards, guidelines, and para-meters. Where there is any kind of guideline recommended by an organization such as a medical society, a dialysis provider that deviates from that recommendation runs the risk that a jury later will view the guideline as setting the "standard of care". This risk can be reduced by documenting the reasoning behind any decision the provider makes to adopt its own, different standards, with particular reference to risks that can be reduced and benefits that can be increased by taking a different route [33].

At the same time, implementation of published guidelines or standards is no guarantee against liability. Juries can and do reject such guidelines, particularly if they are convinced by the patient's expert witnesses that the guidelines do not consti-tute a proper standard of care. Hence, a caregiver should base any decision to *follow* a set of guide-lines upon explicit consideration of whether those guidelines are justified, in light of the caregiver's knowledge, experience, and medical judgment. Any guidelines the provider implements also should leave room for professional judgment. Otherwise, the provider risks violating its own "standard of care" simply by missing a "checklist" item that may not fit the facts of a particular case.

To all appearances, the field of dialysis in many areas lacks any true consensus treatment stan-dards. For example, there does not seem to be universal agreement as to how much dialysis is the "right" amount [38, 39]. Other areas of current contention seem to include management of ane-mia, nutrition for dialysis patients, and vascular access procedures for hemodialysis [40]. One offi-cial of the U.S. Health Care Financing Adminis-tration ("HCFA") has been quoted as seeing a desperate need for practice guidelines, because of a lack of any agreement on what constitutes standard practice [41].

In an environment without clear consensus stan-dards, both sides in a malpractice lawsuit may be able to point to a number of different practices in support of their versions of the proper "standard of care". This makes it all the more important that caregivers base their treatment choices upon care-ful consideration of various alternatives, and famili-arity with the available research.

As this chapter was being written, the National Kidney Foundation (NKF) announced the formulation of guidelines for dialysis treatment [42]. Conceivably some of these guidelines, offered by the NKF's dialysis outcome quality initiative (DOQI) project, will lead to greater uniformity in dialysis treatment. On the other hand, it also is conceivable that various providers will decide to adopt some of the DOQI guidelines and decline to adopt others (at least to the extent HCFA does not incorporate the DOQI guidelines into HCFA's "conditions of coverage") [42, 43].

At some point in a courtroom, the DOQI guidelines undoubtedly will be offered as the "standard of care". The prudent provider should evaluate these guidelines, with their possible use in court in mind, well in advance of any lawsuit. Where a provider differs with the DOQI guidelines, the provider ought to be able to articulate clearly the reasons for this difference, based upon experience, contemporary research, and medical judgment. Similarly, where a provider adopts a DOQI guideline, the provider should be in a position to explain the medical justification for that decision, again by reference to experience, research, and judgment. Whether the decision is to follow or not to follow a given set of guidelines, the provider should base this decision upon an explicit weighing of the various alternative choices.

This is not to say that each guideline offered on an issue in dialysis care, whether from NKF-DOQI or elsewhere, is cause for an elaborate bureaucratic process. Instead, the point is that questions of what is the "standard of care" should be addressed early, in the context of designing practices and procedures of care, rather than later in the context of a court battle. Incorporating concerns about possible liability risks at the "front end" need not add much additional time and effort to the process of setting a clinic's or unit's processes and procedures, and doing so can build in some measure of protection against later legal actions. Should the issue eventually come before a jury, the caregiver who has implemented carefully-considered guidelines will be in a stronger position to defend his or her reasonableness, and compliance with the standard of care, than one who operated without the benefit of such guidelines.

CONCLUSION

Even at their best, quality assurance systems will not eliminate lawsuits, and will not eliminate jury decisions against ESRD treatment providers. In terms of *reducing* the risks posed by lawsuits, however, quality assurance should be viewed as a powerful tool. Of course, the risk of a lawsuit is only one of several factors to be weighed in the balance in developing quality assurance and other programs for ESRD treatment. Analysis of legal principles and courtroom practicalities cannot take the place of sound medical judgment, but instead should be kept in mind – and used to inform medical judgment – where it is consistent with the medical interests of the patient.

NOTES

[1] There are variations among states in the geographic frame of reference from which the standard of care is drawn. For instance (and oversimplifying for brevity's sake), some states look to the practice in either the same or a similar locality, while other states' courts measure negligence against a nationwide standard of care [6, 8–10]. States also vary in the precise framing of *whose* practices are selected to set the standard of care. For example, courts in one state refer to the "diligence, skill, competence and prudence" practiced by *"minimally competent* physicians in the same specialty or general field of practice", while another state's courts measure the standard of care by reference to "an *ordinarily competent* physician under like conditions" [6, 7, 11]. Where a doctor holds himself or herself out as a specialist, courts may look to standards (typically national standards) applicable within that specialty [1, 9]. A few states also have passed laws that provide for the development of medical practice guidelines, most of which serve only as recommendations that the physician may disregard, but at the risk of the guidelines being offered in court as some evidence of the standard of care [5, 12].

[2] The author, in describing lawsuits brought against dialysis providers, seeks only to illustrate the kinds of allegations that might be made in such a lawsuit. It is not the author's intention to pass judgment on the merits of any of these lawsuits, i.e. to draw conclusions as to who, if anyone, was negligent.

[3] For example, in one case a court instructed the jury that the applicable standard of care was "that degree of skill and knowledge which ordinarily was possessed", at the time of the alleged malpractice, by physicians in the same practice area in the same or a similar locality, "consider[ing] [the physician's] background, training and the care and skill required" of physicians "rendering care under similar circumstances" [10].

REFERENCES

1. Liang BA. Medical malpractice: do physicians have knowledge of legal standards and assess cases as juries do? U Chi L Sch Roundtable 1996; 3:59.
2. Vidmar N. The Randolph W. Thrower symposium: scientific and technological evidence: are juries competent to decide liability in tort cases involving scientific/medical issues? Some data from medical malpractice. Emory L J 1994; 43:885–911.
3. Farber HS and White MJ. A comparison of formal and informal dispute resolution in medical malpractice. J Legal Stud 1994; 23:777.
4. Kozac CS. A review of federal medical malpractice tort reform alternatives. Seton Hall Legis J 1995; 19:599–647.
5. Ouellette v. Mehalic, 534 A.2d 1331, 1332 (Maine 1988).
6. Hall v. Hilbun, 466 So.2d 856, 866, 873 (Miss. 1985).
7. Kacmar DE. The impact of computerized medical literature databases on medical malpractice litigation. Ohio St. Law J 1997; 58:617.
8. Stoia SJ. Vergara v. Doan: Modern medical technology consumes the locality rule. J Pharm Law 1993; 2:107–12.
9. Morrison v. MacNamara, 407 A.2d 555, 560-65 (D.C. App. 1979).
10. Vergara v. Doan, 593 N.E.2d 185, 186-87 (Ind. 1992).
11. McLaughlin v. Sy, 589 A.2d 448, 452 (Maine 1991).
12. Kuc GW. Practice parameters as a shield against physician liability. J Conn Hlth Law Policy 1995; 10:439.
13. LEXIS/NEXIS: GENFED library, COURTS file; STATES library, COURTS file; VERDCT library, ALLVER file.
14. Szymanski v. Hartford Hospital, 1993 Conn. Super. LEXIS 715, 1 (March 17, 1993).
15. Ellis v. Bio-Medical Applications of South Arlington, Inc., Case No. 342-123569-89 (Texas Tarrant County Court), reported in North Texas Reports 1992, May 1992, p. V-72, available in LEXIS/NEXIS, VERDCT library, ALLVER file, November 29, 1997.
16. Perryman v. Rosenbaum, Case No. 86-3453 (Georgia De-Kalb County Superior Court), verdict date June 5, 1991, reported in The Georgia Trial Reporter 1991; 4(5): 212, available in LEXIS/NEXIS, VERDCT library, ALLVER file, November 29, 1997.
17. Smith v. Cathy-Cook, Case No. TC 000 659 (California state court), verdict date June 10, 1996, reported in Verdictum Juris Press, available in LEXIS/NEXIS, VERDCT library, ALLVER file, November 29, 1997.
18. Natelli v. Ferrante, Docket No. L-0295-90 (New Jersey Union County Court), verdict date Jan. 9, 1991, reported in New Jersey Verdict Review & Analysis 1992; 12(9), available in LEXIS/NEXIS, VERDCT library, ALLVER file, November 29, 1997.
19. Schumacher v. Martin, No. L-555-93 (Summerset County New Jersey), verdict date Dec. 14, reported in New Jersey Jury Verdict Review & Analysis 1996; 16(12), available in LEXIS/NEXIS, VERDCT library, ALLVER file, November 29, 1997.
20. Unidentified plaintiff v. unidentified defendant, verdict date Oct. 22, 1987, reported in New York Jury Verdict Review & Analysis 1987; IV(12), available in LEXIS/NEXIS, VERDCT library, ALLVER file, November 29, 1997.
21. Fitchett v. Estate of Reilly, Case No. 93-C-025 (new Hampshire Belknap County Court), verdict date June, 1994, reported in Medical Litigation Alert 1994; 3(3), available in LEXIS/NEXIS, VERDCT library, ALLVER file, November 29, 1997.
22. Gultz v. Ungaro, Case No. 95-6375 (Broward County, Florida), verdict date April 30, 1997, reported in Medical Litigation Alert 1997; 5(11), available in LEXIS/NEXIS, VERDCT library, ALLVER file, November 29, 1997.
23. Sage WM, Hastings KE and Berenson RO. Enterprise liability for medical malpractice and health care quality improvement. Am J Law Med 1994; 20:1–28.
24. Einaugler v. Supreme Court of New York, 918 F.Supp. 619, 621-623 (E.D. N.Y. 1996), aff'd 109 F. 3d 836 (2d Clr. 1997).
25. Seal v. Bogalusa Community Medical Center, 665 So.2d 52, 52-53 (La. App. 1995).
26. State of Louisiana v. Joint Commission on Accreditation of Hospitals, Inc., 470 So.2d 169, 171-72 (La. App. 1985).
27. Velandia M, Fridkin SK, Cardenas, V et al. Transmission of HIV in dialysis centre. Lancet 1995; 345:1417–22.
28. Weiss v. Goldfarb, 295 N.J. Super. 212, 216-19, 233, 684 A.2d 994, 996-98, 1005 (1996), rev'd on other grounds, 154 N.J. 468, 713 A.2d 427 (1998).
29. Kadzielski L, Weingarten S and Schroder G. Peer review and practice guidelines under health care reform. Whittier Law Rev 1995; 16:157–76.
30. Pfifferling J-H. Ounces of malpractice prevention; improving physician behavior. Physic Exec 1994; 20:36.
31. Press I, Ganey RF and Malone MP. Satisfied patients can spell financial well-being. Healthcare Financial Manag 1991; 45:34.
32. Lester GW and Smith SG. Listening and talking to patients: a remedy for malpractice suits? Western J Med 1993; 158:268.
33. Cohn B, Ehrhardt ME and Phillips M. Protecting yourself from malpractice. Patient Care 1990; 24:53.
34. Burda D. Five future areas of liability risk haunt providers. Hospitals 1986; 60:48–50, 52.
35. Orentlicher D. Health care reform and the patient-physician relationship. Hlth Matrix 1995; 5:141–80.
36. Crawford L. Preparing a defendant physician for testimony before a jury: attitudes can be as important as facts. Med Malprac Law Strat 1996; (August):1.
37. Hallam K. Jurors won't listen to doctors they dislike. Med Econ 1996; 73:178.
38. Owen WF Jr., Lew NL, Liu Y, Lowrie EG and Lazarus JM. The urea reduction ratio and serum albumin concentration as predictors of mortality in patients undergoing hemodialysis. N Eng J Med 1993; 329:1001–6.
39. Cohen P. Predictors of mortality in patients undergoing hemodialysis correspondence. N Eng J Med 1994; 330:573–4.
40. Wheeler D. Nephrologists focus on quality of care for chronic renal failure. Lancet 1996; 348:1370.
41. Inglehart JK. The American health care system – the end stage renal disease program. N Engl J Med 1993; 338:366–71.

42. National Kidney Foundation. National kidney foundation releases new guidelines for dialysis care. PR Newswire Oct. 15, 1997.

43. Gardner J. Dialysis outcomes in works: HCFA may set quality, practice guidelines for ESRD program. Mod Healthcare 1997; Feb:64.

7. Quality criteria for the clinical record

SUSAN WILLIAMS, KIM PIERPOINT AND CORRINE ALGRIM BOYLE

Quality improvement initiatives in the clinical dialysis setting require the tracking and trending of data which can be used to identify, analyze and improve patterns of care and patterns of outcomes. Improving clinical outcomes is dependent on the availability of reliable clinical data for analysis and feedback to the renal care team. Designed properly, the dialysis facility clinical record can facilitate timely and accurate communication of patient care information to the renal care team, promote quality of service provided, and contribute to both qualitative and quantitative evaluation of care.

Clinical records vary from the official medical record of the patient to a multitude of unofficial, yet vital, forms and tracking systems. The intent of these systems is to allow the clinician to monitor the many variables associated with management of acute and chronic dialysis patients and to meet reporting requirements of governmental and regulatory agencies. As the financing and delivery of health care continues to evolve in the direction of managed care, the facility-based clinical record needs to keep pace. This means that dialysis facility managers should continuously evaluate the relevance and usefulness of its clinical record-keeping system to support innovation and improvement in the organization and delivery of high-quality care while continuing to meet regulatory reporting requirements and externally-mandated quality improvement initiatives.

Since becoming a federal program in 1974, End Stage Renal Disease (ESRD) has been subject to many regulations and quality compliance initiatives. The more recent initiatives have the most impact on the dialysis facility in terms of reporting requirements. The Joint Commission of Accreditation for Health Care Organizations (JCAHO) initiated the Agenda for Change in 1987 [1]. This plan required hospitals, and therefore hospital-based dialysis units, over a five year period to implement Continuous Quality Improvement (CQI) [2] as the quality management process in all facilities. In a separate effort, the Forum of ESRD Networks and the Health Care Financing Administration (HCFA) in 1994 implemented the HCFA ESRD Core Indicator Project [3].

Fortunately, some regulatory agencies are switching focus from quality assurance to quality improvement. Most notably, HCFA's new framework for quality emphasizes outcomes assessment and continuous quality improvement as the foundation of its new Health Care Quality Improvement Project [4]. This involves transition from case by case review to population-based assessment of care and has placed greater emphasis on the quality and availability of data in the dialysis clinical record. As ESRD quality improvement activities move in the direction of Outcomes Assessment, the reliance on data for measurement, monitoring and feedback to the clinicians for use in their Continuous Quality Improvement programs will be pivotal to improvements in the process of clinical care.

In the future, it is reasonable to expect the evolution of ESRD Quality Improvement Activities in the U.S. will continue to be driven by initiatives such as the National Kidney Foundation's Dialysis Outcomes Quality Initiative (DOQI) [5] and the ESRD Core Indicator Project. The interest in ESRD quality improvement programs is expanding worldwide and some countries have enacted requirements for quality improvement for all facilities.

L.W. Henderson and R.S. Thuma (eds.), Quality Assurance in Dialysis, 2nd Edition, 73–80.
© 1999 *Kluwer Academic Publishers. Printed in Great Britain*

DATA OVERLOAD

The clinical record provides data for evaluation and documentation of the quality and appropriateness of care delivered. It is also the document relied upon to support administrative and financial requirements such as billing and external quality reporting mandates. Many reporting requirements historically have influenced not only the amount of data, but the kind of data kept by the dialysis centers. Proliferation of data reporting requirements has led to the use of numerous forms to manage patient care over an extended period of time. *Data overload* among staff, therefore, is not uncommon. When this happens, staff become less concerned about the accuracy and legibility of what they are recording simply because of the volume of data collection activities they are required to perform on a daily basis. If the volume of data is allowed to build without systematic organization and dissemination, it is not useful to clinical staff. Without knowing where to look for specific information on a patient, staff may not refer to previous documentation to assist them in assessments of current problems, let alone use the data to search for opportunities to improve. For example, in some situations tests are repeated unnecessarily because the original results could not be found in time. This has a negative impact on the efficiency and effectiveness of care, increases the cost of providing the dialysis treatment and is frustrating to staff.

PLANNING FOR INFORMATION MANAGEMENT

Searching for better ways to provide dialysis treatment is not new to dialysis professionals. A search for opportunities to improve care should not require intensive detective work to uncover meaningful trends in the process or outcomes of care. Trends should be easily identified through proper management of the data collection and evaluation process. This is why having a well-planned approach to information management is essential for dialysis facilities today. One solution to the documentation issue is automation of the clinical record [6–8]. In fact, the information management plans in many dialysis settings include some level of computerization. This is appropriate. However, before rushing to automate the various administrative, business and clinical processes, the dialysis facility manager's first task is to conduct a thorough evaluation of current practices. If these practices don't already work on paper, automation may make a marginal manual documentation system worse.

What must occur is the design, implementation and testing of both the clinical and administrative processes upon which the dialysis facility operates. This is the same process which needs to take place in a facility with or without computer support. The following six questions should be asked by every dialysis manager to identify sources and uses of information, and where areas of duplication and gaps exist:

1. What data is being collected now and why?

2. How is the data used?

3. Who is collecting the data?

4. When is the data collected?

5. What forms are used in the process and do they make sense?

6. What data should be collected that currently is not collected?

WHAT DATA IS BEING COLLECTED NOW AND WHY?

Medical Record

The central data repository of clinical information collected in the unit is the dialysis medical record [9]. The contents of the dialysis medical record are influenced by many legal, regulatory, accrediting and policy directives. The following list is a composite of some of these directives. Reporting requirements have been divided into recommended and optional; these may differ from unit to unit depending on the location and are intended as a guideline and may not be all inclusive.

Table 7.1. Medical records

Recommended

– Intake admissions data (patient profile)	– Pre and post dialytic assessment	– Infection rates
– Patient informed consents	– Intradialytic flow sheet	– Medication record
– Patient bill of rights	– Medical directives (living wills)	– Laboratory and diagnostics
– Patient grievance procedure		– Patient education and rehabilitation
– Physician orders	– Viral surveillance	– Access record
– Problem list	– Consults	– Discharge summary
– History and physical	– Transfusion record	
– Modality selection	– Nursing, social worker, Dietitian assessments	
– Patient care plan by dialysis team individualized	– Dialysis adequacy	
– Long term care plan	– Narrative records/progress notes	

Optional

– Chart checklist	– Pre dialysis checklist	– Health maintenance record
– Research protocol		

Facility Records

In addition to the patient medical record, many unofficial records must be maintained by the facility in order to meet license, certification, accreditation and legal requirements. Many of these records support the systems necessary to run the units, maintain equipment or staff the patient care area and each, once again, may vary in their requirements depending on the location of the facility.

These lists can serve as a starting point for facility managers to use in creating their own master list according to their specific needs which can then be used to develop a database.

HOW IS THE DATA USED?

The data is used for regulatory compliance, clinical decision support, and to support quality improvement initiatives. Quality improvement initiatives ideally strive to exceed minimal expectations and attain optimal outcomes [10]. Assessment of state, federal, and institutional requirements for documentation help to establish the

Table 7.2. Facility records

Recommended

– Water treatment records	– Occurrence reports	– Machine maintenance records
– Credentialing records	– Medical by-laws	– Morbidity mortality data
– Standards of practice	– Home supply records	– Infection control
– Individual orientation records	– Reuse records	– Quality improvement program
– Facility mandatory inservice	– Performance appraisals	– Hazardous waste program
Records:	– Policy and procedures	– On call records
Fire/safety	– Staff meeting records	– Patient satisfaction surveys
CPR	– Governing board minutes	
Infection control	– Billing records	

Optional

– Mission statement	– Research protocols	– Patient classification system
– Career ladder records	– Continuing education	– Annual report
– Operational directives	– Organizational chart	– Staffing patterns

---

framework for the clinical records system. Once the minimum requirements are identified, one can explore the need for expansion, modification or reduction of current documentation or record keeping systems. The goal should be to reduce unnecessary paperwork and unnecessary recording. A good documentation system should support proactive planning for quality improvement.

Dialysis centers are required to have a quality monitoring program in place, but may not know how to direct the documentation system toward quality improvement [11, 12]. Since the medical record is the central document in all dialysis facilities, monitoring the quality of care through documentation should begin with the medical record.

The most common standards used in monitoring the medical record is the standard of clinical pertinence. Clinical pertinence can be determined when a set of criteria are met which demonstrate that the care rendered addressed the individualized medical needs of the patient. One method of monitoring clinical pertinence of the dialysis medical record is to establish a standard set of criteria and the expected rate of completion. A review of the medical records of the dialysis population then can be assessed for trends where those standards are not being met. Examination of the variance from the expected rate through statistical analysis will determine if the variance is significant [13]. If there is indication that the variance should be explored, use of cause and effect or flow diagram tools can be implemented to work toward a solution and to point out opportunities for improvement [14]. The example in Table 7.3 demonstrates a standard set of criteria by which the clinical record can be measured for quality in the dialysis setting.

WHO IS COLLECTING THE DATA?

The people who collect the data are usually patient care staff who are invested in improving the outcome of what they do for patients. Since time allotted for patient care is increasingly scarce in the clinical setting, data collection processes – whether manual or automated – should not detract from the caregiver's primary responsibility. The type of data collected should support the care

Table 7.3. Clinical pertinence standard

The clinical record documentation will reflect individualized appropriate medical treatment

Clinical pertinence criteria
1. The history and physical provides adequate information to assess the condition of the patient and begin the process of diagnosis and treatment
2. Diagnostic and therapeutic orders are documented
3. Clinical observations and results of treatment are documented
4. Reports of procedures and tests are documented
5. Diagnostic impressions are documented
6. Progress notes adequately reflect the patient's condition and course of treatment
7. Plans are developed for follow-up care and discharge instructions pertinent to the care of the patient
8. Conclusion-final disposition of the patient's condition is documented
9. Instructions and patient education are documented
10. Signature of the physician is present
11. Handwriting is legible
12. Consultations and referrals are documented
13. Documentation is appropriate for the medical situation
14. Abnormal study results are addressed

given from a legal as well as a treatment perspective. Therefore, the data should be concise, accurate, timely, legible, factual and clinically pertinent [15]. The data collection method developed for the clinical dialysis setting should promote these criteria. Additionally, it should be streamlined to achieve efficiency in the daily work of all patient care providers.

WHEN IS THE DATA COLLECTED?

Often, data is collected when reporting forms are due. This means that it is collected retrospectively and in reaction to external pressures rather than at the point of service delivery. One advantage of computerization is in the technology of data entry. Voice recognition devices, laptop computers, and other forms of data input make point of service data collection relatively easy. The value of point of service entry is that data is immediately available to the clinical care team for reference and decision support.

WHAT FORMS ARE USED IN THE PROCESS AND DO THEY MAKE SENSE?

The first step in answering this question is to conduct an inventory of all forms. If information is not recorded so that it can be readily found and used efficiently, cause and effect diagramming and process flow diagramming can depict the relationships between the steps required to produce a complete record or to identify points where the process of charting becomes cumbersome and breaks down. Using a process flow diagram to map the processes of forms design, data collection and analysis will help identify where improvements in the system are necessary before moving toward automation. Flow diagramming is an excellent tool to use when determining the effectiveness or efficiency of a system [14].

The forms should be tested over a period of time. Data recorded should be reviewed for its accuracy and validity. The facts relating to the patient's care should be recorded in a timely manner and in an organized format so that there is a clear chronological picture of what has happened to the patient during the course of the treatment by each provider. The people who use the documentation system are the best individuals to ask for input when designing a new form or an entire system. If the system is simple, user-friendly, flexible and designed with future improvements in mind such as computerization, the system will be used. The forms themselves should be organized and printed so as to guide the user in a sequential manner from the assessment of patient care through planning, implementation and evaluation. This process then sets the data collection in a logical sequence for monitoring quality improvement opportunities.

WHAT DATA SHOULD BE COLLECTED THAT CURRENTLY IS NOT COLLECTED?

This question can best be answered by first examining the clinical setting and care delivery model utilized in the unit, and then defining information needed to support them.

Influences of the Clinical Setting

The clinical setting influences the type of data necessary for an effective documentation system. The dialysis treatment location and acuity level of the patient directly influence planning for documentation systems. The acutely ill, chronic and home patient have many similar core data elements. On the other hand, each of these groups of patients have a set of data which is unique to their setting and care requirements. In addition to the location and acuity of the patient population, the need to interface with other health care providers also influences the design of the documentation system. In the hospital setting, the dialysis record must be part of the centralized medical record system. In the free-standing dialysis clinic, mechanisms must be in place for the communication of clinical data between the center and other health systems which provide support to the nephrology team for the care of the patient. The home dialysis record must support an even broader network of health care providers such as the patient's local physician, community health agencies and home equipment and supply companies.

Influences of the Care Delivery Model

A case management care delivery model is increasingly utilized by both providers and managed care organizations to organize and deliver services to the chronically ill in managed care settings. Whether situated in the facility, hospital or nephrology office, the case manager is charged with defining and achieving expected outcomes within acceptable levels of resource utilization. The objective is to prevent catastrophic onset of illness through early detection, patient education, and care coordination. Having the right information at the right time is essential in helping case managers find and refer patients early.

The information needs of a case management care delivery model applied to chronic populations such as ESRD differ significantly from traditional settings. This is because ESRD information systems have evolved around isolated clinical or financial transactions such as billing or external reporting requirements. Traditional systems are centered around outcomes reporting. These are important, but limited to evaluating patient status.

A case management model founded on principles of continuous quality improvement requires that we analyze outcomes as part of the continuous feedback loop. Successful implementation of practice guidelines, such as DOQI, depends on our ability to measure and report variance from established norms and to adjust our clinical decisions and care plans accordingly. This approach expands the facility's information requirements as well as its ability to analyze and use it. Some of those information needs include the following:

- Early intervention protocols, researched-based practice guidelines and critical pathways

- Variance analysis and reporting capability

- Electronic linkages between the payer, providers, and disease manager within tight security parameters to ensure patient confidentiality

- Incorporation of patient education, self-care, and satisfaction tools

- Disease-specific data repositories

This approach to information management will enable case managers to continually monitor outcomes and to refine clinical practice guidelines and protocols based on scientific process.

WHERE TO BEGIN: THE MEDICAL RECORD

The most familiar document in the clinical setting is the patient's medical record. It is a tool for communication between professionals about the care of the patient. It serves as a diary of chronological facts pertaining to the diagnosis and course of the treatment and serves as a reservoir of data for evaluation of the comprehensive treatment of the patient. A good medical record is a map of the what, when, and how a patient received care [16]. The medical record also acts as the one permanent record of care and treatment of the patient from admission to discharge. A well kept record can assist the provider in the care process and the outcomes of care. On the other hand, a poorly kept record can make anyone appear to have given poor care [15].

A good medical record provides an accurate account of what has happened to the patient with evidence of interventions, rationale by the provider and response to the intervention by the patient. The medical record also serves as a tool from which useful data for research and development of new approaches to patient management can be obtained. Given potential uses for the medical record, security measures are required to protect patient confidentiality [17]. Medical records should be kept in an area which can be secured from the general public and only individuals with official business and approved releases should be allowed to use the records for any purpose.

Both of the lists of records found in the dialysis setting have many common data elements. Because the number of reporting requirements have grown over time, much of the information is repeated from form to form. Reducing the amount of recording by staff through an organized and efficient information system is the first step in ensuring quality of care in the dialysis unit.

Information systems which streamline the process of recording, interfacing and integrating the data will lead to better and more efficient use of the records by staff in their care of the patient. Without a streamlined information system, quality programs become unmanageable, discouraging and eventually ignored.

Once the information systems for recording and maintaining patient data have been established, these records will be key tools or sources for tracking and trending of data and quality improvement activities [18].

THE CLINICAL RECORD AND QUALITY MONITORING: PRACTICAL APPROACHES

The nursing process is one example where a systematic approach of problem analysis is used to determine the plan of care and evaluation of the clinical outcome. In research, the problem solving process is orderly and disciplined to acquire reliable information and to analyze that information in an orderly manner. The Deming industrial model and later adaptations of Deming for health care by Batalden and Vorlicky require that there is a definitive plan [19]. This plan will guide an organization to establish standards of quality, monitor the organization's ability to uphold the standards and ultimately to improve upon the standards.

The goals of quality monitoring are:

1. To assure identification and correction of system wide and unit based problems.

2. To promote care that is cost effective and clinically effective.

3. To promote optimal patient care through the ongoing assessment of all aspects of care, together with the correction of identified problems.

4. To identify and reduce risk factors while at the same time managing known risks.

5. To meet the requirements of external agencies.

Two established models for monitoring quality in ESRD care today are the JCAHO 10 Step model [20] and the HCFA/Network RoadMap [4] which is a seven step approach for systematically identifying, designing, implementing, and evaluating a process improvement project. Changes in both models have already occurred and over time the models will continue to evolve as the principles of outcomes assessment become refined in the health care setting.

The steps outlined by the HCFA/Network roadmap are:

1. Make a commitment to improve care.

2. Clarify current knowledge of the process performance and write an opportunity statement.

3. Describe and analyze the basic process and identify sources of variation (process analysis).

4. Search for root causes of variation and select an area for improvement.

5. Design and implement an improvement trail.

6. Evaluate the improvement trail.

7. Act on the results.

Each of these models focuses on improving the process of care; therefore documentation should support the goals of quality monitoring and assist the quality improvement team in their evaluation process. Other tools are available to offer guidance such as CQI Applications to Renal Therapy pro-

vided by Baxter Healthcare Corporation [21, 22].

Quality improvement is an analytical process and requires critical thinking on the part of the individuals involved. Critical thinking by staff should lead to actions which promote successful experiences. A team working together can be more creative and innovative than one individual working alone toward a solution. The analytical process for the team can include brain-storming which is free from professional barriers or the stigma of organizational hierarchy. This type of team process will lead to better problem solving and efficiencies will increase.

The most important resource group for designing a clinical documentation system is the members of the dialysis team who must use the forms and provide the patient care on a daily basis. Input from all disciplines and the patient is imperative to fully address every issue pertinent to the quality standards desired. The patient's perception of the quality of services they receive should also be included [23]. The most common method of obtaining patient data is from patient satisfaction surveys [24]. These surveys must be administered carefully in the chronic dialysis population in order to protect anonymity and promote honest feedback. If done correctly, the information derived from the survey will be invaluable to the quality monitoring programs.

In summary, models for implementing quality improvement programs in the renal setting are readily available. Each model depends on a reliable data system to drive systematic tracking, trending and analysis of the care processes and patient outcomes.

CONCLUSION

The importance of the clinical record in the dialysis setting cannot be emphasized enough. As demonstrated through various examples in this chapter, a valid clinical record is essential to providing accurate and pertinent data for monitoring patterns of care and patterns of outcomes. Clinical data is required for evaluation of the processes of care through measurement, monitoring, analysis, and feedback to the clinical team. As a result, the quality improvement program in use at the facility can simultaneously evaluate quality, assess, prevent and reduce risk, implement cost-effective resource management measures, and identify and combat potential problems. Integration of the design of the clinical record system with the quality improvement program will ensure ongoing success of improving patient outcomes. A well organized, streamlined, interactive clinical record system is the key to a successful continuous quality improvement program.

REFERENCES

1. The Joint Commission Guide to Quality Assurance, 1988: The Joint Commission on Accreditation of Healthcare Organizations, Chicago.
2. Conway-Welch C. Entering a new era of quality care. ANNA J 1989; 16:469–71.
3. 1996 Annual Report ESRD Core Indicators Project. Department of Health and Human Services Health Care Financing Administration Health Standards and Quality Bureau, January 1997.
4. A Guide for Improving the Quality of Care of Dialysis Patients, the National Anemia Cooperative Project, U.S. Department of Health and Human Services: Health Care Financing Administration, July 1996.
5. National Kidney Foundation-Dialysis Outcomes Quality Initiative Clinical Practice Guidelines, American Journal of Kidney Diseases. September 1997: vol 30, no 3, supp 2, October 1997: vol 30, no 4, supp 13.
6. Pollak VE, Peterson DW and Flynn J. The computer in quality control of hemodialysis patient care. QRB 1986; 202–10.
7. West E. Designing information systems to increase quality care. Computers in Healthcare, Sept 1990.
8. Kaiser LR. Anticipating your high tech tomorrow. Healthcare Forum, 12–20, Nov/Dec 1986.
9. Harbert G. A national model for ESRD patient medical records. Nephrol News Issues 1994; May:40-42.
10. Laffel G and Blumenthal D. The case for using industrial quality management science in health care organizations. J Am Med Assoc 1989; 262Z:2869–73.
11. Bednar B and Neff M. Preparing for inspection: a tool to maximize quality and minimize risk. ANNA J 1990; 17:159–64.
12. Rajki KL, Feltman BA and Smeltzer CH. Assessing the quality of nursing care in a dialysis Unit. ANNA J 1985;12(1).
13. Schyve PM and Prevost JA. From quality assurance to quality improvement. Psych Clin N Am 1990; 13:61–71.
14. McDonald JC and Newton GA. The patient flow management model: a process for quality assurance. Hlth Rec Manag 1990; 10:32–43.
15. Professional Liability Program, Farmers Insurance Group of Companies, Keeping the Record Straight: Guidelines for Charting, QRC Advisor 6(3): 7–9, Jan 1990.
16. Mogli GD. Role of medical records in quality assurance program. Am Ro 1989; 30:11–15.
17. Chasteen JE. For the record. Dent Assist 1987; Sept/Oct:23–6,
18. Donabedian A. The quality of care: how can it be assessed? J Am Med Assoc 1988; 260:1743–8.
19. Walton M. The Deming management method. New York: Putnum Publishing Group, 1986.
20. Joint Commission on Accreditation of Healthcare Organizations, 1988: Accreditation Manual for Hospitals, Chicago.
21. Peritoneal Access Management Utilizing Continuous Quality Improvement, Baxter CQI Applications to Renal Therapy, Renal Division, Baxter Healthcare Corporation, 1997.
22. Peritonitis Management Utilizing Continuous Quality Improvement, Baxter CQI Applications to Renal Therapy. Renal Division, Baxter Healthcare Corporation, 1995.
23. Louden TL. Customer perception counts in quality assurance. Hospitals 1989; Jan 20:84.
24. ANNA, Quality Assurance for Nephrology Nursing, First ed, 1989.

8. The impact of global vigilance reporting requirements on the quality of dialysis products and services

PAMELA McDONNELL AND RICHARD S. THUMA

INTRODUCTION

In the past several decades, increased regulation of the drug and device industry has significantly impacted the way manufacturers develop, manufacture, market and monitor medical products. As the distribution of medical products expands globally, so also the need for industry and regulators to understand product safety and performance on a world-wide basis. The resulting depth and specificity of quality system requirements have led to significant demands on both industry and governmental agencies.

Governments have implemented new policies and programs to address issues of quality of medical care. These programs and policies have many objectives, but among the most important are those aimed at containing costs and managing care.

In a classical sense, the scope of quality assurance encompasses a large number of activities and systems for maintaining the quality of patient care. However, Quality Assurance neither promises nor guarantees error-free health care. It has, within the provider side of the business, the goal of building confidence and faith in the quality of the care being rendered. Achieving error-free health care at all times is impossible. O'Leary says that "an effective quality assurance program is not an end in itself; rather, it is a means for maintaining and improving health care".

The drivers for governments to enact local laws to regulate medical devices, drugs, and equipment vary widely. Four major purposes might be proposed: First, it is important to identify providers whose delivery of care is sor far below an accep-

table level that immediate actions are needed to ensure patient safety.

Second, if QA programs identify suppliers with products and services determined to be unaacptable, those suppliers can be the subject of concentrated attention with the objective of correcting the problems and bringing products up to an acceptable level.

Third, regulations focus on improving the average quality of products and services provided. This objective embraces the concept of continuous improvement. By encouraging a large number of suppliers to continually improve their products and processes.

Fourth, and last, QA may motivate and assist suppliers and providers to achieve high levels of quality as a competitive advantage. Programs may identify excellent suppliers who serve as models for Best Demonstrated Practices.

Today, in many countries, vigilance and surveillance requirements are global in scope; and the requirements are defined more specifically by law as well as in standards, regulations and directives. This expansion in the depth to which industry is regulated has had some very positive outcomes, but has also presented some challenging problems. In many cases, it is the challenges and obstacles that have driven the trend toward mutual collaboration between regulators and industry from around the world.

There are two very good examples of effective industry/regulator collaboration:

The International Conference on Harmonization (ICH) represents an effort between industry and regulators from North America, Europe and

L.W. Henderson and R.S. Thuma (eds.), Quality Assurance in Dialysis, 2nd Edition, 81–92.
© 1999 *Kluwer Academic Publishers. Printed in Great Britain*

Japan. This collaborative effort resulted in the development of and issuance of international guidelines The guidelines themselves include harmonized definitions relating to drug development and pharmaco-vigilance. They also contain, a standardized approach to Periodic Safety Update Reports (PSUR). The PSUR is a regulatory submission containing an aggregate collection of information regarding the pharmaceutical being reported. Information contained in the PSUR includes:

- Reference to all registration numbers by country and dosage as well as outlines of specific indications per country;

- Core Data Sheet which includes all product characteristics and indications, contraindications and specificities per country;

- A summary of any market withdrawals or suspensions, failure in obtaining renewals, restrictions on distribution, and changes in indications or formulation;

- A summary of changes to the safety information, i.e. new contra-indications, precautions, warnings, adverse drug reactions (ADRs), or insertions;

- An estimate of the population exposed to the drug and interpretation of results;

- Detailed case histories of the adverse events reported during the time period covered by the report;

- An analysis of all literature referencing the drug;

- A listing of any pre- and post approval studies initiated and adverse events encountered during the study period;

- An overall safety evaluation and conclusion.

For medical devices, similar harmonization efforts have been made. The most well known of these is the Global Harmonization Task Force (GHTF) and ISO TC210. This Technical Committee (TC) and task force have developed a standardized nomenclature for device reporting called MEDDRA. There is considerable effort to adopt the MEDDRA nomenclature globally. This would greatly simplify both Industry and Regulators ability to compare information on a regional and country basis.

These efforts and continuing trends toward collaborative rule making between industry and regulators will no doubt continue. It is clear that the efforts reflect the mutual recognition of the need for appropriately regulated medical products, as well as the mutual concern regarding promulgation and implementation of meaningful and effective regulatory requirements.

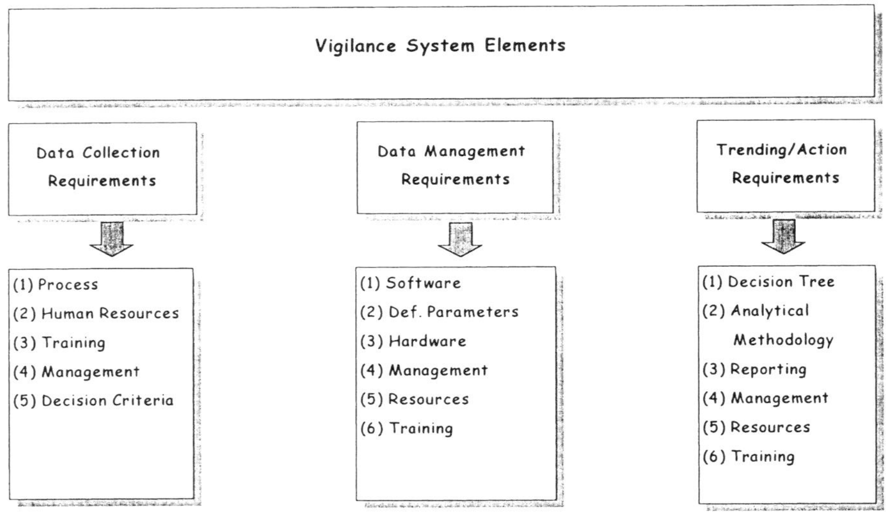

Fig. 8.1. Elements of a generalized vigilance system.

As mentioned, the road to international vigilance compliance has not been easy – the additional administrative burden on industry and regulators has been significant. Figure 8.1 is a generalized vigilance system diagram. Today, the search for additional solutions to efficiently and effectively deploy and manage global vigilance continues. Electronic solutions that meet current needs are difficult to deploy in all geographic areas. Establishing effective systems globally are often hampered by the differences in cultures, governmental requirements and technical and organizational infrastructures. However, the initiatives aimed at harmonizing requirements is a critical step that will further all of our efforts to meet the rapidly changing global requirements.

DEFINITIONS

Surveillance is defined as those activities that monitor all aspects of product performance in the market, both pre- and post-market approval. Examples of surveillance activities would include product complaint management, device tracking, formal post-market studies, pre-market studies, and et cetera.

Vigilance, or vigilance reporting, is often used generically to reflect the subset of surveillance activities that may result in, or require, submitting a regulatory report to a governmental agency. Specifically, vigilance activities or regulatory reporting reflect those types of surveillance data that suggest an adverse event or potential adverse event has occurred. Reports of deaths, serious injuries, or in the case of medical devices, near incidents (Europe) or reportable malfunctions (U.S.), or periodic safety update reports (pharmaceuticals), are examples of "vigilance" reporting.

Medical Device includes disposable medical devices, durable medical equipment, as well as accessories to medical devices or durable medical equipment.

Rather than provide the myriad variations of existing reportable event definitions – definitions relating to terms such as "serious", "unexpected", permanent impairment, and etc. – refer to country or region specific standards, regulations or references. For example, ICH guidelines define terms relating to reportable events for pharmaceuticals,

and harmonize these definitions. Other applicable references include the U.S. Code of Federal Regulations, Japan's Pharmaceutical Affairs Law, Europe's Medical Device Directive, Australia's Guidelines for the Registration of Drugs, and many more. The point being, that country-specific nuances between reporting criteria and definitions are so varied, one must refer to the current country specific references relating to the products marketed to obtain definitions.

REGULATORY ENVIRONMENT

Governmental agencies have introduced vigilance and product surveillance requirements that impact the particular region governed, and in many cases, also impact other countries or regions where the same product is marketed.

Key drivers behind the expansion of reporting and surveillance requirements include ensuring products are safe and effective for use. In some cases, the impetus behind revisions or additions to regulatory reporting requirements is linked with a significant safety issue identified by the analysis or receipt of, surveillance or vigilance data by a manufacturer or regulatory agency. Timely, comprehensive analysis of vigilance and surveillance data provides manufacturer and regulators with useful information to continuously improve quality systems and prevent potential safety or product problems, as well as providing a mechanism to validate and monitor the suitability and effectiveness of the quality systems in place.

Furthermore, as information access has become more rapid, governmental bodies and manufacturers' have determined that they can only provide assurance of safety and effectiveness to their public if they fully understand whether products are performing as intended on a world-wide basis, rather than focusing solely on a country or region specific view.

MANUFACTURING AND PRODUCT DEVELOPMENT ENVIRONMENT

This rapid progression towards global awareness on the part of regulatory agencies and manufacturers presents many challenges to companies that do business on a global basis. One of the challenges is accommodating the financial impact of the regulations. In a highly regulated industry like the pharmaceutical and medical device industries, the incremental expenses associated with vigilance reporting are significant. Table 8.1 represents FDA's estimate of the expenses to manufacturers for reporting. Industry believes the figures given are very significantly underestimated.

Table 8.1. U.S. government's estimate of total cost to industry to implement vigilance reporting systems (in $ millions)

Industry segment	One-time expense	Annual expense	Total expenses
User facilities	8.93	19.31	28.24
Manufacturers	0.19	12.22	12.41
U.S. agents for foreign manufacturers	0.0	0.13	0.13
Total costs	9.12	31.56	40.77

Furthermore, to be successful in the marketplace and to maintain compliance with regulations, manufacturer's must:

1. Develop effective quality systems that are global in scope and are aligned with the differing requirements of regulatory agencies.

2. Develop and implement effective systems for collecting global adverse event data for all approved medical devices and pharmaceutical products.

3. Develop and implement effective systems for collecting information on adverse events or alleged failures relating to products undergoing clinical trials or market evaluations prior to regulatory approval.

4. Develop methods for keeping up to date on the rapidly changing regulations globally.

5. Develop a system of vigilance that communicates each reportable adverse event or malfunction (for devices) to appropriate country regulatory bodies within required time frames.

6. Assure that reporting and investigation occurs within the time frames specified by the various countries.

7. Develop methods to report adverse events and reportable malfunctions (medical devices) to countries where a manufacturer markets similar products.[1] This communication should take place time proximate to the date at which a manufacturer determines the event involves their product and there appears to be a relationship between the reported event and the manufacturers product.[2]

As a management review tool, analysis of product surveillance and vigilance data is one source of feedback regarding the effectiveness of related quality systems. For example, root cause analysis of an adverse event or product problem may lead to consideration of labeling changes, supplier or manufacturing process problems, user error, etc.

As a consequence, vigilance and surveillance systems are usually linked with internal processes that capture and document company decisions

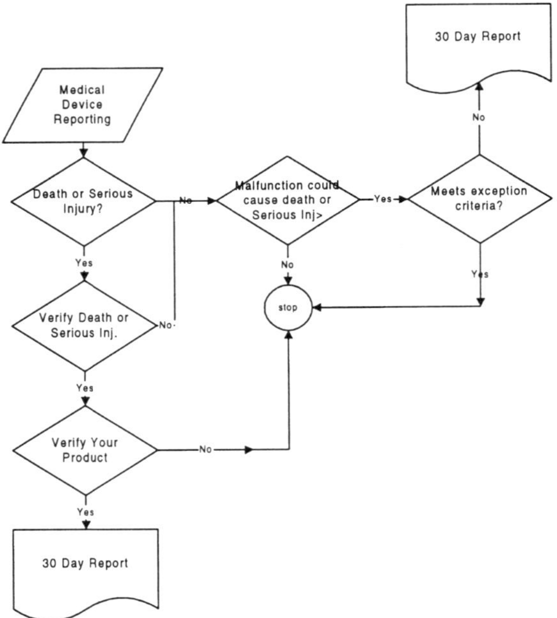

Fig. 8.2. Simplified decision tree for determining reportability and type of report required to comply with FDA regulations.

regarding these data, particularly if associated with any corrective or preventive action (see Figure 8.2). Systematically linking vigilance and surveillance processes with corrective and preventive action processes will ensure quality systems are continuously improved, and suitability verified (some might use the word "validated").[3]

Effectively linking analysis of surveillance and vigilance data with appropriate corrective and preventive action is a critical dimension of quality system requirements and continuous improvement. Figure 8.3 is a diagram of an integrated product surveillance system.

Inter-regional Environment

In the global market place, many regions or countries not only require surveillance and vigilance reporting related to product performance in that region, but also require that a manufacturer report vigilance data that occurs outside the region. The evolution of "inter-regional" reporting requirements has required that manufacturers accommodate these requirements in their quality systems from product inception, to market approval, and throughout the product's life cycle. Requirements vary from country to country and are generally linked with the nature of the medical or medicinal product, for example, the products classification or intended use. Vigilance reporting requirements as well as surveillance requirements are more stringent for implantable devices, or what industry often refers to as critical devices.

The challenges presented by inter-regional surveillance and vigilance requirements are not insignificant: Manufacturers must have processes in place to ensure that surveillance and vigilance information is captured, documented, investigated, and disseminated to the various countries or regions where the same product is marketed. As mentioned previously, requirements for surveillance and vigilance reporting should be considered throughout a product's life cycle and manufacturers should incorporate these requirements into the product development, regulatory, clinical and marketing plans.

Integrated Complaint System

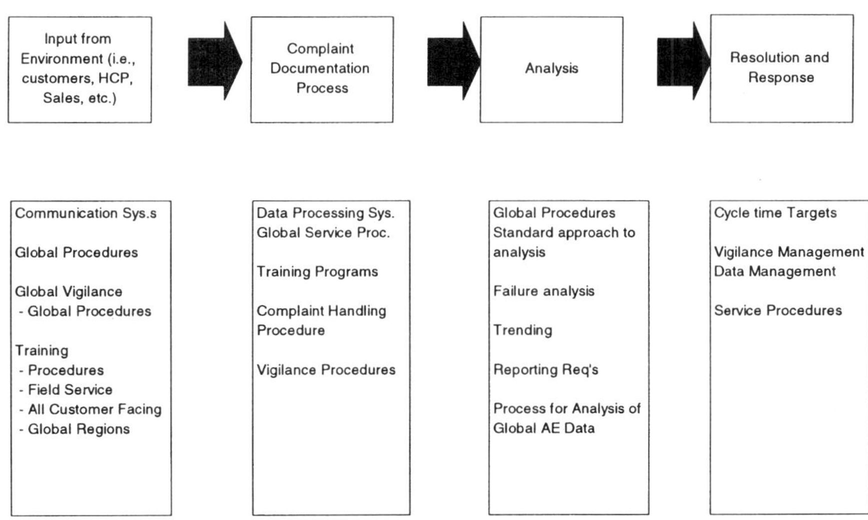

Fig. 8.3. An example of elements comprising an integrated product surveillance system.

                                   Pamela McDonnell and Richard S. Thuma

VIGILANCE REPORTING

Vigilance reporting for medical devices is now required in Japan, Europe and the United States. It is anticipated that vigilance reporting will be required in Canada sometime during the summer in 1998. As industry expands in the global marketplace, particularly in third-world countries, or those regions where reporting requirements are not well defined as yet, manufacturer's need vigilance quality systems that are flexible and effective in order to keep pace with the evolving regulatory requirements. See Table 8.2 for a summary of regional requirements.

Historically, companies in the pharmaceutical industry have had to comply with vigilance requirements for a longer period of time than those operating in the Medical Device markets. Pharmaceutical companies have also had more experience accommodating requirements for accumulation and reporting of global safety data. Global compilation and analysis of device vigilance and safety data is a more recent regulatory-requirement and has caused many manufacturers to scramble in their attempts to come into compliance. Those companies that have used the Pharmaceutical Industry as a model, have had an easier time.

Table 8.2. Vigilance reporting requirements by geographic region

Region	Regulation	Governing agency	Type of products	Scope	Requirements
United States	Food, Drug & Cosmetic Act	Food & Drug Administration (FDA)	Pharmaceuticals and medical devices	Pharmaceuticals and devices manufactured in the U.S. or imported to the U.S., as well as pharmaceuticals manufactured and distributed outside the U.S., but similar in formulation to pharmaceuticals with a U.S. NDA	Surveillance requirements as requested by FDA; vigilance reporting for medical devices and adverse event reporting for pharmaceuticals
	Safe Medical Device Act of 1990				
	Safe Medical Device Act as amended, 1992				
	Proposed 'Sentinel' system				FDA proposes to use a selection of the healthcare community to report directly to monitor product safety and manufacturer's compliance with vigilance reporting requirements
Europe	Medical device directive	Competent authorities	Medical devices	Inter-regional	Incidents (deaths, serious injuries), 'near incidences'. Labeling that is mis-leading or inadequate to protect patient safety, significant regulatory actions taken as a result of
		EMEA	Pharmaceuticals	Country-specific, except with regard to PSUR reporting and product registration, or re-registration	Reporting of adverse drug reactions and periodic safety update reports

Table 8.2.(cont)

Region	Regulation	Governing agency	Type of products	Scope	Requirements
Japan	Post-market surveillance (PMS)	Japan Ministry of Health & Welfare (JMHW)	Devices	Country specific, except with regard to significant regulatory actions involving similar products marketed outside Japan	
		Japan Ministry of Health & Welfare (JMHW)	Pharmaceuticals	Inter-regional	Adverse drug reactions as well as periodic safety update reports
Canada		Health & Protection Branch (HPB)	Pharmaceuticals	Country specific	
		Health & Protection Branch (HPB)	Devices	Regulations not yet in effect	
Australia/ New Zealand			Pharmaceuticals		
U.S., Europe Canada, Japan	International Conference on Harmonization (ICH): guidelines		Pharmaceuticals	Inter-regional	The ICH guidelines standardize approaches to pharmaceutical product development, clinical trials and safety reporting

Initiatives to standardize vigilance reporting and analysis are evident in the ICH (International Conference on Harmonization) guidelines that have been developed over the past few years. Efforts to standardize classification of devices and reporting of device problems are underway in the device industry as well. To date, those efforts to standardize have involved only regions where regulatory requirements for vigilance have been in place for some time, e.g. the United States, Canada, Europe, and Japan.

Until a more universal approach to vigilance is defined for all products, it is incumbent on Industry to develop effective means to collect, document, investigate, analyze and disseminate adverse event information world-wide. Simply put, industry needs to stay abreast of what to report, how to report, when to report, and where.

WHAT TO REPORT

One of the more obvious obstacles to success in the vigilance process is the means by which a company stays abreast of regulatory reporting requirements in each country or region where they do business. What is reportable in one country may not be reportable in another.

Until harmonized requirements are more widely deployed, industry must rely on expertise either within the regions where they do business, or through other mechanisms, to establish what types of events must be reported, both within the region where the event originated, as well as to other regions that may require "reciprocal" reporting. Reciprocal reporting reflects those regions that require safety information relating to reportable events that involve similar products marketed in other regions.

                                    Pamela McDonnell and Richard S. Thuma

HOW TO REPORT

Currently, report formats and data elements still vary. ICH guidelines harmonize many of the pharmaceutical reporting requirements, but are still not fully adopted. PSUR format and data elements are an excellent example of the advantages of adopting a harmonized approach to vigilance. In areas where ICH is not yet adopted, or device vigilance is the focus, industry benefits by identifying core reporting data elements and formats from a global perspective to standardize vigilance processes to the extent possible. This is necessary from the standpoint of harmonizing business practice to minimize administrative burdens, and is particularly important when a company elects to adopt an electronic solution for data management.

It is incumbent on industry to understand country specific requirements in order to fully comply with international vigilance requirements. I would again refer you to current country specific laws, regulations, standards or directives for direction on appropriate compliance in this area.

WHEN TO REPORT

In order to determine how quickly vigilance information must be distributed globally, understanding existing reporting time frames is essential. Reporting requirements, in terms of time, vary from country-to-country and between regions (see Tables 8.3, 8.4 and 8.5).

To accommodate the differences, one approach would be for manufacturers to establish quality systems that ensure vigilance information is disseminated to their geographically dispersed organizations within sufficient time to ensure each region- or country-based unit can review and determine reportability prior to reporting deadlines. It is important to establish on a country or region specific basis, the minimum reporting time frames based on existing regulatory requirements. Once established, the company can use that information to set standards for dissemination of potentially reportable events.

For example, in Australia, serious unexpected drug reactions should be communicated within 72 hours to the Therapeutic Goods Administration

Table 8.3. Requirements for expedited local reporting of serious adverse events – selected countries – investigational drugs

Country	Unexpected	Expected	Related	Not related	Time frame
Australia	Y	NY	Y	N	Within 72 hours
Denmark	Y	Y	Y	Y[6]	Immediate
France	Y	Y	Y	N	7 calendar days for death or life threatening; else 15 days
Germany	Y	Y	Y	N	15 calendar days
Italy	Y	Y	Y	N	3 days for serious adverse 6 days for serious expected Every 6 months for all others
Japan	Y	N	Y	N	7 days for death or life threatening; 15 days all other serious ADRs
Spain	Y	N	Y	N	5 working days for fatal or life threatening; 15 days for others
U.K.	Y	N	Y	N	7 calendar days for death and life threaening; full report 15 days for all events
United States	Y	N	Y	N	3 working days for death and life threatening; 10 working days for all other SAEs

Table 8.4. Some country requirements for expedited local reporting of serious adverse events marketed products

Country	Unexpected	Expected	Related	Not related	Time frame
Australia	Y	N	Y	N	Within 72 hour of receipt
Austria	Y	Y	Y	N	Immediate (within 15 calendar days)
Belgium	Y	Y	Voluntary	N	Within 15 days
Denmark	Y	Y	Y	N	15 calendar days
France	Y	Y	Y	N	15 working days
Germany	Y	Y	Y	N	15 calendar days
Italy	Y	Y	Y	N	3 days for serious adverse 6 days for serious expected Every 6 months for all others
Japan	Y	N	Y	N	15 days or 30 days for SAEs attributed to cancer or lack of efficacy
Spain	Y	N	Y	N	15 days
U.K.	Y	Y	Y	N	Within 15 calendar days
United States	Y	N	Y	N	Within 15 working days

Table 8.5. Some country requirements for reporting of foreign adverse events on marketed products

Country	Unexpected	Expected	Related	Not related	Time frame
Australia	Y	N	Y	N	Within 72 hours if significant safety issue or action initiated by another regulatory authority
Austria	Y	N	Y	N	No time limits
Belgium	Y	N	Y	N	Within EU: not to be transmitted Outside EU: 15 calendar days
Denmark	Y	N	Y	N	Within EU: report in PSUR Outside EU: 15 calendar days
France	Y	Y	Y	N	Within EU: none Outside EU: 15 working days
Germany	Y	Y	Y	N	15 calendar days
Italy	Y	N	Y	N	15 days (2 days if company notified more than15 days after incident) for all serious unexpected reactions; every 6 months for all other serious expected reactions
Japan	Y	N	Y	N	15 days for all SAEs 30 days for SAEs attributed to cancer or lack of efficacy
Spain	Y	N	Y	N	Within EU: report in PSUR Outside EU: 15 days
U.K.	Y N(ex EU)	Y(EU)	Y	N	Within EU: within 15 calendar days Outside EU: unexpected SAE within 15 calendar days
United States	Y	N	Y	N	Within 15 working days

(TGA) [2]. In the U.S., serious unexpected drug reactions are reported to FDA [3] within 15 days. A critical element of "when to report" is staying abreast of changes in reporting requirements. Many approaches may be used, but again, it incumbent on industry to establish quality systems that incorporate timely updates to their policies and procedures as requirements change.

WHERE TO REPORT

Because of the continued evolution of reporting requirements, vigilance quality systems must also consider how to stay abreast of NEW reporting requirements in regions where none may currently exist. For example, an adverse drug reaction involving a drug product marketed in the U.S., Europe, Japan and Canada should be disseminated to each of those regions, regardless of which of the four regions received the initial report. Vigilance systems must accommodate the inter-regional reporting requirements that exist today, and be updated routinely for expansion of regulations in other global markets.

However, it is confusing enough for manufacturers to understand what needs to be reported just within one region. Most business units develop simple flow charts to facilitate the decision process. Figure 8.4 represents one such chart.

Efficient communication of vigilance information is one key to compliance with reporting requirements, and has resulted in significant efforts on the part of industry to employ computer-based approaches to that enables global access to adverse event information. The use of computers, the Internet, and other strategies to streamline access to safety information has had a positive impact on the product development and regulatory approval cycle times.

Reduction of time-to-market continues to be a critical success factor in today's competitive environment. The obsession with continued reductions of cycle times will, no doubt, continue to fuel advances in data processing, data management, and information retrieval.

The following is a discussion of regional requirements in Europe that highlights the need to effectively integrate global vigilance information.

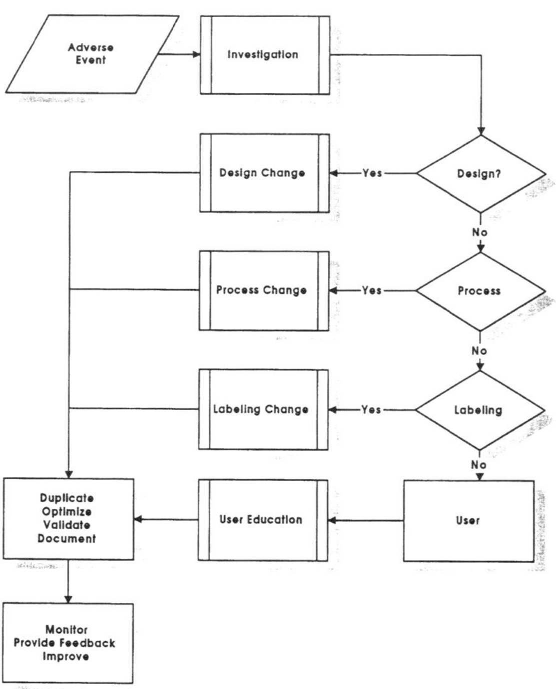

Fig. 8.4. Product change driven by root cause analysis of adverse event information

PHARMACEUTICALS

Pharmaceutical products in Europe are governed by the European Agency for the Evaluation of Medicinal Products (EMEA).

Currently, each country in Europe has specific requirements for market approval (registration) and periodic updates regarding the safety and efficacy of the particular pharmaceutical product a manufacturer has on the market. These requirements vary slightly from country to country, and reporting time periods are based on the products initial approval date to market. ICH guidelines have not yet been promulgated legally within the European Union, although some manufacturers have adopted the ICH recommendations regarding PSUR data elements.

Within the European Union, PSUR reports are expected to reflect global safety information for the drug formulation. This includes safety information from clinical studies, as well as spontaneous reports of adverse events received post-product approval.

In Europe, spontaneous reports of serious unexpected adverse drug reactions (post market authorization) are reported within proscribed time frames within the country where the event occurred, as well as in the country where the product was manufactured.

Europe is also governed by the Committee for Proprietary Medicinal Products (CPMP). This agency functions in the following capacities:

- Coordination of the evaluations of medicinal products subject to market authorization procedures;

- Transmission of various assessment reports and labeling for those medicinal products;

- Coordination of a pharmaco-vigilance system;

- Coordination of the verification of manufacturers compliance with GMP, GLP and GCP's;

- Recording the status of marketing authorizations;

- Assisting in the maintenance of a public data base on medicinal products;

- Assisting the community of Member States in providing information to healthcare professionals and general public about medicinal products; and,

- Providing advice on the conduct of tests and clinical trials needed to register the medicinal products.

The CPMP also prepares opinions for the EMEA on any questions about the evaluation of medicinal products and may set up working parties or expert groups to aid in their mission [4–6].

MEDICAL DEVICES

The Medical Device Directive introduced device vigilance reporting requirements that require a manufacturer to report deaths, serious injuries (incidents) and "near incidents" (product malfunctions that could lead to deaths or serious injuries) to the competent authority within the country where the event occurred. These reports must be made within 30 days of a manufacturers knowledge that a reportable event has occurred. In addition, incidents are generally also communicated to the notified body that originally approved the product for market throughout the EU (CE marking).

The Medical Device Directive (MDD) also requires manufacturers to report situations where product labeling is either misleading or inadequate to protect patient safety. Significant regulatory

actions taken as a result of vigilance activities are also reportable, even if the event occurs outside the EU.

Generally speaking, any vigilance report that occurs on a product approved for sale within the EU, regardless of whether the event occurred outside the EU, should be reviewed to determine if the reported event meets vigilance reporting requirements in the EU. This review should be conducted in sufficient time to allow the manufacturers European authorized representative to meet reporting time frames established by the MDD.

SUMMARY

In conclusion, the growth of global vigilance reporting has had a largely positive impact on the quality of goods and services supplied on a global basis and on the process of developing and bringing new medical products to market.

The efforts expended by manufacturers in developing quality and regulatory reporting systems to comply with global vigilance requirements have been prodigious. However, effective use of such surveillance and reporting systems and the data they provide can drive continuous improvement in product development, clinical trials, and product related services. Standardizing approaches to vigilance reporting and providing real-time access to the data can offer assistance in cycle-time reduction.

On the other hand, it is imperative that Industry work hard with governments and regulating bodies to harmonize the reporting and data collection requirements. Without harmonization, the aspect of having to comply with so many differing, not to mention changing, requirements is daunting, indeed.

NOTES

[1] Once a manufacturer establishes that a reportable event has occurred, whether adverse event or reportable malfunction (medical devices) the information should be communicated immediately to allow other countries that have reporting requirements to meet prescribed time frames.

[2] Some regulations require reports even though a clear causal relationship has not been established. Reference country or region specific regulatory reporting requirements to ascertain compliance obligations.

[3] The sentence reflects current regulatory environment where it is expected that industry will initiate appropriate corrective and preventive action and will ensure the effectiveness of that action – hence the term "verify" or "validate".

REFERENCES

1. O'Leary D. Quality assessment: moving from theory to practice. J Am Med Assoc 1988; 260:1760.

2. Australian guidelines for registration of drugs, vol. 1, July 1994.

3. Code of federal regulations. 21CFR314.80.

4. Anon. A brief guide to the EC rules governing medicines, 5th edition. European Federation of Pharmaceutical Industries' Association, April 1994.

5. Sauer F. A new and fast drug approval system in Europe. Drug Inf J 1997; 31:1–6.

6. Jones K. Wider perspectives of European medicines control. Drug Inf J 1996; 30:1–7.

7. Federal register. 1960; 50(237):53577–606.

9. Regulatory environment and government impact on the quality of dialysis products

STEVEN HOFF AND RICHARD NEWMAN

ABBREVIATIONS

510(k), a premarket notification to the FDA for a medical device; CBER, Center for Biologics Evaluation and Research; CDER, Center for Drug Evaluation and Research; CDRH, Center for Devices and Radiological Health; CFR, Code of Federal Regulations; CPMP, Committee for Proprietary Medicinal Products; EEA, European Economic Area; EEC, European Economic Community; EMEA, European Agency for the Evaluation of Medicinal Products; FDA, Food and Drug Administration; GCP, good clinical practices; GLP, good laboratory practices; GMP, good manufacturing practices; ICH, International Conference on Harmonization of Technical Requirements for Registration of Pharmaceuticals for Human Use; IND, investigational new drug application; MDD, medical device directive; MRA, mutual recognition agreement; NDA, new drug application; PMA, premarket approval application (class III medical devices in the U.S.)

INTRODUCTION

Governmental efforts to regulate renal dialysis product manufacturers focuses on three general areas: product registration, regulatory inspections and postapproval surveillance. Product registration is commonly associated with regulatory submissions to the various governmental agencies, where the quality of product design, performance, clinical studies and other information are used to establish the safety and effectiveness of those products. Regulatory inspections help drive the quality of processes within the industry and the overall quality systems and implementation of the good manufacturing practices (GMPs). Postapproval surveillance provides the long-term quality impact on the industry by requiring industry to understand the performance and reliability of their products in the end-user's hands.

During the 1990s there have been some major changes in the way the drug and device industries are regulated. For the renal dialysis manufacturers, these changes have had a significant impact on how dialysis-related products are developed, manufactured and marketed. In some cases the rules have become more restrictive, while others have become more flexible. Local regulations have seen remarkable changes as the global community has sought to harmonize the process of drug and device development and registration. This has led to the issuance of many new guidance documents and concensus standards through which the dialysis product developers can more clearly understand the current requirements and processes for new product development and registration. While the industry will go through a distinct and perhaps difficult period of reassessing the product development process as the new regulatory initiatives are implemented, it will become apparent that what were thought to be very difficult hurdles for global product development ten years ago will become achievable realities for the dialysis product manufacturers.

In the past there were many roadblocks to the rapid development of quality products for renal dialysis, with the need to comply with each nation's regulatory requirements. Duplication of effort and attemped leveraging of various data-

L.W. Henderson and R.S. Thuma (eds.), Quality Assurance in Dialysis, 2nd Edition, 93–104.
© 1999 *Kluwer Academic Publishers. Printed in Great Britain*

bases for multnational product registrations were often fraught with delay, excessive expenditures and frustration. With the regulatory requirements and registration review backlogs of the past, many of the industry's relationships with government agencies could be described as tenuous, even adversarial.

This chapter will present some of the recent changes in the regulatory areas which significantly impact the manufacturers of renal dialysis products, with a focus on product registrations and government inspections. The third area which impact product quality, postapproval surveillance, is addressed in the chapter "Global vigilance as a government-mediated method for monitoring quality of dialysis products".

REGULATORY ENVIRONMENT

International harmonization of regulatory requirements is having an enormous impact on the quality of new product development, manufacturing and registration. This is best demonstrated by two movements: The CE Mark for medical devices throughout Europe, and the International Conference on Harmonization of Technical Requirements for Registration of Pharmaceuticals for Human Use (ICH) between Europe, Japan and the United States. In addition, the appearance of Mutual Recognition Agreements (MRA) between various nations will extend the harmonization process into other areas affecting the quality of dialysis products.

DEVICES

In the past, medical devices, such as hemodialysis machines and dialyzers, were registered in individual countries, each having a set of specific registration requirements. Some relief in this process has occurred with the advent of the CE Mark, which harmonized the registration of medical devices in the European Economic Area (EEA).

The concept of the CE Mark was brought into existence in June 1993, when the Council of European Communities issued the Medical Device Directive (MDD), which has been transposed into national laws throughout the European Economic

Area, comprising 18 countries (Table 9.1) [1, 2]. The purpose of the EEA's adoption of the MDD is to allow the healthcare industry to benefit from the advantages of a single European market, which allows their CE marked products to circulate freely in the EEA, without additional technical constraints issued by the various Member States. The MDD harmonizes these European requirements along with device certification and the inspection procedures for manufacturers to ensure the highest degree of safety and product quality of the medical devices throughout the EEA.

Table 9.1. European economic area nations

Austria	Greece	The Netherlands
Belgium	Iceland	Norway
Denmark	Ireland	Portugal
Finland	Italy	Spain
France	Liechtenstein	Sweden
Germany	Luxembourg	U.K.

The MDD came into full effect on June 13, 1998. At that time all medical devices in Europe (EEA) must bear the CE Mark, which signifies conformity to the essential requirements of the MDD [2]. These essential requirements for new products cover a number of areas, for example, product design, materials, testing, manufacturing, software and labeling.

The guarantee of conformity to the Essential Requirements of the MDD is provided by the interaction between the manufacturer and a third party, the Notified Body. The Notified Bodies are organizations which are recognized by the Member States to conduct device evaluations and inspections of the quality systems of the various manufacturers.

The manufacturer is held responsible for the quality, safety and effectiveness of their medical devices, which is enforced through the manufacturer's written declaration of conformity and commitment to keep all technical information available for inspection by the Notified Bodies and national authorities.

With the issuance of the Medical Device Directives, the European Commission mandated that European technical standards be harmonized according to the essential requirements of the MDD. As a result, many new technical standards have been issued, which have been applied across the medical device industry in Europe and in other global regions. Of major impact was the requirement for a full quality assurance system (Annex II of the MDD, 93/42/EEC), which included design controls for new medical device products. The International Organization for Standardization established the specific requirements for Quality Systems, through the issuance of the ISO 9000 series of standards.

The European harmonization of the medical device regulations has influenced revisions of regulatory requirements in other countries, including Canada and the United States. Canada changed their device regulations to include a risk-based classification system and eleven principles of safety and effectiveness, which was patterned after the Essential Requirements of the European Medical Device Directive. These regulations became effective in July, 1998. Canada is also pursuing a Mutual Recognition Agreement with the European Union for medical device registrations [3].

In the United States, new legislation affecting the medical device industry was passed as the Safe Medical Devices Act (SMDA) of 1990 and the Medical Device Amendment of 1992. Along with the new regulations and programs that were implemented by FDA at the Center for Devices and Radiological Health (CDRH), the medical device industry understood that they were expected to submit higher quality submissions. This led to a significant backlog of submission reviews, which, in turn, led to several years of frustration between FDA and industry. However, in 1994, Congress provided for an increase in staffing, and along with several management initiatives, CDRH has brought the submission backlog to essentially zero, with the average review time dropping from 184 days (1994) to about 98 days (1997) [4].

With the Medical Device Amendments, extensive revisions of the Good Manufacturing Practices (GMP) regulations became effective in June 1997 under the Code of Federal Regulations (21CFR 820), Quality System Regulation. This was FDA's first GMP revision since 1978, and included changes to ensure that the new regulation was compatible with ISO 9000. The earlier GMPs had not covered design control, and the SMDA of

1990 authorized the FDA to bring preproduction design control and validation under its purview. Human factors are an important part of quality assurance programs and are used to help decrease the likelihood of user errors, especially in light of the increase use of medical devices by lay people. If these defects could be identified early in the development process, then large savings in resource and monetary expenditures could be expected [5, 6]. As written, the design control section of the regulation (21CFR 820.30) describes requirements which are both broad and flexible. They do not tell a manufacturer how to design a product, but how to document the design phase (Table 9.2) [7]. Thus the new regulations open the door to FDA inspection of the product development process, and manufacturers need to have procedures in place to document this process.

Several publications describe these design control requirements and how to go about implementing this process [5–11]. The expected benefits of the new harmonized GMPs are to provide a more global medical device quality standard, which will make global marketing more readily possible. They also ensure better documentation and procedures for designing, purchasing and servicing of medical devices. The new design controls require a lot of effort to implement, but will be a benefit to engineering by potentially decreasing development times and indentification of design errors earlier, where they are more inexpensive and easier to correct [12].

Currently, in the face of budget cuts from Congress, CDRH is moving more toward a risk-based approach to their work, with selective focusing of effort on high-risk, high-impact products. They propose to shift the reviewer efforts from the lower-risk 510(k)s to PMA applications, pre-1976 devices, device reclassification, and technically complex 510(k) submissions. "Low risk" 510(k)s could be sent to third party reviewers or exempted from review altogether [13]. As part of the effort, FDA has exempted 573 generic type devices since 1976, and is currently evaluating the remaining Class I devices for exemption. Reclassification is also being considered for many Class II and III devices. After FDA's review of the medical device classifications, all Class III medical devices will require the submission of a PMA for product registration, which in general is a much more

Table 9.2. Design control requirements (21CFR 820.30)

Item	Manufacturers are to establish and maintain the following
Design development planning	Plans that describe and reference the design and development activities and define responsibility for implementation
Design input	Procedures to ensure that the design requirements relating to a device are appropriate and address the intended use of the device.
Design output	Procedures for defining and documenting design output that allows adequate evaluation to conformance to design input requirements.
Design review	Procedures to ensure that formal documented reviews of the design results occur at appropriate stages.
Design verification	Procedures for verifying the device design, and confirm that design output meets the design input requirements.
Design validation	Procedures for validating the device design to ensure that devices conform to defined user needs and intended uses.
Design transfer	Procedures to ensure that the device is correctly translated into production specifications
Design changes	Procedures for identification, documentation, validation, verification (if needed), review and approval of design changes before their implementation
Design history file	A design history file for each type of device

demanding exercise, containing significant manufacturing and clinical information. In March, 1998, CDRH issued a new guidance document, "A New 510(k) Paradigm", which presents optional approaches to the registration of new medical devices, in order to conserve their reviewer resources [14]. Under the "New 510(k) Paradigm", Class II devices could be reviewed by FDA using the traditional method under section 510(k) of the Food, Drug and Cosmetic Act. However, two alternatives would also be allowed. First, the "Special 510(k): Device Modification" would use some criteria from the Quality System regulations and have a 30 day review period. The second alternative, the "Abbreviated 510(k)", would use special controls and consensus standards for 510(k) review. These alternatives can provide some relief to device manufacturers, but again, some up front effort may be required in order to put in place the necessary "special controls and consensus standards".

Other proposals include a revision of the Medical Device Reporting (MDR) management and reduction in the number of routine inspections, with a new focus on compliance and enforcement inspections [13].

In June, 1997, after five years of negotiations, the FDA and EU concluded their work on a Mutual Recognition Agreement (MRA) regarding inspections and product assessments for drugs and medical devices, where the FDA would recognize EU third parties or Conformance Assessment Bodies (CABs), which would conduct quality system audits and premarket reviews to FDA standards [15–18]. Also, the EU would accept FDA inspections and premarket reviews that used EU standards. The EU Member State authorities and FDA would maintain their authority to ensure the health and safety of their respective populations. A three year transition period will be used, where joint confidence building programs between FDA, EU authorities and CABs will be conducted to educate all parties on clearance procedures for medical devices and inspection standards for drugs and devices. The FDA and EU will conduct an equivalence assessment at the end of the transition period and determine what next steps should be taken under the MRA.

This was a very difficult MRA to negotiate. However, through the combined efforts of the government authorities in the U.S. and EU and strong support from industry groups, the aggreement was finalized [17, 18]. During the implementation of the MRA, FDA expects to be able to move inspectors from European assignments to other regions and to increase inspection coverage in the area of bulk pharmaceuticals. While this "framework agreement" is limited in scope, it does represent an important step toward harmonization of regulatory activities related to the drug and device industry [19].

DRUGS

The working environment of the global pharmaceutical industry has undergone some revolutionary changes during this decade, with the formation of the European Union, the "reinvention" of U.S. government and the FDA, and perhaps most importantly, the work of the International Conference on Harmonization of Technical Requirements for Registration of Pharmaceuticals for Human Use (ICH).

Europe

The activation of the Maastrict Treaty in November of 1993 transformed the European Community into the European Union. In the same year a new pharmaceutical registration system was opened, with the European Agency for the Evaluation of Medicinal Products (EMEA) as its authority in London. The essential function of the EMEA is to provide the best scientific advice about the evaluation of the quality, safety and efficacy of medicinal products. Through the Committee for Proprietary Medicinal Products (CPMP), the EMEA coordinates the evaluations of medicinal products subject to the market authorization procedures; transmits various assessment reports and labeling for these medicinal products; coordinates a pharmacovigilance system; coordinates the verification of compliance with GMP, GLP and GCPs; records the status of marketing authorizations; assists in the maintenence of a public database on medicinal products; assists the community and Member States in providing information to healthcare professionals and general public about medicinal products, and provide advice on the conduct of tests and clinical trials needed to register the medicinal products. The CPMP also prepares opinions for the EMEA on any questions about the evaluation of medicinal products and may set up working parties or expert groups to aid in their mission [20–22]. The EMEA also supervises the drugs through the use of guidelines on GMP, GLP and GCPs.

The primary objective of the new drug registration system was to ensure the highest degree of public safety and to promote the free movement of pharmaceuticals within the European Union, without national boundries. The new marketing authorization applications (MAA) are assessed in the areas of quality, safety and efficacy, under a single requirements pathway for European drug approval. The European Union harmonization process used to bring the registration system into being became effective on January 1st, 1995. The full set of rules governing medicinal products in Europe is provided in a series of Directives promulgated since 1965 [20].

United States

Within the United States, there is a movement to make government work better. For the FDA, this means reducing unnecessary regulatory burdens, but at the same time it is expected that the protection of the public health will be maintained at the expected high standards. The reinvention of drug and medical device regulations should mean a faster review process for new products and decrease the regulatory requirements for industry [23, 24]. For example, some of the proposed changes for the pharmaceutical industry include:

- Some additional manufacturing changes which can be made without FDA preapproval, that do not affect drug product quality or performance.

- Eliminate requirements for environmental assessments. FDA has proposed an increase in the number of categorical exclusions.

- Expanding export opportunities for unapproved drugs to 21 developed countries, even without an open IND in the U.S.

- Allow the use of electronic records and signatures in place of paper [25]. This could simplify record-keeping and reduce the time required to file an application or other regulatory documents.

- FDA has issued public statements in several forums, which clarifies how FDA determines the effectiveness of new drugs. In some appropriate cases a single, large, well-designed, multicenter study may be sufficient to support the approval of a drug. For this approval to be successful, the study results must be strong. A statistically marginal result would not be convincing.

- Expanding and standardizing computer technology used by the FDA in the review of new products, which should help industry identify compatible software and document management systems.

- Harmonize international standards for the review of drugs.

Changes like these can decrease the product development times and the total time to market for drug products, by reducing the total requirements and duplicative efforts.

In November, 1995, the FDA's Center for Drug Evalulation and Research (CDER) announced reorganization plans to improve its overall effectiveness and divided its drug development oversight and application review efforts between two offices: the Office of Review Management (ORM) and the Office of Pharmaceutical Science (OPS). Several other functions were also reorganized. The ORM is responsible for all new drug development oversight and market application review efforts except chemistry and human biopharmaceutics and for postapproval monitoring of marketed drugs. Within ORM, the Office of Drug Evaluation has increased its number of reviewing divisions from 10 to 14. This has effectively reduced the number of applications per division, increased the focus on a smaller number of drug groups per division, and decreased the "funnel-effect" of the final sign-off process for various applications [26].

The Office of Pharmaceutical Science (OPS) is responsible for chemistry and human biopharmaceutical related topics in the NDA review process. The OPS also reviews generic drug applications and conducts testing and research activities related to the drug review process. Within OPS, CDER created the Office of New Drug Chemistry, which combines the chemistry and manufacturing review process. With these efforts and the impact of the Prescription Drug User Fee Act of 1992 (PDUFA), CDER has been able to very noticeably improve the review process (Tables 9.3 and 9.4).

Backlogs have been greatly reduced; applications are reviewed within expected timeframes,

Table 9.3. Improved CDER review process

New drug applications	Approvals	Median total time to approval (months)
1993	70	21.4
1994	62	19.0
1995	82	16.5
1996	131	15.4
Efficacy supplement approvals		
1993	48	19.0
1994	50	12.0
1995	69	16.0
1996	118	13.9
Manufacturing supplement approvals		
1993	848	8.2
1994	1065	7.7
1995	1024	5.9
1996	1422	5.4

Table 9.4. FDA review backlog (number of overdue applications)

	New NDA	Efficacy supplements	Manufacturing supplements
1993	39	56	575
1994	35	55	202
1995	11	34	65
1996	2	2	10

and the FDA review culture has changed to reflect a new timeliness and thouroughness. With the implementation of the PDUFA requirements, the FDA feels that they now provide a predictable and accountable review process.

CDER has also made a commitment to improved communications within FDA and with the pharmaceutical industry. This led to the formation of the Office of Training and Communication (OTCOM). Some of the communication initiatives with industry include:

- CDER Internet site

- Video-conferencing capabilities

- Fax-on-Demand service for immediate access to publications, guidance documents and other information

- Public workshops, such as Marketing on the Internet, Clinical Safety Data and Project Management Training

- Industry training on Scale-Up and Post-Approval Changes (SUPAC)

- Increased formal interaction with trade and health professional organizations

- Increased CDER staff participation at public meetings.

FDA has been working with the European Community, Japan, and the North American Free Trade Agreement (NAFTA) partners to harmonize drug testing and development standards [19]. This type of effort can increase the safety and quality of imports into the United States and can help new products gain more rapid entry into various global markets. A cost savings to industry should be realized with having only a single standard to meet versus a national standard for each country. For the FDA, they maybe able to be more efficient in the use of its resources, by sharing the work load and increased cooperation with other countries.

One example of the cooperative efforts with other global regions is the Mutual Recognition Agreement (MRA), which was discussed above, as it applies to medical devices [15, 19]. With regard to drugs, the MRA would allow the exchange of inspection reports on pharmaceutical production facilities. In this case, the FDA and European Union regulatory agencies would see to it that domestic facilities would be inspected and ensure that they are in GMP compliance with the regulations of the country to which they export. The MRA covers pharmaceutical inspections of production facilities for prescription and nonprescription (OTC) drugs and biologics, intermediate products, bulk pharmaceuticals and certain veterinary products. When an inspection is requested, the appropriate regulatory agency will have 45 days (preapproval) or 60 days (postapproval) to conduct the inspection and issue the report. As with the medical device provisions of the MRA, this cooperative agreement will greatly reduce the number of foreign inspections that need to be conducted by the FDA and the various EU agencies, thereby gaining a large cost savings and better utilization of limited resources. Under this MRA,

a three year transition period will also be used with regard to pharmaceutical inspections, which will be used by all parties to gain confidence in the equivalence of each other's inspection capabilities.

The U.S. Congress enacted the Food and Drug Adminstration Modernization and Accountibility Act (FDAMA) on November 9, 1997 [27]. Some provisions of this legislation which may impact the renal dialysis product industry include:

- Mutual Recognition Agreements and Global Harmonization are restated as continuing goals between the U.S. and Europe.

- Contracts for Expert Review of part or all of medical device applications will be legislated.

- Device Performance Standards will allow manufacturers to submit a declaration of conformity to a recognized standard. The supporting data will not be submitted with this type of abbreviated 510(k) premarket notification, thus allowing a quicker review time.

- Improving collaboration and communication on PMAs through more timely meetings with FDA to review clinical trial requirements or application review status.

- Certainty of review timesframes will be established for 510(k)s at 90 days and 180 days for PMAs. All review and determinations must be made within these timeframes, and restarting or extending the review clock will not be allowed.

- The number of required clinical trials may allow for one adequate and well-controlled trial to establish effectiveness, under appropriate situations.

- Exemption of certain devices from premarket notification requirements. All Class I and an FDA issued list of Class II devices will be exempt. Manufacturers may also petition the FDA for exemption of these requirements.

- Drug and Biologics Data Requirements may be reduced, as FDA will issue guidance on abbreviated study reports for NDAs.

- PDUFA was reauthorized for an additional five years.

- Commitment to File Supplemental Application: Incentives for Research: This would allow manufactures to disseminate information about an off-label use for their drug, biologic or device, if they have submitted a certification that the studies needed to support a supplemental application will be filed within a prescribed period of time after the initial dissemination of the information.

Some of these topics have appeared in this discussion as FDA initiatives, and the purpose of this legislation was to give some formality to them.

Internationally, probably the greatest factor to change the regulatory environment as it impacts the renal dialysis product industry was the International Conference on Harmonisation of Technical Requirements for Registration of Pharmaceuticals for Human Use (ICH), which was formed in 1989/1990 between the European Union, Japan and the United States [28]. This unique project brought together the regulatory authorities and experts from the pharmaceutical industries of the three regions. The overall purpose was to find ways to harmonise technical guidelines and requirements for drug product registrations, with the objective of a more economical use of human, animal and material resources and the elimination of unnecessary delay in the global development and registration of new drugs, while keeping an appropriate level of quality, safety and efficacy of these products. The conference was cosponsored by six groups:

- European Commission (EU)

- European Federation of Pharmaceutical Industry Associations (EFPIA)

- Japanese Ministry of Health and Welfare (JMHW)

- Japan Pharmaceutical Manufacturers Association (JPMA)

- United States Food and Drug Adminstration (FDA)

- Pharmaceutical Research and Manufacturers of America (PhRMA)

In addition, representatives of the International Federation of Pharmaceutical Manufacturers Associations (IFPMA), the World Health Organization (WHO), the European Free Trade Association (EFTA) and the Canada Health Protection Branch were also present.

Harmonization topics were selected by the ICH Steering Committee, on the advice of Expert Working Groups (EWG) and on the basis of a Concept Paper, which identified the primary objectives of the process [29]. These topics were sent through a five step process, which briefly included:

1. **Expert working groups** held discussions and drafted documents (guidelines, recommendations, policy statements, points to consider), which were sent to the Steering Committee.

2. **The consensus draft** was then forwarded by the six cosponsors in the Steering Committee to the regulatory agencies in the three regions. These agencies then had a formal consultation process over a six month period to develop comments on the consensus draft.

3. **Formal consultation outside the ICH** produced comments, which were collected and exchanged between the regulatory bodies, and a designated Regulatory Rapporteur amended the draft document. The revised draft was referred to the ICH EWGs for sign-off.

4. **The final draft** was discussed by the Steering Committee and signed-off by the three regulatory participants in the ICH. The document was recommended then for adoption to the three regional regulatory agencies.

5. **Implementation** was the final step in the harmonization process and included the incorporation of the various recommendations or documents into the domestic regulations.

During this harmonization process, the ICH held four conferences to discuss the work of the various Expert Working Groups. The final conference was held in July, 1997 in Brussels, with 1,600 delegates attending the meeting. Also, attendance by regulatory authorities and industry based outside the three regions was very prominent, and this demonsrated the importance and influence of

Table 9.5. ICH guidelines: quality and efficacy

Quality guidelines

Stability

Q1A	Stability testing of new drug substances and products
Q1B	Photostability testing of new drug substances and products
Q1C	Stability testing requirements for new dosage forms

Analytical validation

Q2A	Validation of analytical procedures: definitions and terminology
Q2B	Validation of analytical procedures: methodology

Impurities

Q3A	Impurities in new drug substances
Q3B	Impurities in new drug products
Q3C	Impurities: residual solvents (draft)

Specifications

Q6A	Specifications for new drug substances and products (draft)
Q6B	Specifications for biotechological products (draft)

Biologic-biotechnology products

Q5A	Viral safety evaluation
Q5B	Genetic stability
Q5C	Stability of biotech products
Q5D	Derivation and characterization of cell substrates (draft)

Efficacy guidelines

E1	Extent of population exposure to assess clincal safety
E3	Structure and conduct of clinical study reports
E4	Dose response information to support drug registration
E5	Ethnic factors in acceptability of foreign clinical data (draft)
E7	Studies in support of special populations: geriatrics
E8	General considerations for clinical trials (draft)
E9	Statistical principals for clinical trials (draft)
E10	Choice of control group in clincal trials (draft)

Clinical safety data management

E2A	Definitions and standards for expedited reporting
E2B	Data elements for transmission of individual case safety reports (draft)
E2C	Periodic safety update reports

Good clinical practices (GCP)

E6	Consolidated guideline
E6A	Addendum on investigator's brochure
E6B	Essential documents

Safety guidelines

Carcinogenicity

S1A	Carcinogenicity: need for carcinogenicity studies
S1B	Carcinogenicity: use of two rodent species (draft)
S1C	Dose selection for carcinogenicity studies of pharmaceuticals

Table 9.5. (cont.)

Genotoxicity

S2A	Genotoxicity: specific aspects of regulatory genotoxicity tests
S2B	Genotoxicity: a standard battery for genotoxicity testing (draft)

Toxokinetics and pharmacokinetics

S3A	Toxicokinetics: assessment of systemic exposure in toxicity studies
S3B	Pharmacokinetics: repeated dose tissue distribution studies

Toxicity testing

S4	Single dose and repeat dose toxicity tests
S4A	Repeat dose toxicity tests in non-rodents (draft)

Reproductive toxicology

S5A	Detection of toxicity to reproduction for medicinal purposes
S5B	Reproductive toxicity: toxicity to male fertility

Biotechnology products

S6	Safety studies for biotechnological products (draft)

Regulatory guidelines

M1	Medical terminology – MEDDRA Version 2.0
M2	Electronic standards for the transfer of regulatory information and data (ongoing)
M3	Timing of preclinical studies in relation to clinical trials (draft)

the ICH process in the global pharmaceutical industry [28]. The first phase of the ICH process has produced an impressive list of tripartite harmonized guidelines (Table 9.5). Many of these have been implemented in the three regions.

Because of the worldwide interest in the ICH process, the Steering Committee agreed to a broader base for the next stage of harmonization, and they have produced a discussion paper on a Common Technical Document [28, 30]. With the development of common guidelines for technical data, the next logical step would be the harmonization of the format and content of the Medicines Approval Application (MAA) in all three regions. In July, 1995, the Pharmaceutical Research and Manufacturers of America (PhRMA) suggested the Common Technical Document as an ICH topic, and the Steering Committee requested a comprehensive comparison of the registration requirements in the three regions. The regional pharmaceutical manufacturer's associations produced a final report for the Steering Committee in July, 1997. The expected benefits from the development of the Common Technical Document include:

- More logical order of submitting documents in the MAA

- Reassessing exactly what information is vital to an MAA

- Minimizing the review time by regulatory agencies

- Minimizing the need for extra resources to produce assessment summaries

- Facilitating exchange of regulatory information; encourage joint regulatory reviews and mutual discussions of MAA assessments in the three regions

- Facilitate the exchange of documents, tables and summaries for those companies that work globally.

- Improve procedures by which questions and deficiency letters can be addressed by experts in different regions.

- Agreement on a defined terminology

- Make electronic submissions easier to prepare

- Assure implementation of ICH agreements

It was decided that Expert Working Groups on Quality, Safety and Efficacy would be created to continue working on the Common Technical Document, with the expectation that a final consensus would be achieved early in the year 2000. The development of the Common Technical Document is going to be a lengthy and perhaps difficult process [28, 30, 31].

IMPACT ON THE REGULATORY ENVIRONMENT

The 1990s have witnessed an unprecedented movement in the gobal regulatory environment toward harmonization of the regulatory requirements for pharmaceuticals and medical devices. This has had special impact in the European Union, Japan and the United States, and it is clear that additional countries are taking a keen interest and are expected to join in the evolution of the regulatory environment as we open the next century. These international regulatory efforts have brought forth a revised set of GMPs, which now include product design controls. This is expected to enhance the quality of medical devices. Also, the implementation of the ICH guidelines will aid the pharmaceutical industry to develop new drugs under essentially one set of rules, thereby decreasing the confusion and difficulties of bringing new products into the various global regions. And with the use of MRAs between various countries, the renal dialysis product manufacturers can expect a more useful inspection process by regulatory agencies. All of these changes in the regulatory environment will significantly impact the quality of new renal dialysis products introduced into the clinical setting in the years to come.

The ability to achieve harmonization of the regulatory environment will be greatly impacted by the growth of available communication technologies, especially the creative utilization of the World Wide Web (Web) for Internet and corporate Intranet activities. Already, the access to information on the Web is remarkable (Table 9.6), with new websites appearing continuously.

The increased use of electronic document management and electronic regulatory submissions will also impact the product registration process, as the need for paper documents declines. Much work is still needed in this area, with consensus agreements on hardware and software requirements and the harmonization of the standard information format and content in the Common Technical Document.

As with any major change, these new opportunities to improve the regulatory environment bring waves of anxiety, confusion and discomfort, as companies and regulatory agencies need to alter their accepted ways of doing business and adopt the new regulatory intiatives. New industry initiatives will be required, involving global communication paradigms, global regulatory and product development strategies, and perhaps, outsourcing of highly specialized product development functions [32]. This will require a high dose of extra effort and expenditures of monies and resources. However, the expected outcomes and benefits

Table 9.6. Regulatory related websites

		http://www
Regulatory sites		
EMEA	European Agency for the Evaluation of Medicinal Products	eudra.org/emea.html
FDA	Food and Drug Administration	fda.gov
FDLI	Food and Drug Law Institute	fdli.org
HCFA	Health Care Financing Administration	hcfa.gov
HIMA	Health Industry Manufacturers Association	himanet.com
ISO On-Line	International Organization for Standardization	iso.ch/welcome.html
IEC	International Electrotechnical Commission	iec.ch/
ICH	International Conference on Harmonization of Technical Requirements for Registration of Pharmaceuticals for Human Use	ifpma.org/ich1.html
RA info	Regulatory Affairs Information	medmarket.com/tenants/rainfo/rainfo.htm
RAPS	Regulatory Affairs Professional Society	raps.org>
Pharmaceutical		
APPS	Americal Association of Pharmaceutical Scientists	aaps.org
Avicenna		avicenna.com
DIA	Drug Information Association	diahome.org/
MED Market		medmarket.com/medmarkt.html
NIH	National Institutes of Health	nih.gov
Pharm InfoNet		pharminfo.com/
PharmWeb		pharmweb.net
Renal		
ASN	American Society of Nephrology	asn.online.com
E-Neph	E-Neph	eneph.com
NKF	National Kidney Foundation	kidney.org
Renalnet	RenalNet	ns.gamewood.net//renalnet.html
USRDS	United States Renal Data System	med.umich.edu/usrds/

could far exceed the initial period of effort and difficulty as the Renal Dialysis Industry should be able to realize shorter product development timelines in all of the major global markets, with concommitant savings in many areas of product development. Instead of multiple internal efforts to meet the many national requirements for product registration, the new system may eventually allow a one time effort to develop a single technical dossier that will permit product registration on a global basis.

REFERENCES

1. Council of European Communities, Medical Device Directive, 93/42/EEC, Brussels, Belgium, June 1993.

2. Verdonck P, editor. The medical device directives. Passport to the future. Baxter World Trade, Brussels, Belgium, 1995, pp. 14.

3. Morton M., Canadian medical device proposal includes new requirements for premarket notification. RA Focus 1996; 1(11):10–11.

4. Burlington DB. New directions in medical device regulation. An FDA progress report. FDA, Center for Device Evaluation and Radiological Health, Rockville, MD, September 8, 1997 (Internet http://www.fda.gov/cdrh/medev/medevreg.html).

5. Sawyer D. Do it by design. An introduction to human factors in medical devices. FDA Guidance, CDRH, Rockville, MD, December 1996.

6. Freedman DP and Weinberg GM. Handbook of walkthroughs, inspections, and technical reviews, 3rd edition. NY, Dorset House, 1990:12.

7. Kahan JS. FDA's revised GMP regulations. The road to global improvement? Med Dev Diag Indust 1994; 16:128–32.

8. Riley WJ and Densford JW III. Processes, techniques and tools: the how of a successful design control system. Med Dev Diag Indust 1997; 19:74–80.

9. FDA. Design control guidance for medical device manufacturers Rockville, MD., FDA, CDRH, 3/1997.

10. FDA. Medical device quality system manual. A small entity compliance guide. Rockville, MD, FDA, CDRH.

11. The quality system compendium. Arlington, VA, Assoc Adv Med Instrum 1996.

12. Oliver DP. Ten techniques for trimming time to market. Med Dev Diag Indus. 1997; 8:58–65.

13. Dickinson JG. In its bold new course, FDA needs industry help. Med Dev Diag Indust 1997; 19:52–5.

14. FDA. A new 510(k) paradigm: alternative approaches to demonstrating substantial equivalence in premarket notifications. Rockville, MD, FDA, CDRH, 3/98.

15. United States of America – European Community mutual recognition agreement of conformity assessment. Sectorial annex on medical devices, US/EC Final Draft 6/5/97.

16. Segal DE and Rubin PD. Mutual recognition agreement between the United States and European Union signals new era of device and drug regulation. RA Focus 1997; 2:20–1.

17. Wechsler J. Modernization in China and an MRA at home. Pharmaceut Techol 1997; 9:16–28.

18. Wechsler J. Electronic submissions and harmonized inspections. Appl Clin Trials 1997; 6:16–22.

19. FDA Talk Paper. FDA's Negotiations with EU, 6/16/97 (Internet: http://www.fda.gov/bbs/topics/ANSWERS/ANS00802.html)

20. Anon. A brief guide to the EC rules governing medicines, 5th edition. European Federation of Pharmaceutical Industries' Associations, April, 1994.

21. Sauer F. A new and fast drug approval system in Europe. Drug Inform J 1997; 31:1–6

22. Jones K. Wider perspectives of European medicines control. Drug Inform J 1996; 30:1–7.

23. FDA. Reinventing regulation of drugs and medical devices. April, 1995. (Internet: http://www.fda.gov/po/reinvent.html).

24. FDA backgrounder. Reinventing drug and medical device regulation, 5/5/96. (Internet: http://www.fda.gov/opa-com/backgrounders/reinvent.html).

25. Anon. Electronic records; electronic signatures, final rule. Electronic submissions. Establishment of public docket, Notice. Fed Reg 3/20/97; 62 (54):13430–66.

26. FDA. Center for drug research and evaluation. Report to Industry 1996. 2/10/97.

27. U.S. Congress. Senate bill S.830: Food and drug administration modernization and accountability act of 1997.

28. Harman R. ICH 4 – the end of the beginning. Reg Affairs J 1997; 8:713–4.

29. Anon. The ICH process for harmonisation of guidelines, IFPMA, 1997. (Internet: http://www.ifpma.org/ich4/html).

30. Miller D. International conference on harmonization: the end or just the beginning. RA Focus 1997; 2: 6–9.

31. Möller H. A common technical document of quality: a nightmare or reality? RA Focus 1997; 2:10–11.

32. Colburn WA, McClurg JE and Cichoracki JR. The strategic role of outsourcing. CROs and the outsourcing phenomenon. Appl Clin Trials 1997; 6:68–75.

10. Global spectrum of quality assurance in the provision of dialysis

ROBERT ALLEN

The term spectrum can be defined as a continuous range which extends to opposite extremes. With this is mind, it is not surprising to note if one were to examine the global spectrum of quality in the field of dialysis, they would discover the range of quality is as broad and diverse as the cultural differences between the various nations and their inhabitants. Certainly, it is important to define and understand what quality is before it can be examined which in itself creates another dilemma as quality is interpreted differently by everyone.

DEFINING QUALITY

The Dialysis Outcomes Quality Initiative (DOQI) in the U.S. recently was charged with the responsibility to define quality dialysis care. The findings are currently being published as the renal community worldwide waits patiently in anticipation. According to Brown [1], the position of this initiative pronounced the following message: "ESRD patients receiving dialysis must be treated in a holistic manner by a qualified and adequately staffed multidisciplinary healthcare team, which includes the patient as a responsible member of the team. The care delivered must be predictable, comfortable, compassionate and should maximally increase life expectancy and reduce the need for hospitalization. To this end, patients must be active and informed participants in all aspects of their care, including the choice of treatment modality. As active members of the healthcare team, they must in turn be responsible and accountable for treatment outcomes, insofar as they are psychologically and physically capable". This is a powerful statement that for the first time clearly places some of the responsibility for quality on the

patient as well as the rest of the healthcare team. Translating this idea to the rest of the world has been and will continue to be difficult in regions where patients lack resources and opportunities for education and therefore, may have poor understandings of their disease. Additionally, in many countries some members of the healthcare team also lack education and practical skills and are not on par with healthcare workers in other further developed nations. Often the only professional member of the healthcare team may be the physician.

In recent years, the U.S. has recognized the need for quality assessment, quality assurance and continuous quality improvement in the ESRD program. This has been driven by the numerous federal and state agencies that govern the delivery of the care for patients receiving therapy. Additionally, several kidney organizations have devoted their annual meetings to issues related to quality of care and to clinical practice guidelines [2]. Governments in other countries are also now beginning to recognize the importance of developing quality health care systems. In a recent publication, Dr B. Charra further commented, "Prescribing an optimal dialysis is rather easy, delivering it is far more complicated. The delivery of an optimal dialysis depends in large part on the nursing team" [3]. In order to evaluate quality it is also necessary to examine data. Data is an integral part of the CQI process and should be used to teach and never to judge [2]. However, this is a difficult concept to convey in the international market when data is often presented in a comparative format. To achieve success on this front it is important to deliver a convincing representation to all participants and it is necessary to elicit their mutual cooperation in the sharing of data. The

L.W. Henderson and R.S. Thuma (eds.), Quality Assurance in Dialysis, 2nd Edition, 105–109.
© 1999 *Kluwer Academic Publishers. Printed in Great Britain*

results of this data can be utilized as an effective tool to motivate providers to improve their clinical results in the absence of regulatory of financial barriers. The goal of data collection on a global basis should be for expressed purpose of sharing information that permits patients and providers to benefit from the vast experience of others and to use the data to improve clinical outcomes which may in turn reduce program cost.

What Indicators or Criteria Should be Monitored?

The question of who will be placed on renal replacement therapy, whether HD or PD, is common across many countries. Some additional concerns are: who should be placed on a transplant waiting list and why? The prescription for dialysis is often another area for continued interest and research including which dialyzer, size, methodology and treatment time to employ. Hospitalization rates, cause, and frequency are important quality indicators to monitor. Complications associated with dialysis such as access malfunctions, adverse patient occurrences, peritonitis and mortality should also be monitored as an indictor of quality. Let us not forget about the quality of life assessments often performed by patient survey instruments which may provide useful information from the patient's perspective regarding the quality of care.

MORTALITY AS A INDICATOR OF QUALITY

The literature clearly demonstrates that mortality among ESRD patients varies significantly between countries, within countries and between facilities. Mortality is very difficult to study due to the variables in demographics and co-morbidity however, researchers continue to attempt to adjust their statistics to improve crude mortality data. Port attempted to compare the mortality rates of patients in the U.S. to those of Europe and Japan and concluded that higher mortality rates in the U.S. could not be explained by international differences in patient age, gender, race, or treatment modality [4]. Experience with one multinational dialysis provider in 15 countries including Europe, Asia and Latin America has demonstrated the national data systems in many coun-

tries vary so greatly that the integrity of the data may be questionable. With this said, is it reasonable to compare results when evaluating incomplete or unreliable data? Certainly, conclusions are often suggested and extrapolated based on available data consequently the summary generalizations may be incorrect.

In recent years, the European community has developed several Data Protection Laws that have made data collection and the sharing of data challenging for ESRD researchers. The only source of information regarding renal replacement therapy in Germany was provided by the EDTA registry. In 1985 the new data protection law in W. Germany led many nephrologist to voluntarily withdraw their participation with the EDTA registry [5]. With the drop in response rate to 50% the validity of data for Germany has been compromised. At this time, there appears to be no common data source which is compiling information on patients or renal replacement providers in Europe. The UK also seems plagued by the data protection laws it has developed. While it is understandable to ensure confidentiality of medical records for patients it seems to be conflicting with the process to improve quality which relies so heavily on the evaluation of clinical outcomes. It is evident at this time that overcoming the security issues while ensuring patient confidentiality and anonymity is the first step toward resuming the sharing of outcome results.

Observations in South America

Latin America is typically a region of the world that provides healthcare to a large population group that are poorly educated and also economically deprived. Additionally, many of the countries in this part of the world have governments that do not provide full reimbursement to providers of ESRD services. Furthermore, the quality of healthcare services available to the population may also be not up to par with other developed nations in N. America and Europe. It is also safe to express the opinion that the level of training, skill, knowledge or expertise of healthcare professionals and support personnel also mirror the preceding statement referring to the quality of care. With this said, what is the patient's general perception and opinion of the quality of care that they receive? To answer this question, facilities will generally utilize a patient satisfaction survey instrument. In general, the survey results reviewed by one multinational company reveal that patients are generally satisfied with the level of care they receive. Certainly this conclusion was limited to a very small pool and may not be indicative of the rest of the world. Physicians in Latin America are often considered infallible by patients and they are not likely to be concerned with issues related to malpractice in these countries where professional liability concerns are rare. Mortality is commonly accepted as the "will of God" and rarely the consequence of poor medical care in these nations dominated by Catholic faith. Many Latin Americans do not consider life or the ideology of prolongation of life as precious as it is in N. American and European countries.

PRACTICAL PROBLEMS

Generally speaking, measuring quality in many dialysis facilities is complicated by reimbursement constraints, increasing operating cost, and the burden of compliance with existing reporting requirements [2]. In the U.S. the greatest majority of dialysis patients are entitled to health care coverage through the Medicare system or through private insurance companies. Additionally, many of the ancillary services associated with the delivery of optimal ESRD care are also reimbursed to the provider. For example, the treatment of anemia is supported by the reimbursement of erythropoetin and iron preparations. Therefore, ESRD patients commonly receive the treatment they need for the management of anemia without the restraint cost. Conversely, in many Latin America and some Far East countries the national health insurance programs may not be available to all citizens and the reimbursement for renal replacement therapies is limited. With limited funding many patients do not receive the necessary ancillary medications much less the quantity of dialysis prescribed. In areas where funding is not available only individuals with personal wealth can afford a regular course of therapy. This is particularly true of many countries in the Far East. Consequently, it is impossible to achieve the minimum adequacy standards of quality dialysis that are commonly

recognized on a global basis. Anemia control as mentioned earlier is easier for the practitioner to manage with the availability, administration and reimbursement of erythropoetin. Without sufficient reimbursement structures in place and/or inadequate erythropoetin supply, it is extremely challenging for practitioners to achieve the minimum quality standards that are recognized worldwide for ESRD patients. To complicate this issue the literature is well documented with evidence that suggest that improved urea reduction ratios or Kt/V results has a direct impact on improving hematocrit levels. Physicians often feel their hands are tied as they struggle against these odds.

NUTRITION

Research conducted by Dr. Lowrie in the U.S. concluded that there was a direct correlation between serum albumin levels and mortality. Physicians worldwide recognize this important correlation but are often impotent to change or influence this clinical indicator in regions where malnutrition is prevalent. Clearly, there are many patients that are clinically malnourished in parts of the world where insufficient food supplies is a way of life. How can a practitioner combat this situation which is often compounded by poverty? Maslow's Hierarchy of Needs asserts that the basic necessities of life are first and foremost to one's survival. Maintaining one's quality of life is often secondary to survival and so, it is not uncommon to observe patients in poor nutritional states with low serum albumin levels. To combat this problem many facilities and physicians exercise humanitarian efforts and provide food supplementation to their patients that are impoverished regardless of the facility's financial condition. Some patients look forward to receiving their dialysis treatment three times a week in anticipation of also receiving the only meals they may enjoy during the week.

COSTS ASSOCIATED WITH DELIVERING QUALITY

In the U.S. there is no definite direct connection between reimbursement for ESRD services and the quality of care according to Rutherford [6].

However, some experts seem to correlate the increase in mortality to reimbursement pressures. "Undoubtedly, there exist a level of reimbursement below which quality will be affected adversely although that level has not been documented exactly" [6]. Clearly, the costs of a CQI program should be considered by all to be the "cost of conducting business". The questions most often raised are: who will pay for the staff training, data collection, analysis and the computerized record systems? When you consider the cost of a providing renal replacement service along with the level of reimbursement available and the financial limitations and education of the patients in many countries it is easy to understand why it is so difficult to make significant improvement in the quality of care that is delivered.

One must also be cognizant of the amount of total healthcare dollars spent per person in many countries is significantly lower than other developed countries.

The computer can play a unique and valuable role in addressing the concern for quality of patient care by keeping account of the many variables and the flow of information that occurs in treating patients with chronic diseases [7]. The use of computer systems in the healthcare environment was originally designed for the processing of administrative functions and has only recently been that they have been used to analyze outcomes. Traditionally, this task has been abstracted manually in an unsystematically organized medical record. The manual system of data collection and analysis is a very time consuming and expensive process which may not appear on the surface to generate much added value. It has also been observed that instituting computerized medical records in many countries is a monumental challenge for many reasons. Again, the cost benefit may not be supported by the reimbursement system and the level of skill and knowledge of personnel to operate systems is generally very limited or not present at all. To achieve the desired end results facilities may need to start with the teaching of basic operations a computer system.

Implementation of a CQI program does entail cost. Wright noted that, "While the individual employees are encouraged to increase their productivity by expanding their knowledge and skills and then implementing those skills in a daily practice, the cost of training and education can be substantial" [8]. Wright also reported that the cost of implementing a CQI process in his organization included not only the personnel time and the computer equipment but it also required his facility to invest in newer generation dialysis equipment and more expensive dialyzers in order to achieve the improved adequacy results. This assessment is probably true for most practitioners that are struggling to improve quality in their organizations. As clinical staff gain increased experience more patients will actually achieve the prescribed prescriptive goals. Wright further emphasizes that this process takes time, repetition and the total commitment of the leadership within the dialysis unit. The process often takes several years and may be complicated as the natural human tendency is to change to the old way of doing things and to resist the new way until it has been an equally ingrained habit.

BENEFITS

The potential rewards of instituting CQI programs are great and beneficial to many but most of all to the patients suffering with chronic renal failure. The patients stand to gain the most from improved outcomes, lower mortality and fewer hospitalizations which may in turn translate to increased revenues for ESRD providers. Introducing a continuous quality improvement program is often met with a great deal of anxiety from the clinical staff. In order to initiate a CQI program and process successfully it is important for facilities to drive out the fear and to break down the barriers that may exist surrounding this way of behaving. Vlchek suggests that facilities start by strengthening their communications and to be honest about problems occurring in dialysis units with each person [9].

WHO SHOULD LEAD THE EFFORT?

The position expressed by several experts in the field suggest that the primary responsibility for furthering the effort of quality assessment, assurance and improvement lies with the nephrology community. They further suggest that physicians and nursing professionals acquire the skills and expertise in clinical measurements of quality. Vlchek also pointed out that the most valuable outcome for his organization that he witnessed was the major improvement in staff morale [9].

CHACO

A fabulous example of Continuous Quality Improvement in motion can be observed in the isolated interior of Argentina in the province named Chaco. In this region, a facility has integrated a successful CQI ideology completely into their organization. The leaders of this organization received formal training in the United States where Total Quality Management (TQM) was first introduced in the early 1980s. Armed with the knowledge and the desire to improve the overall operations of their organization two physicians set out in 1983 on a mission to accomplish the goal of improving quality. Fourteen years later, they are quite proud of their accomplishments and their facility is a model example for others. Each member of their staff is fully committed to working on quality and each week the entire staff reviews their individual performance to identify opportunities of improvement. Even the cleaning personnel are considered integrated team members and together they celebrate their successes. Periodically the local newspapers will feature photos and captions which illustrate both patient and employee satisfaction with the organization. This leads to employee and patient retention and improved operating efficiencies. This facility emulates what Vilchek noted when he stated that, "CQI delivers a way for every employee to bring their ideas and skills forward for the betterment of the entire operation. When a person's ideas are solicited and responded to, the individual feels their opinion is valued and appreciated" [9].

Future

According to Rutherford, The future looks bright for ESRD and the CQI process has proven to be effective for the ESRD population. Healthcare can and will be transformed with this focus on quality. In order for quality improvements to occur within various countries, it will be necessary for the respective federal governments to initiate coordinated strategies and to provide the leadership, support and funding to promote this effort [2]. As providers and consumers become more knowledgeable about the end stage renal disease process and the care delivered they will begin to demand higher quality in technology and treatment. It is up to the renal community to provide the tools and educational resources that support the effort to improve the quality of renal replacement therapy worldwide to all the stake holders. Together this collaborative force can make a difference.

BIBLIOGRAPHY

1. Brown W. Defining quality dialysis care. Dialysis Transplant 1996; 25:810–29.
2. Scheier R. Measuring managing and improving quality in the end-stage renal disease treatment setting: committee statement. Am J Kid Dis 1994; 24:383–8.
3. Charra B. Ensuring quality in dialysis therapy. ETDNA 1997; 23:40–4.
4. Port FK. Variations in patient outcomes between the United States and other countries. Presented at the Institute of Medicine conference on measuring, managing, and improving quality in the end stage renal disease treatment setting, Washington, D.C., September 21–22, 1993.
5. Frei U. Quality assurance in renal replacement therapy. Nephrol Dialysis Transplant 1996; 11:1937–8.
6. Rutherford W. End stage renal disease a proving ground for quality improvement in health care. Semin Nephrol 1997; 17:218–25.
7. Pollak V. The computer in quality control of Hemodialysis patient care. Qual Rev Bull 1986; 12:202–10.
8. Wright L. Improving outcomes for maintenance hemodialysis patients by using continuous quality improvement. Dialysis Transplant 1996; 25:346–53.
9. Vlchek D. A blueprint for re-engineering implementing CQI in a large dialysis chain. Nephrol News Iss 1996; 10:26–31.

11. Clinical quality of the patient at onset of dialysis treatment

T. ALP IKIZLER AND RAYMOND M. HAKIM

The mortality rate of treated ESRD patients remains high in United States (24% per year) [1]. The life-expectancy of treated ESRD patients is 20–25 years less than the normal age-sex-race matched U.S. population over the age of 45. Despite recent advances in our understanding of the uremic state and improvements in the science and technology of renal replacement therapy, the prognosis of this patient population remains poor. Moreover, the health care cost of treating the U.S. ESRD program exceed $8 billion annually.

Several recent studies suggest that the clinical status of the end-stage renal disease (ESRD) patients at the time of initiation of dialysis may substantially affect their subsequent clinical outcome while on maintenance dialysis. The clinical status of the ESRD patients at the onset of dialysis treatment can be explained as a reflection of several subjective and a few objective parameters relative to the extent of the uremic state and can also be regarded as the criteria to initiate maintenance dialysis. These subjective parameters are often influenced to a great extent by the patient's perception of his or her quality of life. Clearly, the goal of any therapy, including dialysis, must be improvement of the patient's well being and quality of life. In this respect, over the past few years, a number of studies have sought to determine methods to slow the progression of renal failure and delay the onset of terminal renal failure, thus avoiding the need for dialysis. These efforts have been promulgated in the interest of saving money, both for patients and society at large, and to prevent the patient from being exposed to the "unpleasant experience" of dialysis; these studies have had an impact on the indications and rationale for starting dialysis. However, application of therapy must be at a time when the real risks of delaying the therapy outweigh the perceived benefits of withholding it.

In this chapter, we will attempt to provide the most appropriate approach to preserve the well-being of the patients with advanced chronic renal failure (CRF) prior to and at the time of initiation of chronic dialysis therapy. Specifically, an overview of the proposed association of clinical status at the onset of initiation of maintenance dialysis therapy with subsequent clinical outcome while on dialysis will be presented. The general considerations for appropriate care of the CRF patient prior to initiation of dialysis, as well as the criteria to initiate dialysis will be discussed. We will finally emphasize the adverse effects of malnutrition at the start of dialysis and the importance of monitoring nutritional parameters as a guide in the decision to initiate dialysis. The ultimate goal of such an approach is to improve the clinical outcome of ESRD patients while on dialysis.

ASSOCIATION OF CLINICAL STATUS AT THE ONSET OF DIALYSIS WITH SUBSEQUENT OUTCOME

A number of studies have suggested that the clinical status of the ESRD patients at the time of initiation of dialysis affects their subsequent clinical outcome while on chronic dialysis. The severity of uremic symptoms as well as the biochemical findings related to the extent of metabolic and hormonal abnormalities, the nutritional status of the patient, and the readiness of the patient for chronic dialysis at the onset on dialysis are the most clinically significant factors that are related to this association.

Serum albumin (SAlb) concentration has been a

L.W. Henderson and R.S. Thuma (eds.), Quality Assurance in Dialysis, 2nd Edition, 111–123.
© 1999 Kluwer Academic Publishers. Printed in Great Britain

commonly used estimate which correlates with outcome in multiple patient populations, including ESRD patients. It is not only a marker of nutritional status, but also a reliable index of the degree of illness of the patient. In this regard, The United States Renal Data System (USRDS) recently analyzed subsequent mortality of patients presenting for dialysis with different levels of SAlb concentrations [2]. In this study of approximately 3,500 patients, the risk of death was substantially higher for patients starting dialysis with a SAlb concentration lower than the "reference" population (SAlb between 3.6 to 4.0 g/dL). It should be appreciated also, that patients with SAlb concentrations greater than 4.0 g/dL had statistically significant lower risk of death than the reference population (Figure 11.1a). It is important to note that low SAlb is an independent risk factor for mortality and not just a reflection of underlying co-morbid conditions. Similar findings were demonstrated with serum creatinine concentrations (Figure 11.1b). Interestingly, there is an inverse correlation between serum creatinine levels at the initiation of dialysis and subsequent outcome, namely low levels of serum creatinine are associated with higher mortality. The explanation for this is probably the fact that serum creatinine is a surrogate marker for lean body mass and hence nutritional status. The importance of SAlb at initiation of dialysis is also underscored by unpublished data by Lowrie, based on a large number of patients starting dialysis. As shown in Figure 11.2, life table analysis shows a marked decrease in survival in patients starting dialysis with SAlb levels less than 4.0 g/dL, and is clearly worse the lower the initial SAlb. In a study from Japan, Iseki and colleagues have shown that low serum albumin, hyperkalemia, and hyponatremia at the time of initiation of dialysis were all associated with increased mortality risk in a cohort of 1,491 incident hemodialysis patients [3]. Similar data have been published with regard to serum prealbumin at the time of initiation of dialysis [4].

Our own experience suggests that similar association also exists with regard to morbidity, in particular hospitalization and length of stay. Specifically, in an analysis of several biochemical parameters including SAlb and serum creatinine at the time of initiation of dialysis in a cohort of 99 ESRD patients, we have found that patients with

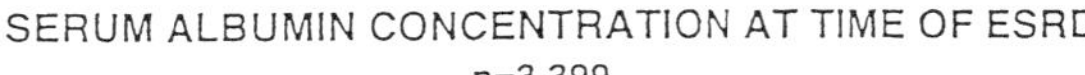
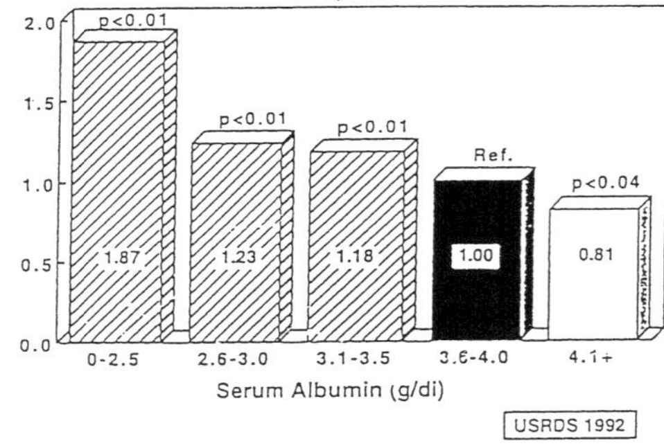

a

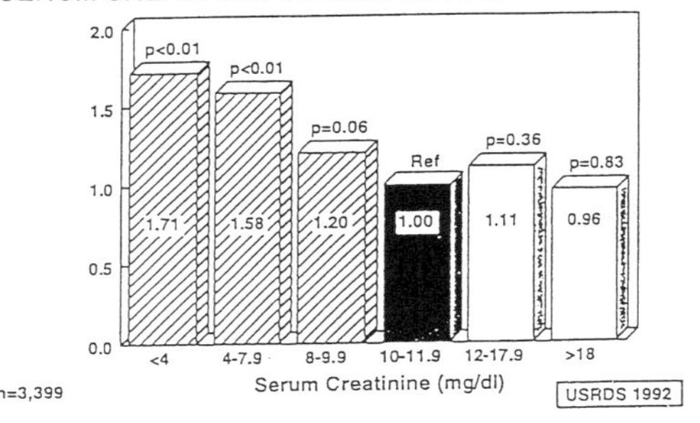

b

Fig. 11.1 (a) Relative risk of mortality in dialysis dependent patients as a function of serum albumin concentration at initiation of end-stage renal disease. Data based on cohorts in 1986–1987. (b) Relative risk of mortality in dialysis dependent patients as a function of serum creatinine concentration at initiation of end-stage renal disease. Data based on cohorts in 1986–1987.

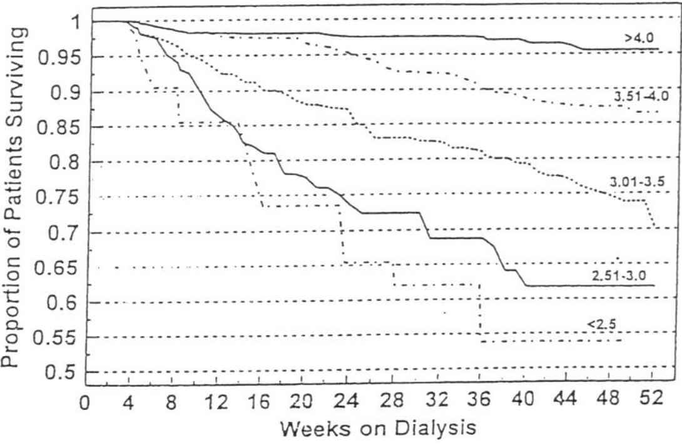

Fig. 11.2. Life-table analysis of patients initiating dialysis with various levels of serum albumin (g/dL).

SAlb less than 4.0 g/dL at the time of initiation of dialysis had significantly higher number of admissions, length of stay and higher hospital charges during the subsequent 12 months while on dialysis compared to patients with SAlb higher than 4.0 g/dL. Similar results were obtained when patients were grouped according to their serum creatinine concentrations. Patients with serum creatinine less than 8.0 mg/dL at the time of initiation of dialysis had significantly higher number of admissions, length of stay and higher hospital charges as compared to patients with serum creatinine higher than 8.0 mg/dL at the time of initiation of dialysis.

Although the majority of these studies cited above reflect the outcome of patients initiating hemodialysis, most studies of peritoneal dialysis patients also indicate a correlation of poor clinical status at the time of initiation with increased morbidity and mortality. Indeed, the results of a large multi-center study (CANUSA) provided convincing evidence that several estimates of nutritional status including serum albumin, subjective global assessment (scoring of four items: weight loss in the previous six months, anorexia, subcutaneous fat, muscle mass), normalized protein catabolic rate (to reflect dietary protein intake), and percent lean body mass were all correlated directly with patient survival. Higher estimates of all these parameters were consistently associated with improved survival [5].

In summary, there is ample evidence to suggest that multiple parameters reflecting the clinical status of the ESRD patients at the time of initiation of dialysis are associated with subsequent clinical outcome while on dialysis. Although these parameters may reflect a variety of different clinical conditions, the nutritional status of the ESRD patient seem to be a key factor in determining the outcome.

GENERAL CONSIDERATIONS FOR APPROPRIATE CARE OF THE PATIENT PRIOR TO INITIATION OF DIALYSIS

Referral

The appropriate care of the CRF patient prior to initiation of dialysis is complicated and requires careful attention to multiple confounding factors.

Table 11.1 summarizes several important aspects of general considerations for appropriate care of the patient prior to initiation of dialysis Before we discuss the general care of the CRF patient prior to and at the time of initiation of dialysis, an important issue that needs consideration is the time of referral of the renal patient to the nephrologist. Given the complexity of their disease and associated complications, it is of critical importance that CRF patients should be followed by a nephrologist especially at the advanced stage of their disease. Unfortunately, the importance as well as the potential value of early referral of CRF to the nephrologist is not well recognized. With the current financial constraints imposed by managed health care providers, patients are being asked to utilize a "gatekeeper" who constrain their referral to nephrologists, but for most cases it is the lack of awareness among traditional referral resources that delays referral to the nephrologist.

Late referral is defined as the referral to the nephrologist less than 6 months prior to initiation of renal replacement therapy. It is a common occurrence seen in approximately 30–50% of

Table 11.1. General considerations for appropriate care of the patient prior to initiation of dialysis

A) Timely referral to the nephrologist

B) Appropriate management of uremic complications
   - Fluid and electrolyte abnormalities
        Avoid fluid overload and excessive salt intake;
        Avoid hyperkalemia
   - Metabolic acidosis
        Keep $tCO_2 > 18$ mEq/L
   - Renal osterodystrophy
        Keep $PO_4 < 6.0$ mg/dL; PTH < 300 pg/mL; avoid
        aluminum containing antacids
   - Cardiac disease and hypertension
        Prevent LV hypertrophy and CAD; treat
        hypercholesterolemia if indicated
        Maintain a blood pressure of < 120 mmHg systolic
        and 80 mmHg diastolic
   - Anemia
        Keep Hct 33–36%

C) Timely placement of vascular access (preferably arterio-enous fistulae)

D) Patient education

E) Timely (healthy) initiation of dialysis

ESRD patients. Several studies have suggested that early referral has significant medical and economic advantages. Khan and colleagues have shown that 2-year patient survival with early referral was 59% compared to only 25% with late referral [6]. Campbell et al. reported that 1-year mortality was 39% in urgent referrals (< 1 month), 19% in intermediate referrals (1–4 months) and 6% with early referrals (> 4 months) [7].

Late referral is frequently associated with worse symptoms of uremia. Jungers et al. reported that in 65 patients who were referred late (< 1 month), 57% had severe hypertension, fluid overload or pulmonary edema, 90% needed emergency dialysis, and 60% had serum bicarbonate < 16 mEq/L at the time of initiation of dialysis [8]. Mean serum albumin was 3.5 ± 0.57 g/dL in this group. On the contrary, in 153 patients who were referred early (> 6 months), only 15% had severe hypertension, fluid overload or pulmonary edema, 4% had serum bicarbonate < 16 mEq/L and mean serum albumin was 3.86 ± 0.35 g/dL in this group.

The referral pattern also has significant financial implications. In the study by Campbell, the cost of hospitalization during initiation of dialysis was $23,633 for late referral compared to $4,980 for early referral [7]. Jungers et al. estimated that for each patient referred late, there is 0.2 million French Francs excess cost compared to patients referred early [8].

In summary, there is as yet no established guidelines and patterns for referral of renal failure patients to the nephrologist. Late referral of CRF patients predispose them to medical and financial disadvantages. It is clear that timely referral of CRF patients will enable the nephrologist to provide the appropriate care to the patients and the improve the clinical quality of the patient at the onset of dialysis.

Complications of Renal Failure

As the CRF patient progresses to ESRD, several complications of renal failure develop in these patients. These include multiple disorders of metabolism and organ-system functions. It is critical to define and appropriately manage these complications in a timely fashion in order to assure the clinical quality of the patient at the onset of dialysis. We will briefly discuss the most significant of these complications with regard to their importance on the subsequent outcome while on dialysis.

Fluid and Electrolyte Abnormalities

Abnormalities in fluid and electrolyte homeostasis are common complications of progressive renal disease. Sodium imbalance is usually seen when GFR is less than 10% primarily due to the tubular dysfunction. Most of the patients are on diuretic therapy as they approach ESRD. The dose should be adjusted not only to avoid fluid overload and possible pulmonary edema but also to prevent hypovolemia if vomiting, fever, diarrhea, or gastrointestinal bleeding occur. Potassium metabolism is also altered in patients with advanced renal failure. Patients are at higher risk of hyperkalemia from dietary indiscretion or hypokalemia if they are on diuretic regimen or suffer from vomiting and/or poor nutrition. Patients with certain underlying diseases such as diabetic nephropathy or interstitial nephritis are more prone to hyperkalemia. Finally medications especially angiotensin converting enzyme inhibitors increase the risk of hyperkalemia. Both sodium and potassium abnormalities can be adequately managed by appropriate dietary counseling and close follow-up during the late stages of renal disease and undesirable outcomes including cardiovascular complications leading to emergent initiation of dialysis can be avoided.

Metabolic Acidosis

Metabolic acidosis is another important complication of advanced renal disease that may affect the clinical status of the CRF patient at the time of onset of dialysis. Metabolic acidosis may develop from a number of reasons including the kidney's inability to excrete hydrogen ions as well as decreased filtration of phosphate and sulfate compounds. An important consideration in advanced renal failure patients is that recent studies indicate that metabolic acidosis promotes malnutrition in renal failure patients by increased protein catabolism [9, 10]. Studies by Mitch et al. have suggested that muscle proteolysis is stimulated by an ATP-dependent pathway involving ubiquitin and proteasomes during metabolic acidosis [11]. More recently, Ballmer et al. reported that metabolic acidosis of 7 day duration, induced with high doses of NH4Cl significantly reduced albumin synthesis and induced negative nitrogen balance in otherwise healthy subjects [12]. Acidemia can also have negative effects on the bone metabolism and predispose the CRF patients to worsening of bone disease.

Metabolic acidosis can be treated by sodium bicarbonate supplementation. Treatment should be initiated when serum bicarbonate concentration falls below 18 mEq/L. However, special attention should be given to avoid sodium overload and worsening of hypertension. In addition, concomitant use of aluminum containing phosphate binders and citrate containing preparations to treat acidemia is contraindicated since citrate increases aluminum absorption and predisposes the patient to acute aluminum intoxication. It has also been shown that correction of metabolic acidosis actually improves muscle protein turnover and increases the sensitivity of the parathyroid glands to calcium in dialysis patients [13]. Therefore, there is evidence suggesting that correction of metabolic acidosis may be both nutritionally and metabolically beneficial in renal failure patients and large scale studies are warranted to confirm these observations.

Renal Osteodystrophy

Another foreseeable complication of advanced renal disease is development of renal osteodystrophy. The kidney plays an important role in mineral homeostasis, by maintaining external balance for calcium, phosphorus, magnesium and pH. A combination of factors play a role in the development of renal osteodystrophy. As GFR falls to levels less than 20%, hypocalcemia develops due to hyperphosphatemia, decreasing renal synthesis of $1,25(OH)_2$ vitamin D (calcitriol) and worsening hyperparathyroidism with resistance to peripheral actions of PTH. The resulting conditions such as osteitis fibrosa, osteomalacia, mixed and adynamic bone lesions are important and long-term complications that subsequently affect renal failure patients while on dialysis.

In early renal failure, phosphorus control can be achieved by moderate dietary phosphorus restriction. This usually increases calcitriol to near normal levels. Calcitriol also enhances the absorption of calcium from the gut to avoid hypocalcemia. Once GFR is less than 20 to 30 mL/min, phosphorus restriction is not enough to stimulate calcitriol production and phosphorus binding agents are required. Use of aluminum containing binders should be avoided as much as possible since it is known that the absorption of this metal can predispose the dialysis patients to aluminum related osteomalacia. Calcium carbonate is the most commonly used phosphate binder. It is most effective when given with meals. Since there is a patient-to-patient as well as within patient variability from meal to meal, the dose frequency and timing should be adjusted for each individual meal. For CRF patients who have low calcium concentrations and/or PTH levels that are high (>300 pg/mL), early low dose of calcitriol should be considered. This approach may alleviate the symptoms and development of renal osteodystrophy. However, the patients must be monitored closely for hypercalcemia and hyperphosphatemia.

Cardiac Disease and Hypertension

Cardiac disease is two to five times more prevalent in ESRD patients who are on maintenance dialysis and has been shown to be the leading cause of death in this patient population. Systolic dysfunction, left ventricular (LV) hypertrophy and dilatation are independent predictors of mortality in dialysis patients [14]. Coronary artery disease and cardiac failure are also independent predictors of outcome in dialysis patients. These also account for a significant degree of comorbidity in ESRD patients. Interestingly, recent studies suggest that CRF patients who are not yet on dialysis also develop abnormalities in left ventricular (LV) structure and function. These abnormalities worsen as renal function declines. A recent study showed that 27% of CRF patients with creatinine clearances higher than 50 mL/min had LV hypertrophy whereas this figure increased to 45% in CRF patients with creatinine clearance less than 25 mL/min. Another study reported LV hypertrophy in 39% of CRF patients at the time of initiation of dialysis. Interestingly, there is an approximately 2 year lag period between the apparent adverse effects of LV hyperthrophy and dilatation and initiation of dialysis.

Hypertension has also been shown as an independent risk factor for both development of cardiac disease and clinical outcome in ESRD patients. Increase in mean arterial pressure was independently and significantly associated with the presence of concentric LV hypertrophy, change in LV mass index and cavity volume, and the development of de novo cardiac failure and/or ischemic heart disease in ESRD patients [15]. It is also known that blood pressure control is a key factor in controlling the progression of renal disease [16].

There are no randomized clinical studies to assess the effects of prevention or management of risk factors for cardiac disease for outcome of ESRD patients. However, given the strong relationship between cardiac disease and clinical outcome, such an approach should be considered reasonable, especially at a stage prior to initiation of dialysis. Despite the fact that there are no clear guidelines for the level of control needed to minimize risk for cardiac disease in CRF patients, the following guidelines should be considered: maintaining a blood pressure of < 120 mmHg systolic and 80 mmHg diastolic, no smoking, good long-term blood glucose control in diabetic patients, and PTH < 300 ng/L. The optimal level of cholesterol in patients with advanced renal failure is unclear. However, every patient should be evaluated individually for increased risk of cardiac disease as well as evidence of malnutrition prior to and at the time of initiation of dialysis and cholesterol levels should be managed accordingly. For patients without any signs of malnutrition, maintaining serum cholesterol below 200 mg/dL is advisable. Patients with known coronary artery disease should be placed on appropriate antiplatelet and antiischemic therapies. Finally, advanced anemia is also a risk factor for cardiac disease. Management of anemia in advanced renal failure is discussed below.

Anemia

Progressive anemia is an invariable consequence of chronic renal failure. Although several factors such as uremic inhibitors, shortened erythrocyte survival and iron deficiency have been postulated, inappropriately low erythropoietin production is by far the major cause of anemia of chronic renal failure. Erythropoietin production is directly related to the amount of residual renal function and as renal failure progresses, there is an increased likelihood of developing anemia due to the inability of the kidneys to produce sufficient amounts of erythropoietin [17].

The symptoms related to anemia usually develop when hematocrit decreases to 30% or less. This level of anemia usually corresponds to a mean serum creatinine of 6 mg/dL. However, there is considerable patient-to-patient variation. Many symptoms of anemia are similar to the symptoms related to chronic uremia and may be very difficult to distinguish clinically. These include weakness, fatigue, anorexia, decreased exercise tolerance, difficulty with concentration and memory, and sexual dysfunction. In severe cases or in patients with underlying coronary artery disease, dyspnea and chest pain can also occur. Chronic anemia and associated tissue hypoxia results in development of LV hypertrophy and consequently diastolic dysfunction and myocardial ischemia.

Treatment of anemia of chronic renal failure by recombinant human erythropoietin (rhEpo) has shown that many of the symptoms and complications of anemia can be improved substantially. There is evidence to show that correction of anemia results in improvement in LV hypertrophy in CRF patients. There is also significant improvement in exercise capacity, cognitive function as well as endocrine function with correction of anemia.

The recommended initial dose of rhEpo in predialysis patients is 80 to 120 U/kg/week in two to three divided doses to achieve target hematocrit. On the other hand, the appropriate target hematocrit in CRF patients is not well-established. The current recommendation is in the range of 33 to 36%. It is also critical to maintain adequate iron stores to achieve appropriate response to rhEpo. Serum iron stores should be checked with appropriate tests and patients should be started on oral iron supplementation when needed.

Vascular Access

The leading cause of morbidity in ESRD patients who are on hemodialysis is vascular access associated morbidity. In its latest report, the USRDS estimates that in 1995, the cost for access morbidity is approximately $7,871 per patient per year at risk, and an annual global cost to Medicare that represents 14–17% of total spending for hemodialysis patients per year at risk [1]. Importantly, this access related morbidity leads to a significant reduction in the quality of life of dialysis patients.

An important issue is that epidemiologic data analyzed by the USRDS from HCFA data and other sources clearly demonstrate that lack of appropriate timing of vascular access placement substantially contributes to subsequent access failure. In 1993, approximately half of the patients starting ESRD therapy in the U.S. have had no permanent access placed or attempted before initiation of dialysis therapy for ESRD, and 27% have a temporary catheter 30 days *after* initiation of therapy. In fact, only 25% of patients have had a permanent access placed 30-days before initiation of dialysis therapy [1]. Collins et al. have recently shown that not only access outcome, but *patient outcome* strongly correlates with the timing of access placement [18]. The relative risk of mortality in patients who had accesses placed 6 months or more before initiation of therapy was one half the mortality risk of patients who have had accesses placed less than one month before ESRD therapy.

Despite the almost universal acceptance of its long-term superiority as a vascular access method, the frequency of placement of AV fistulae in the U.S. is small and declining [19]. In all patients who do not have a living related transplantation available and planned, the placement of an A-V fistula no later than at a time the creatinine reaches 4 mg/ dL or when creatinine clearance is approximately 25 mL/min should be advocated. This early placement not only allows time for fistulae to develop, but even if it does not mature, it may dilate the venous system sufficiently to improve the eventual success of the PTFE graft. Importantly, having the AV fistula (with appropriate education and instruction) preserves that arm from repeated venipuncture for blood drawing that leads to sclerosis of the veins. Frequent monitoring of the "maturity" of the fistulae, along with exercises to develop the fistulae and ligation of run-off veins if necessary should help in the development of these accesses.

Patient Education

There is growing evidence to suggest that behavioral interventions that combine patient education and psychological support can exert a beneficial effect on morbidity and mortality after initiation of chronic dialysis therapy. It has been documented that implementation of a dedicated ESRD Clinic at the predialysis stage would result in an increased proportion of individuals who continue to work after initiation of dialysis. It is also likely that predialysis education can increase illness-related knowledge and may also extend the predialysis period as suggested in a recent study.

Many patients have misconception about dialysis, and they fear the unknown. It is likely that a large proportion of them have not seen a dialysis machine prior to initiation of dialysis. Often the range of therapy options is also not discussed adequately with the patients. An early educational process which includes sessions at the dialysis unit will increase the likelihood of better acceptance of the dialysis process. During these sessions, patients and care givers should discuss the different options of renal replacement therapy, and select the therapy that is most appropriate for the individual patient's medical and social needs. Finally, a dietitian and a social worker should be involved extensively during the education process for preparation of the patient for initiation of dialysis.

GENERAL CRITERIA FOR INITIATION OF DIALYSIS

The considerations discussed above are aimed at managing the pre-dialysis patient with optimal care and maintaining the best clinical status until the patient needs to be initiated on chronic dialysis. The indications for initiation of dialysis have been accepted since the mid-1960s, before the recent emphasis on prolonging conservative therapy. The decision to initiate dialysis in patients with progressive renal failure can be considered under two criteria (Table 11.2). "Absolute indications" include the development of life threatening or irreversible events, i.e. pericarditis, fluid overload and pulmonary edema unresponsive to simple measures, hypertension poorly responsive to treat-

Table 11.2. Traditional indicators for initiation of dialysis

A) Absolute indicators
  - Pericarditis
  - Fluid overload and pulmonary edema unresponsive to simple measures
  - Hypertension poorly responsive to treatment
  - Advanced uremic encephalopathy and/or neuropathy
  - Clinically significant bleeding diathesis
  - Persistent severe nausea and vomiting

B) Relative indicators
  - Anorexia progressing to nausea and vomiting (characteristically early in the morning)
  - Moderate fatigue and weakness
  - Decreased attentiveness, memory and cognitive tasking
  - Persistent and severe pruritus
  - Depression and poor interpersonal relationships
  - Malnutrition (see Table 11.3)

ment, advanced uremic encephalopathy and/or neuropathy, clinically significant bleeding diathesis, and persistent severe nausea and vomiting. Most nephrologists would agree that the time course to these life-threatening events is not predictable and to delay initiation of dialysis until such indications are present places the patient at unnecessary risk of mortality and leads to morbidity with prolonged hospitalization.

Measurement of Renal Function

Apart from these "absolute indications", many nephrologists consider specific target values of renal function as indicators for initiation of dialysis. This is not only because Medicare has guidelines for reimbursement according to these values but also there are no established guidelines for this process. It is therefore important to review the appropriateness as well as the limitations of using these measurements in the context of starting ESRD therapy for progressive renal failure.

The above mentioned target values for initiation of dialysis may consist of a particular value of serum creatinine (Scr) or its reciprocal, blood urea nitrogen (BUN), or urinary creatinine clearance. The problems inherent in the measurement of Scr, BUN and creatinine clearance, particularly in patients with reduced renal function is discussed in detail elsewhere [20]. Differences in the extent of

tubular secretion, extrarenal elimination, and rate of generation of creatinine and urea, as well as composition of the diet make assessment of true renal function by such measurements in patients with chronic renal disease unreliable. More importantly, creatinine is appropriately recognized not simply as a measure of renal function but also as a measure of somatic mass; thus a low serum creatinine may reflect loss of muscle mass due to reduction in physical activity or dietary intake as much as improvement of renal function. Similarly, maintenance of a particular value of serum creatinine may reflect a loss of muscle mass rather than a delay in the progression of renal failure.

Variations in the extent of creatinine homeostasis are seen not only between different individuals, but in the same individuals as a function of the progression of renal failure. Glomerular filtration rate (GFR) determined by ^{125}I-iothalamate may vary greatly at the same level of serum creatinine. Other studies utilizing inulin clearance demonstrated markedly low GFRs in the face of normal or near normal serum creatinine [20]. Finally, it has been shown that with depressed renal function, creatinine clearance overestimates true GFR by as much as 100% [21].

These considerations therefore warrant that the documentation of renal function be ascertained by one of several newer filtration markers such as ^{125}I-iothalamate, ^{99m}Tc-DTPA or ^{51}CR-EDTA. In many areas, these sophisticated markers of GFR are not available. Although creatinine clearance overestimates GFR, urea clearance underestimates GFR and reasonable estimation of renal function can be ascertained by measuring simultaneously the 24 hour creatinine and urea clearances and averaging the two values [2]. Thus, taken individually serum creatinine, BUN or creatinine clearance may not provide the "objective" criteria to determine renal function and must be used cautiously and certainly not as exclusive criteria for the decision to initiate dialysis.

With those problems in mind, is there a target GFR at which patients should be considered for initiation of dialysis? Studies in the past measured renal function at initiation relying on Scr concentration or creatinine clearance. Mean "renal" survival time in 108 patients from the time patients reach a Scr between 9.5 and 10.0 m/dL to the initiation of dialysis (based on development of overt uremic symptoms) is approximately 10 ± 1.2 months [22]. Twenty five percent of the patients who reached a Scr of 10 mg/dL, needed initiation of dialysis within 3 months from achieving this level of renal failure.

Other studies have shown similar levels of renal function (as determined by creatinine) prior to initiation of dialysis. In a study based on HCFA form 2728, it was suggested that, in more than 1,700 patients, the mean creatinine at initiation of dialysis was 9.1 ± 4.5 mg/dL (median 8.2 mg/dL), but in diabetics, the mean was 8.1 mg/dL and median was 7.8 mg/dL [2]. Jungers indicated that, independent of the degree of protein restriction, the average creatinine level at initiation of dialysis was approximately 10 mg/dL [23], although in a more recent study from the same group, a slightly lower value of serum creatinine at initiation of dialysis was found [8]. These authors also found a more rapid rate of progression than the previous study: the interval between a Scr of approximately 5.6 mg/dL to dialysis was 15.4 ± 0.8 months and only 6.3 ± 0.4 months for patients once they reached a creatinine of approximately 8 mg/dL.

No studies have looked at the true GFR as measured by iothalamate clearance, inulin clearance or other isotopic measures at the time of initiation of dialysis, although ongoing studies as part of the Modification of Diet in Renal Disease (MDRD) study may perhaps answer this question in the future. Be that as it may, it is not clear that any particular level of creatinine or BUN is an appropriate marker for the initiation of dialysis. Measurements of averaged urea and creatinine clearance or more accurate determination of GFR that do not rely solely on creatinine would obviate the problem of reduced muscle mass and other variations affecting serum levels. As noted earlier, measurements of renal function by any means, should be considered only as supportive evidence and used in conjunction with the overall assessment of the patient, and in particular clinical signs and symptoms indicating the onset of malnutrition.

Finally, it is also instructive to consider the equivalence of dialytic clearance and residual renal function as a guide to initiation of dialysis; in other words, how much of an equivalent amount of excretory function of the kidney does hemodialysis replace? Assuming a urea clearance of 300 mL/minute for a high-flux dialyzer at a blood flow rate of approximately 400 mL/minute, the weekly urea clearance, based on 4 hours of dialysis, 3 times per week is 216 L; averaged on a continuous basis, this is equivalent to a clearance of urea of 21.4 mL/minute. Similar considerations for creatinine (assuming a dialytic clearance of 200 mL/minute) show that dialysis with the above regimen represents an average of 14.3 mL/minute of creatinine clearance. In addition, the availability of high-flux dialyzers or hemofilters, with pore sizes that allow for diffusion or convection of middle molecules with molecular weights greater than 15,000 daltons, provides closer approximation of native renal function. Clearly, the continuous function of the native kidneys and their multiple other functions in contrast to the discontinuous nature of intermittent hemodialysis makes such an analysis a very simplified comparison; nevertheless, the model allows a frame of reference for consideration of initiation of dialysis.

Relative Indications

The more commonly accepted criteria, so called "relative" indications, reflect a general but fairly severe decline in the quality of life of the patient. Indeed, it was reported that signs and symptoms of 118 patients starting dialysis has shown that 61% of the patients had anorexia and weight loss, 58% had generalized weakness, 49% encephalopathy and 41% nausea and vomiting [2]. It should also be noted that development and expression of these "relative" signs and symptoms in patients with slowly progressive renal disease is variable and may be accepted by the patient and family and not brought to the attention of the physician. Patients with slowly progressive renal failure often adjust their ability to perform tasks and downgrade their sense of well-being and habits as renal failure progresses. Further, some of the medications required by patients with chronic renal failure may have side-effects that mimic uremic symptoms. Conversely, the partial correction of anemia by treatment with erythropoietin may improve the patient's CNS and cardiovascular symptoms and sense of well being without affecting the extent of uremia [24]. Finally, in many, there may be no "major" event that precipitates the need for initiation of dialysis. Thus, it may be useful to identify other markers of uremia that are less subjective and/or equivocal, to avoid jeopardizing the health of the patient. Indeed, an important concept in these discussions is that the initiation of dialysis should occur in an effort to improve the quality of life and rehabilitate the patient to full potential, not just to prolong a less than optimal survival. It is our view, based on a critical review of available data, that the signs and symptoms of malnutrition should be considered as objective criteria for initiation of dialysis and are important early indicators.

NUTRITIONAL STATUS AS A MARKER FOR INITIATION OF DIALYSIS

The rationale to consider the signs and symptoms of malnutrition as criteria to initiate maintenance dialysis relies on the well-established fact that uremic malnutrition combined with low residual renal function at the time of initiation of dialysis effects outcome in ESRD [2, 4, 25, 26]. This subject is discussed in detail earlier in this chapter. It is important to note that all parameters considered to reflect the clinical quality of the ESRD patient at the time of initiation of dialysis are either markers of nutritional status themselves or closely related to nutrition. There is now evidence to suggest that signs and symptoms of malnutrition can be seen in CRF patients as they lose their residual renal function prior to initiation of dialysis.

Although anorexia has been recognized as one of the hallmarks of advanced uremia, the level of renal failure at which it occurs and the extent of anorexia have not been adequately documented. Results of the MDRD feasibility study (similar to the full MDRD study but smaller in scope, without blood pressure randomization and carried out for only one year) contain important information on this issue [27]. It should be noted that patients with pre-existing evidence of malnutrition, proteinuria ≥ 10 g/day, insulin dependent diabetes, heart or liver failure were excluded from this and the subsequent full study. In this selection of "healthy" CRF patients, positive correlations were found at baseline between the true GFR (determined by I^{125}iothalamate) and actual and reported protein and calorie intake, albumin concentration,

body weight, transferrin, and urine creatinine to height ratio. Thus, at entry into the study i.e. before assignment to different dietary group, the lower the GFR the worse the biochemical markers of malnutrition. In all dietary groups, the estimated actual energy intake was significantly (20%) lower than prescribed intake.

In an abstract presenting results of the full MDRD study, Kopple and co-workers reported on the nutritional status of 1,687 patients evaluated during the initial baseline visit of the study [28]. They again found that lower GFR was significantly associated with reduced protein intake. Decreased GFR was also significantly associated with reduction in caloric intake, body weight and muscle area, percent body fat, urine creatinine, serum albumin, and serum transferrin. They concluded that the preliminary signs of protein and calorie malnutrition began rather early in the course of chronic progressive renal failure and became more evident when the GFR was less than 10 mL/min.

In a previous study of patients with progressive azotemia, Hakim and Lazarus reported decreased food intake even with no dietary instructions to restrict protein or calories [22]. This decrease was thought to reflect a combination of anorexia and alteration in the smell and taste of foodstuffs. It was noted that the avoidance of food often applied to meat products with patients "instinctively" avoiding these high protein foods even without dietary counseling. However, it was also noted that there was no decrease in the serum albumin of such patients as they moved from mild to severe renal insufficiency, suggesting that visceral protein status was preserved (unlikely) or that low serum albumin was a late indicator of malnutrition.

In a prospective analysis of the effects of progression of renal disease in CRF patients [29], Ikizler et al. reported that mean spontaneous dietary protein intake declined from 0.70 ± 0.17 g/kg/day at a creatinine clearance between 25 mL/min and 10 mL/min to as low as 0.54 ± 0.17 g/kg/day when creatinine clearance was less than 10 mL/min. Moreover, declining serum cholesterol, insulin-like growth factor-1, and serum prealbumin were observed with declining renal function. Dietary interventions in these patients were minimal and consisted only in attempts to attenuate the hyperphosphatemia by limiting dairy products.

In a cross-sectional analysis at the time of initiation of dialysis of 680 patients enrolled in a cohort study, CANUSA Peritoneal Dialysis Study group demonstrated a strong association between baseline residual renal function and nutritional status [30, 31]. Finally, in a cross-sectional study, Pollock et al. [32] also reported significant association between dietary protein intake and level of renal function as well as several nutritional parameters in CRF patients prior initiation of dialysis. Overall these observations provide the evidence that worsening level of uremia is a cause of insidious malnutrition in pre-dialysis patients and spontaneous decrease in dietary protein and energy intake can be regarded as an early index of uremia and reasonably should be considered as a marker for initiation of dialysis. Thus, we propose that spontaneous decrease in dietary protein intake should be used as an early index of uremia. At the very least, patients with dietary protein intake of less than 0.8–0.7 g/kg/day should be targeted for frequent follow-up to monitor nutritional status more intensely. Indeed, the report by National Kidney Foundation-Dialysis Outcomes Quality Initiative on Peritoneal Dialysis recommended as such for initiation of dialysis.

Markers of Malnutrition

Since the association between nutritional status and level of renal function as well as their effect on subsequent outcome is established, the challenge is to appropriately monitor the nutritional indices in the pre-ESRD patient. Table 11.3 depicts proposed guidelines for utilization of multiple nutritional indices for decision to initiate dialysis in advanced CRF patients. Since serum albumin concentration, even slightly less than 4.0 g/dL, has such an important effect on mortality and morbidity risk, it is one of the most important markers of malnutrition in the CRF patients. Serum albumin is a very reliable indicator of visceral protein stores. However, its concentration is also determined by several other factors, including the rate of synthesis and catabolism. Serum albumin has a long half-life at 20 days making it a late marker for nutritional status. In addition, the distribution of albumin between extracellular and intravascular spaces may be variable depending on the etiology of renal disease or the presence or absence of fluid

Table 11.3. Indices of malnutrition as criteria for initiation of dialysis

A) Serum albumin concentration – <4.0 g/dL in non-nephrotic patients – <3.8 g/dL in nephrotic patients
B) Serum prealbumin concentration <32 mg/dL
C) Serum transferrin concentration <200 mg/dL
D) Spontaneous dietary protein intake <0.7 g/kg/day
E) Continuous decline in body weight (>10% within 6 months) or low percentage of ideal body weight (<85%)
F) Abnormally low percentage of lean body mass by body composition (using BIA/DEXA/PNAA)

Abbreviations: Bioelectrical impedance analysis (BIA); Dual energy X-ray absorptiometry (DEXA); Prompt neutron activation analysis (PNAA)

overload. In malnourished patients, albumin appears to shift into the intravascular compartment. Finally, low serum albumin may reflect unrecognized inflammatory conditions independent of nutrition [33]. Therefore, serum albumin concentration should be evaluated with caution while assessing the nutritional status of the CRF patients.

Several visceral proteins have a shorter half-life and may be earlier markers of malnutrition. Among these are transferrin (which has a half-life of 8 days instead of 20 days for albumin) and prealbumin, which has a half-life of 2 days. Recent studies of prealbumin in ESRD patients both at the time of initiation of dialysis as well as while on chronic dialysis have shown it to correlate inversely with mortality [4]. An important point to keep in mind while utilizing serum prealbumin is that prealbumin is excreted by the kidneys and its concentration is falsely elevated in patients with advanced renal disease.

Anthropometric measurements have often been used to estimate body composition and nutritional adequacy. Reproducibility of anthropometric measurements is poor and is dependent upon the skill of the observer. There are likewise, no studies which have correlated anthropometric measurements of pre-dialysis patients with clinical outcome.

In the MDRD study, urinary nitrogen appearance (UNA) was a useful tool to measure protein intake in the evaluation of nutritional status. We also follow protein intake of our patients from 24-hour urinary collection according to the methodology described by Maroni et al. [34]. As indicated earlier, studies in patients with chronic renal failure not on supervised protein restriction, have demonstrated that protein intake decreases gradually as renal failure progresses [29]. Spontaneous decreases in urea nitrogen appearance (reflecting decreased dietary protein intake) coupled with decreased creatinine appearance, reflecting decreased muscle mass, may well be easy and readily available indices of early malnutrition that should be sought. In patients on unrestricted dietary protein prescriptions, the finding of a decline in daily protein intake of less than 0.8–0.7 g/kg/day should be viewed with concern. Follow-up should occur as often as once every 3 to 4 weeks and if reduced protein and calorie intake persists, the patient should be started on dialysis. Finally, newer assessment tools such as bioelectrical impedance, dual energy X-ray absorptiometry and prompt neutron activation analysis may be useful to assess body composition and nutritional status in those patients approaching dialysis.

SUMMARY

Multiple studies suggest that the clinical status of the disease patients at the time of initiation of dialysis may substantially affect their subsequent clinical outcome while on maintenance dialysis. Comorbid conditions related to the etiology of the renal failure as well as metabolic and homeostatic disturbances related to renal failure have a significant influence on the well-being and outcome of these patients. These metabolic and homeostatic disturbances include fluid and electrolyte abnormalities, metabolic and hormonal derangements such as acidosis and osteodystrophy, cardiac disease, hypertension and anemia. All of these abnormalities can be managed with appropriate care to minimize their adverse effects. In this respect, timely referral of CRF patients to the nephrologist is an essential part of management of CRF patients.

When considering the timing for initiation of dialysis, advanced uremic symptoms should be anticipated and avoided. Instead, earlier manifestations of the uremic syndrome should be diligently sought and strongly considered as indications for the initiation of dialysis. In particular, we propose that dialysis should be initiated whenever indices of malnutrition develop in patients with CRF. Increased hospitalizations or prolongation of hospitalization related to malnutrition or complications of inadvertent uremia may obliterate any savings of delaying dialysis and more importantly will significantly reduce the quality of life of patients. Most importantly, a team approach, including a nephrology nurse, social worker, dietician, transplant coordinator and nephrologist and a comprehensive educational program are essential to the process of preparing a patient for maintenance renal replacement therapy.

ACKNOWLEDGMENTS

This work is supported in part by NIH Grant #RO1 DK45604-05 and RO1 HL 36015-12, and FDA Grant # 000943-4.

REFERENCES

1. United States Renal Data System. The USRDS 1996 annual data report. 1997; S1–S152.
2. Hakim RM and Lazarus JM. Initiation of dialysis. J Am Soc Nephrol 1995; 6:1319–28.
3. Iseki K, Uehara H, Nishime K, Tokuyama K, Yoshihara K, Kinjo K et al. Impact of the initial levels of laboratory variables on survival in chronic dialysis patients. Am J Kidney Dis 1996; 28:541–8.
4. Avram MM, Mittman N, Bonomini L, Chattopadhyay J and Fein P. Markers for survival in dialysis: a seven-year prospective study. Am J Kidney Dis 1995; 26:209–19.
5. Churchill DN. Adequacy of peritoneal dialysis: how much dialysis do we need? Kidney Int 1997; 48:S2–S6.
6. Khan IH, Catto GR, Edward N and Macleod AM. Chronic renal failure: factors influencing nephrology referral. Quart J Med 1994; 87:559–64.
7. Campbell JD, Ewigman B, Hosokawa M and Van Stone JC. The timing of referral of patients with end stage renal disease. Dialysis Transplant 1989; 18:66–86.
8. Jungers P, Zingraff J, Albouze G, Chauveau P, Page B, Hannedouche T and Man NK. Late referral to maintenance dialysis: detrimental consequences. Nephrol Dial Transplant 1993; 8:1089–93.
9. May RC, Kelly RA and Mitch WE. Mechanisms for defects in muscle protein metabolism in rats with chronic uremia:

the influence of metabolic acidosis. J Clin Invest 1987; 79:1099–103.

10. Mitch WE and Walser M. Nutritional therapy of the uremic patient. In Brenner BM and Rector FC, editors. The Kidney. Philadelphia, Saunders, 1991; 2186.

11. Mitch WE, Medina R, Greiber S, May RC, England BK, Russ PS et al. Metabolic acidosis stimulates muscle protein degradation by activating the adenosine triphosphate-dependent pathway involving ubiquitin and proteasomes. J Clin Invest 1994; 93:2127–33.

12. Ballmer PE, McNurlan MA, Hulter HN, Anderson SE, Garlick PJ and Krapf R. Chronic metabolic acidosis decreases albumin synthesis and induces negative nitrogen balance in humans. J Clin Invest 1995; 95:39–45.

13. Graham KA, Reaich D, Channon SM, Downie S, Gilmour E, Passlick-Deetjen J et al. Correction of acidosis in CAPD decreases whole body protein degradation. Kidney Int 1996; 49:1396–400.

14. Foley RN and Parfrey PS. Cardiac disease in chronic uremia: clinical outcome and risk factors. Adv Renal Repl Ther 1997; 4:234–48.

15. Foley RN, Parfrey PS, Harnett JD, Kent GM, Murray DC and Barre PE. Impact of hypertension on cardiomyopathy, morbidity and mortality in end-stage renal disease. Kidney Int 1996; 49:1379–85.

16. Klahr S, Levey AS, Beck GJ, Caggiula AW, Hunsicker L, Kusek JW et al. for Modification of diet in renal disease study group. The effects of dietary protein restriction and blood-pressure control on the progression of chronic renal disease. N Engl J Med 1994; 330:877–84

17. Knochel JP. Biochemical alterations in advanced uremic failure. In Jacobson HR, Striker GE and Klahr S, editors. The principles and practice of nephrology. Philadelphia, BC Decker, 1991; 682.

18. Collins A, Xia H and Ma J. Pre-ESRD vascular access insertion is associated with improved elderly patient survival. J Am Soc Nephrol 1997; 8:230.

19. Sands J and Miranda CL. Increasing numbers of AV fistulas for hemodialysis access. Clin Nephrol 1997; 48:114–17.

20. Levy AS. Measurement of renal function in chronic renal disease. Kidney Int 1990; 38:167–84.

21. Shemesh O, Golbetz H, Kriss JP and Myers BD. Limitations of creatinine as a filtration marker in glomerulopathic patients. Kidney Int 1985; 28:830–8.

22. Hakim RM and Lazarus JM. Progression of chronic renal failure. Am J Kidney Dis 1989; 14:396–401.

23. Jungers P, Chauveau P, Ployard F, Lebkiri B, Ciancioni C and Man NK. Comparison of ketoacids and low protein diet on advanced chronic renal failure progression. Kidney Int 1987; 32:67–71.

24. Nissenson AR. Epoetin and cognitive function. Am J Kidney Dis 1992; 20:S21–S24.

25. Ikizler TA, Evanson JA, Greene JH and Hakim RM. Impact of nutritional status and residual renal function at initiation of hemodialysis on subsequent morbidity in chronic hemodialysis patients. J Am Soc Nephrol 1996; 7:1319.

26. Tattersall J, Greenwood R and Farrington K. Urea kinetics and when to commence dialysis. Am J Nephrol 1995; 15:283–9.

27. Modification of diet in renal disease study group. Nutritional status of patients with different levels of chronic renal failure. Kidney Int 1989; 36:S184–S194.

28. Modification of diet in renal disease study group. Relationship between GFR and nutritional status-results from the MDRD study. J Am Soc Nephrol 1994; 5:335.

29. Ikizler TA, Greene J, Wingard RL, Parker RA and Hakim RM. Spontaneous dietary protein intake during progression of chronic renal failure. J Am Soc Nephrol 1995; 6:1386–91.

30. Canada–USA (CANUSA) Peritoneal Dialysis Study Group. Adequacy of dialysis and nutrition in continuous peritoneal dialysis: association with clinical outcomes. J Am Soc Nephrol 1996; 7:198–207.

31. McCusker FX, Teehan BP, Thorpe KE, Keshaviah PR and Churchill DN. How much peritoneal dialysis is required for the maintenance of a good nutritional state? Kidney Int Suppl 1996; 56 50:S56–S61.

32. Pollock CA, Ibels LS, Zhu FY, Warnant M, Caterson RJ, Waugh DA et al. Protein intake in renal disease. J Am Soc Nephrol 1997; 8:777–83.

33. Kaysen GA, Stevenson FT and Depner TA. Determinants of albumin concentration in hemodialysis patients. Am J Kidney Dis 1997; 29:658–68.

34. Maroni B, Steinman TI and Mitch NE. A method for estimating nitrogen intake of patients with chronic renal failure. Kidney Int 1985; 27:58–61.

12. Patient and therapy perspectives: choosing the patient "Is better worse?"

C.M. KJELLSTRAND

I believe almost all the differences in mortality that exists between different European regions and the United States, even when age is controlled, are due to different acceptance criteria or transplantation activity. The reason dialysis patient mortality is highest in U.S.A. and the Nordic countries is because they have the highest acceptance to dialysis and the highest transplant rates in the world. If this is true, a worse survival may reflect a better fulfillment of a nephrologist's duties:

Quality assurance in this chapter is defined as a dialysis unit having a morbidity and mortality that is comparable to an acceptable norm. The norm will be derived from large data bases which are constantly updated, provide much detail and also study the interaction and independence between different factors.

I believe quality comparison is one of the most important and neglected areas in modern medicine. I will however in this chapter concentrate on the pitfalls of quality assurance. This is not because of cynicism or a perverse interest in the flaws of science. Rather, if the problem with quality assurance are not considered the following may result:

1. The old and the poor masses may unnecessarily perish because large groups of patients who can be successfully sustained may remain untreated and die too early due to being considered "poor risk".

2. The best physician, humanely striving to take on the old and the sick may be unjustly punished, while the greedy scoundrels, who ruthlessly select out the "best cases" and then deny them transplantation, may be rewarded.

3. Propaganda by business looking hard at the bottom line may unnecessarily escalate the cost of treatment.

I am purposely avoiding rehabilitation as an outcome parameter because dialysis rehabilitation status seems to be influenced more by cultural and economic factors and by patient motivation, than any factor of dialysis itself [1].

Table 12.1 outlines various factors that have been thought to influence the outcome of dialysis patients. In general, physicians have control and sole responsibility only for technical treatment related factors and only some control over patient–treatment related factors.

The purpose of quality assurance in dialysis is to ascertain whether the differences in outcome are due to treatment related factors or due to differences in the pre-existing factors as outlined in Table 12.1. However, it is important to understand that Selection and Transplant rates are also under the control of physicians and these will be the most important factors discussed. Many of these factors appear self-evident to common sense and some of them are also scientifically proven. For example, advancing age leads to shorter survival as do systemic diseases such as diabetes mellitus and multiple myeloma. In rigorous multivariate analysis these two different factors, independent of each other, shorten survival [2–11].

It must also be understood that the interaction of these many factors may be incorrectly interpreted, even when scientifically studied. Almost all studies can be criticized either because the materials presenting detailed patient data were too small and therefore the complicated statistical analysis necessary was not robust, or if the mate-

L.W. Henderson and R.S. Thuma (eds.), Quality Assurance in Dialysis, 2nd Edition, 125–131.
© 1999 *Kluwer Academic Publishers. Printed in Great Britain*

Table 12.1. Risk factors for death in dialysis patients

I. Pre-existing	
1. Demographic	
Age	XXX
Sex	O
Race	XX
2. Social	
Married	?
Family support	?
Area	?
Smoking	?
Alcohol	?
Income	?
3. Diagnosis	
Diabetes	XXX
Hypertensive nephrosclerosis	XX
Systemic disease	XX
PCKD	++
4. Type and duration of renal failure	
Acute	?
Intermediate	?
Chronic	?
Late start	XX
5. Co-morbid conditions	
Chronic heart failure	XXX
Arteriosclerotic heart disease	XXX
Stroke	XXX
Peripheral vascular disease	?
Pulmonary	XXX
Malignancy	XXX
Gastrointestinal	?
Hepatic	?
Hypertension	XX
II. Selection	
6. Generous acceptance	XXX
High transplant rate	XXX
III. Treatment related	
7. Technical	
Late start	XX
Insufficient (Kt/V <90)	XXX
IPD	XXX
CAPD	?
FAST	?
Blood pressure control	XXX
Biocompatibility	?
Water quality	?
Membrane type	?
Reuse	?
8. Patient	
Malnutrition (low BUN/Cr-ratio low BUN, low Chol, low Alb, low BMI, low transferin)	XXX
High CA $\times$ PO$_4$ product	XXX
High interdialytic weight gain	XXX
Inactivity	XXX
Blood pressure control	XXX

XXX, leads to higher mortality; O, of no influence in mortality; ++, leads to lower mortality; ?, influence unknown

rial was large, many patient details provided, were invariably soft. For example, the European Dialysis Transplant Association have no rigorous, good, prospective data on co-morbid conditions besides the diagnosis of kidney disease. Finally there are poorly understood, and as yet unanalyzable shifts or changes in risk factors that occur with time. As patients were studied in one large center, the presence at start of dialysis of arteriosclerotic heart disease, stroke, COPD, malignancy or diabetes all adversely affected survival [4] but when the presence of these factors was studied in the same center in a patient population over the age of 70, they all disappeared as risk factors, advanced age overwhelmed all of them [12].

Finally, whatever the facts are, they will be the subject of wildly different interpretation depending on prejudice and interest. Whatever the merits or demerits of reuse are, the patient on dialysis will regard them with suspicion if he believes it will give him AIDS, but will like it if he believes it causes less damage to his blood. Both the greedy physician and the one who thinks protein coating is advantageous will like it, and the manufacturers of great quantities of cheap dialyzers view it with disdain.

INFLUENCE OF PRE-EXISTING RISK FACTORS

Demographic Risk Factors

Age is a very important risk factor. While life expectancy of both young and middle-aged patients is measured in decades, the mean survival time for patients above age 70 is only 5 years on dialysis [2–12]. However, the relative risk of dialysis, i.e. the chance of dying on dialysis over a 5 year period when compared to non-dialyzed age-matched population decreases with age. Thus young patients aged less than 45 years encounter a 20 times increased chance of dying within 5 years when they go on dialysis compared to only a twofold increase in patients over the age of 75. It is obvious that old age not only overrides other risk factors but also the very risk of dialysis itself [7]. Sex does not appear to be a risk factor, thus there is no difference in survival between men and women in the U.S. [4, 7, 10, 11]. On the contrary, race is of importance in that non-white patients survive better than white [10, 11]. The 5 year probability of surviving for black patients was 41.2% versus 37.4% for white patients, even when adjusted for age, sex and primary disease [11]. This unexpected result may have to do with the low transplant rate in black patients and points to an important role for selection in patient survival [13–15].

Social Risk Factor

There appear to be no good studies of the influence of marital status, family support or on the influence of smoking or alcohol. Income may in a perverse way influence survival on dialysis both in a positive and negative way. One can expect a poor patient to be more often malnourished, an important predictor of poor survival [16–18], but also to be less often transplanted [15], an important factor in improving survival on dialysis, as will be discussed.

Diagnosis

Certain diagnoses are associated with a higher death rate. This includes diabetes and hypertensive nephrosclerosis and some other systemic diseases such as myeloma and amyloid which appear to be associated with a shorter survival. On the other hand polycystic kidney disease appears to be associated with a good outcome [2–12].

Type and Duration of Renal Failure

There appear to be no good studies of this. Intuitively one would guess that a fairly short period of uremia may be associated with less chronic metabolic effects and thus with a "stronger body" starting dialysis.

Co-morbid Conditions

There are many studies that prove that the presence of other diseases may shorten survival on dialysis. Chronic heart disease, atherosclerotic heart disease, strokes, peripheral vascular disease, COPD and malignancies have all been associated with a poor outcome as has severe hypertension [2–11, 21]. Some of these diseases appear to be additive in their ill effect. For example, in one study, non-diabetic patients, younger than 45 years, without risk factor, had a 10% six year mortality, and those with arteriosclerotic heart disease or stroke had a 20% mortality rate but those with both diseases had a 40% mortality rate [4]. It is obvious that to evaluate the influence of all these co-morbid factors and their interrelationships with each other and age requires a large number of very carefully prospectively examined patients. Such material does not exist and may never be in existence.

Malnutrition is an extremely important factor in predicting outcome. Thus, patients who have a low BUN/creatinine ratio, or a low BUN, cholesterol, triglycerides, albumin, BMI or transferrin value have a very high mortality rate on dialysis [16–18].

THE INFLUENCE OF SELECTION AND TRANSPLANTATION

It is quite clear that as patients present to dialysis many factors exist which will predict their survival. It is then equally clear that by careful selection one can greatly influence survival results. We hypothesized that physicians who liberally accept many patients per population were likely to take on many old patients and many patients with degenerative diseases, systemic diseases, or malnourishment. The survival results of such a physician would be "poor" when compared to a more selective and fastidious physician who treated only those who were young, and except for their kidney disease, otherwise healthy. While this is self-evident, it may also appear equally self-evident that simple age matching could avoid many of these problems but things are more complicated than this as will be discussed below. Secondly, we hypothesized that someone who co-operated with a very active tranplant program would also have poor mortality rates. Over 80% of all patients who now start dialysis in the United States and in many other countries with a high acceptance rate, will remain on dialysis and not be transplanted. The chance of receiving a transplant is now falling all over the world as dialysis acceptance rates continue to rise, while tranplant rates have leveled or even declined [19]. Kidneys for transplantation are thus a much more scarce resource than machines for dialysis. Transplantation removes the very best patients, who are the young, without other diseases, and who have a long life-expectancy on dialysis. This results in a worse survival for centers with a high transplant rate when compared to centers where transplantation rates are low.

To investigate this we correlated cumulative 4 year survival in age-matched dialysis patients to acceptance rates for 5 European regions: Latin Europe (France, Spain and Italy), Benelux (Belgium, Netherlands and Luxembourg), German countries (Germany and Austria), the British Isles, Nordic countries (Sweden, Norway and Denmark) and the United States. Similarly, cumulative survival for these regions was correlated to the percent of patients transplanted at 4 years [20]. The results appears on Figure 12.1. In 1985, nephrologists in the U.S.A., where survival was lowest, accepted four times as many patients as British nephrologists and twice as many as in Sweden, Germany and Canada. The transplant rate was twice that in Latin and German countries. The data was also analyzed by stepwise and multiple regression analysis, which gave a much better fit than similar simple linear aggression: R = 0.96, $p = 0.02$ for the equation:

4 year cumulative dialysis survival =
$107 - 0.7 \times$ acceptance rate per million
$-0.4 \times$ percent transplated at 4 years [20].

Thus in this particular analysis over 90% of the differences in cumulative survival between regions were explained by different acceptance and transplant rates, even in age-matched patients. We have in a later model refined this approach and studied it for different age groups and also studied the influence of diabetes. In this newer model acceptance rates and percent patients with diabetes are the most important predictors of long term survival of young patients while transplant rates and acceptance rates appear more important for the old patients [21].

It is evident that acceptance and transplant criteria are important determinants when other factors are held constant, but beyond that probably also represent other factors that may be very difficult to define and to quantitate for a unit. Such factors include clinical impression that encompasses the cumulative sum of or subtle grading of

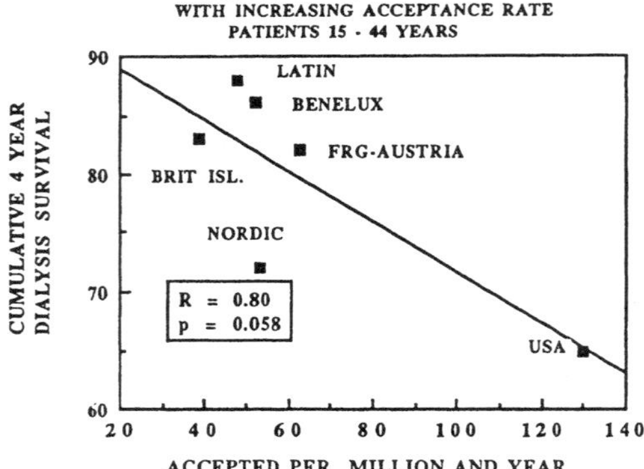

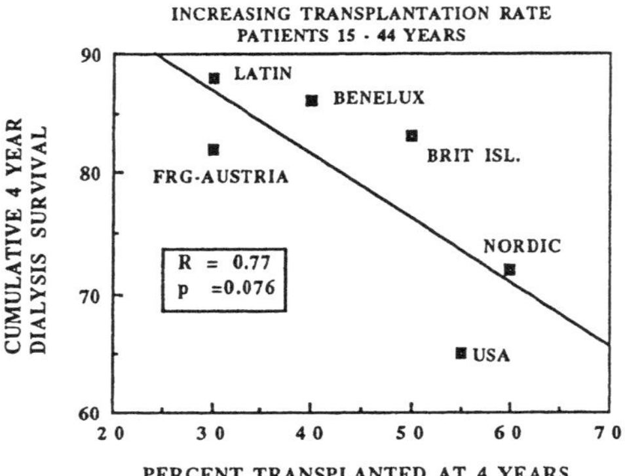

Fig. 12.1. (Top) Linear regression analysis showing the relation between cumulative 4-year dialysis survival for patients age 15–44 and the acceptance rate to dialysis. The more patients that are accepted, the worse is cumulative survival. (Bottom) Cumulative 4-year dialysis survival in relation to the percent of patients transplanted at 4 years. The cumulative survival becomes worse as more patients receive transplants at 4 years. The transplant surgeon takes the young and healthy who show good survival on dialysis and leaves only the old and those with many other diseases who have poor survival. When both acceptance rate and transplant rates are evaluated through multiple regression analysis, over 90% of the differences in cumulative survival are explained. Thus, differences in survival are not dependent on geographical location, but on generosity in acceptance and transplant rates. (From reference 20, reproduced with permission of W.B. Saunders Co.).

co-morbid conditions. These factors are already playing a role in U.S.A. as indicated by an article investigating case mix of patients with end-stage renal disease in profit and non-profit dialysis units

[22]. When 307 patients treated in 5 proprietary, free-standing, profit based units were compared to 3,135 patients treated in non-profit making hospitals, it was found that when the patients were ranked in severity groups based on age, race, primary renal disease and co-morbid conditions, the hospital-based facilities had a higher percentage of patients who were more ill. Thus 60% of the hospital-treated patients were in the 3 groups with the highest severity index but only 50% of the patients in free-standing facilities had such a high index. However, even within each severity group, hospital-based patients had a lower 5 year survival rate than patients in free-standing facilities [8, 22]. One interpretation of these data is that the for-profit units offered better treatment. My interpretation is that their fastidious selection was the cause of the better survival and that the severity indexes used were simply very crude compared to clinical impressions by physicians selecting patients to their profit units. Patient dumping obviously has at its base economic considerations [23]. The old, the sick and the malnourished will cost more, because they are more difficult to care for. When they are dumped on public facilities not only does the survival curve for the fastidious unit shift upwards but the survival curve of the receiving hospital will shift downwards [22, 23]. This gives the twice false impression, that quality is better, when in reality selection is the reason for the improved survival. In a perverse fashion then "better may actually mean worse". Fastidious "good outcome" physicians have not fulfilled their obligations to those who need their services particularly urgently.

One can of course argue that "sick" patients should not be treated at all as the life expectancy is short and the cost relatively high. Actually, when counted in QUALY's hemodialysis for any patient fares very poorly. When the yearly cost is divided by the expected quality of life and its duration the figures become very high [24, 25]. The ultimate extension of this of course is that "the only good patient is a dead patient" and although one can shrug that off as a meaningless cynicism, when this is brought into the clinical arena it is indeed a deadening reality for the old, as the easiest of all selection criteria is age, in itself often used to exclude the old from treatment [26–28].

TREATMENT RELATED FACTORS

Technical

This group of factors is the true matter of investigation for quality assurance:

Is the physician performing technically adequate dialysis?

Many factors enter into this equation, and over some the physician has only partial control as for example late start of dialysis. It has been shown that patients who come with severe uremia to dialysis may have incurable secondary metabolic effects that lead to complications and an increased mortality [29], while those started early do particularly well [30]. To give a patient insufficient dialysis, for example as expressed as Kt/V of less than 0.9 has been associated with a high morbidity [31, 32]. Similarly intermittent peritoneal dialysis is no longer regularly used because of the high complication rate and the high mortality associated with this procedure [7]. Comparable data do not exist for home hemodialysis and what differences exist, appear best explained by different selection criteria [7, 9, 10]. CAPD has the advantage of an even control of uremia and electrolytes but offers the patient Kt/V values that are insufficient for hemodialysis patients [31, 32]. Fast dialysis has also been associated with an increased mortality [33] but much of this appears to be due to the fact that fast sufficient dialysis and short insufficient dialysis are not separated [34]. Another factor though is that fast dialysis, even when thought to be adequate, may in reality more easily become inadequate than slower and longer dialysis. Biocompatibility has been one factor associated with outcome. More biocompatible and open membranes have been thought to lead to less dialysis arthropathy – amyloid. However, the largest study of this problem, comparing the 10 year incidence of these diseases between matched patients on polyacrylonitrile or cellophane membranes has failed to show any statistical significance [35]. Still, many physicians will use the open membrane for patients. The higher cost of this, in a system with a capped budget, results in an erroneously perceived increased quality for some patients but *no* dialysis for others.

Blood pressure control during dialysis is an

important factor for longevity as shown many years ago [36]. Reuse, that has resulted in lethal infection, has invariably been associated with a higher survival or no difference in survival when compared to no-reuse in rigorous studies [8].

PATIENT TREATMENT RELATED FACTORS

These factors are only partially under a physician's control. For example, a high calcium × phosphorus product, malnutrition, "giving up", a high intradialytic weight gain and hypertension are factors over which physicians have only partial control [8]. These factors are only partially influenced by a physician's actions and patient education, but are much influenced by compliance. Inactivity in old patients has also been associated with a high mortality rate. It is not known if inactivity only is the reflection of other underlying factors that simultaneously shorten life and lead to inactivity, or if it is a risk factor itself, that can be influenced by education, physical therapy and training [12].

CONCLUSIONS

The real purpose of quality assurance in dialysis appears to me to be to detect the insufficiencies in technical treatment related factors. Obvious other factors which need to be considered are demographic, social, diagnostic and co-morbid conditions. Other factors complicate the evaluation because of their subtle interaction between technical treatment factors and patient compliance. Such factors are blood pressure and $Ca \times PO_4$ product, nutrition, weight gain and inactivity. Overriding all the previous ones in influencing mortality are generosity in selection and a high transplant rate. Both of these will negatively influence survival of dialysis patients. Therefore "worse may be better" and it does not appear unreasonable to at least consider that a "poor outcome" is indicative that the physician has fulfilled his obligation to a larger number of truly sick patients much better than one whose survival curves look more favorable. Ignoring this fact carries the risk that good physicians will be discouraged, shytsters rewarded and large patient groups remain untreated and die earlier.

REFERENCES

1. Carlson DM, Johnson WJ and Kjellstrand CM. Functional status of patients with end-stage renal disease. Mayo Clin Proc 1987; 62:338–44.
2. Degoulet P, Legrain M, Reach I, Aime F, Devries C, Rojas P et al. Mortality risk factors in patients treated by chronic hemodialysis. Nephron 1982; 31:103–10.
3. Hutchinson T, Thomas DC and MacGibbon B. Predicting survival in adults with end-stage renal disease: an age equivalence index. Ann Int Med 1982;96:417–23.
4. Shapiro FL and Umen A. Risk factors in hemodialysis patient survival. ASAIO 1983; 6:176–84.
5. Vollmer WM, Wahl PW and Blagg CR. Survival with dialysis and transplantation in patients with end-stage renal disease. N Engl J Med 1983; 308:1553–8.
6. Neff MS, Eiser AR, Slifkin RF, Baum M, Baez A, Gupta S et al. Patients surviving 10 years of hemodialysis. Am J Med 1983; 74:996–1003.
7. Hellerstedt BA, Johnson WJ, Ascher N, Kjellstrand CM, Knutson R, Shapiro FL et al. Survival rates of 2,728 patients with end-stage renal disease. Mayo Clin Proc 1984; 59:776–83.
8. Held PJ, Pauly MV and Diamond L. Survival analysis of patients undergoing dialysis. J Am Med Assoc 1987; 257:645–50.
9. Mailloux LU, Bellucci AG, Mossey RT, Napolitano B, Moore T, Wilkes BM et al. Predictors of survival in patients undergoing dialysis. Am J Med 1988; 84:855–62.
10. Silins J, Fortier L, Mao Y, Posen G, Ugnat A-M, Brancker A et al. Mortality rates among patients with end-stage renal disease in Canada, 1981–86. CMAJ 1989; 141:677–82.
11. Renal Data System U.S.A., The National Institutes of Health, The National Institute of Diabetes and Digestive and Kidney Diseases, Division of Kidney, Urologic and Hematologic Diseases, Bethesda, MD. Annual Report, 1989.
12. Westlie L, Umen A, Nestrud S and Kjellstrand C. Mortality, morbidity and life satisfaction in the old dialysis patient. Trans Am Soc Artif Intern Organs 1984; 30:21–30.
13. Kjellstrand CM. Giving life–giving death. Ethical problems with high technology medicine. Acta Med Scand 1988; 725:1–80.
14. Kjellstrand CM. Racial, sexual and age discrimination in renal transplantation. Arch Intern Med 1988; 148:1305–9.
15. Held PJ, Pauly MV, Bovbjerg RR, Newman J, Salvatierra O Jr. Access to kidney transplantation – has the United States eliminated income and racial differences? Arch Intern Med 1988; 148:2594–600.
16. Acchiardo SR, Moore LW and Latour P. Malnutrition as the main factor in morbidity and mortality of hemodialysis patients. Kidney Int 1983; 24:S199–203.
17. Oksa H, Pasternack A and Pasanen M. Serum urea–creatinine ratio as a prognostic index in hemodialysis patients. Clin Neph 1987; 27:125–30.
18. Marckmann P. Nutritional status and mortality of patients in regular dialysis therapy. J Int Med 1989; 226:429–32.

19. Kjellstrand CM and Shideman J. On the impact of and need for chronic dialysis and renal transplantation. Trans Am Soc Artif Intern Organs 1988; 34:328–32.

20. Kjellstrand CM, Hylander B and Collins A. Mortality on dialysis – on the influence of early start, patient characteristics, and transplantation and acceptance rates. Am J Kidney Dis 1990; 15:483–90.

21. Collins A, Kjellstrand CM, Hull A and Parker T. Mortality on dialysis appears directly dependent on the generosity of the nephrologist and the activity of the transplant surgeon. ASAIO 1990; 36:16 (abstract).

22. Plough AL, Salem SR, Shwartz M, Weller JM and Ferguson CW. Case mix in end-stage renal disease. N Engl J Med 1984; 1432–6.

23. Ansell DA and Schiff RL. Patient dumping: status, implications, and policy recommendations. J Am Med Assoc 1987; 257:1500–2.

24. Williams A. Economics of coronary artery bypass grafting. Br Med J 1985; 291:326–9.

25. La Puma J and Lawlor EF. Quality-adjusted life-years: ethical implications for physicians and policymakers. J Am Med Assoc 1990; 263:2917–21.

26. Wetle T. Age as a risk factor for inadequate treatment. J Am Med Assoc 1987; 258:516.

27. Lamm RD. Health care as economic cancer. Dial Transplant 1987; 16:432–3.

28. Callahan D. Setting limits – medical goals in an aging society. New York, Simon & Schuster; 1987.

29. Kjellstrand CMN, Evzans RL, Petersen RJ, Shideman JR, von Hartitzsch B and Buselmeier TJ. The "unphysiology" of dialysis: a major cause of dialysis side effects? Kidney Int 1975; 7:S30–4.

30. Bonomini V, Feletti C, Stefoni S and Vangelista A. Early dialysis and renal transplantation. Nephron 1984; 44:267–71.

31. Lowrie EG, Laird NM, Parker TF and Sargent JA. Effect of the hemodialysis prescription on patient morbidity. N Engl J Med 1981; 305:1176–81.

32. Gotsch FA and Sargent JA. A mechanistic analysis of the National Cooperative Dialysis Study (NCDS). Kidney Int 1985; 128:526–34.

33. Kjellstrand CM. Short dialysis increases morbidity and mortality. Contr Nephrol 1985; 44:65–77.

34. Levin NW. Mortality impacts of shorter dialysis procedures. Kidney Int 1989; 35:254.

35. Brunner FP, Brynger H, Ehrich JHH, Fassbinder W, Geerlings W, Rizzoni G et al. Case control study on dialysis arthropathy: the influence of two different dialysis membranes: data from the EDTA registry. Nephrol Dial Trans 1990; 5:432–6.

36. Lundin P, Adler AJ, Feinroth MV, Berlyne GM and Friedman EA. Maintenance hemodialysis. J Am Med Assoc 1980; 244:38–40.

13. Quality of care in the pre-ESRD period; impact on survival in the first year of dialysis

JAMES TATTERSALL

INTRODUCTION

Most of the recent published data linking quality of care to survival in patients with renal failure have concentrated on the care given after the patient has started dialysis. However, many of the medical problems experienced by dialysis patients and causing death in the early years of dialysis, may be preventable by adequate care in the years before dialysis starts. Dialysis patients generally have significant co-morbidity on commencement of dialysis and the extent of this co-morbidity determines the eventual outcome on dialysis even more than the quality of care given during while the patient is receiving dialysis [1]. Co-morbidity commonly includes hypertensive and ischemic heart disease, [2] generalized vascular disease [3], advanced diabetic complications [4], malnutrition [5] and renal bone disease [6]. These complications are difficult to treat and are largely irreversible. On the other hand, they are largely or completely preventable. Since the co-morbidity is generally established when dialysis starts, it is obvious that we should concentrate our main effort on managing patients in the period before dialysis starts.

No-one would argue with the need for high-quality care in the pre-dialysis period. It is also generally accepted that this care is not generally available for economic reasons. However, one of the main functions of this pre-dialysis care is to halt or slow the progression of renal failure and to prevent or delay the complications of renal failure. Therefore, pre-dialysis care should be highly cost-effective.

Our healthcare systems are overburdened with increasing numbers of poorly re-habilitated dialy-sis patients who are difficult and expensive to treat and have high morbidity and mortality. High quality pre-dialysis care is an economic, practical and ethical necessity if we are to reverse these trends.

CLEARANCE AND Kt/V

Traditionally, renal function has been monitored using blood urea and creatinine concentrations during the period before dialysis starts. Dialysis is started either when the patient develops uremic symptoms or signs or when the blood urea and creatinine concentrations have risen above a certain level. This approach is now known to be flawed. Firstly, the symptoms and signs of uremia are subtle and may not become obvious until the uremic state is well advanced. By this time the patient will almost certainly be malnourished and his chances of survival be compromised. Secondly, their blood urea and creatinine concentrations may not rise as renal function declines. Indeed, patients with the most advanced uremic state may well have blood urea and creatinine concentrations which are not particularly high. This is because the malnutrition which usually results from advanced renal failure causes muscle wasting and reduced protein catabolism, in turn reducing the generation rate of urea and creatinine. In order to separate the effects of solute generation and clearance, it is necessary to measure renal function directly, usually from 24 hour urine collections. In this way, the decision to start dialysis can be made before the patient becomes overtly uremic. These are analogous to the arguments for measuring Kt/

L.W. Henderson and R.S. Thuma (eds.), Quality Assurance in Dialysis, 2nd Edition, 133–142.
© *1999 Kluwer Academic Publishers. Printed in Great Britain*

V in dialysis patients. The appendix outlines some of the methodology and principles of quantifying renal clearance.

THE LINK BETWEEN ADEQUACY AND OUTCOME IN THE PRE-DIALYSIS PERIOD

It is now generally accepted that low urea clearance is associated with increased mortality in dialysis patients [7]. There is also emerging evidence that there is a link between the renal clearance at the time dialysis starts and eventual outcome. The initial blood urea and creatinine levels do not have this predictive power. The CANUSA study [8] demonstrated a significant relationship between Kt/V at the initiation of dialysis and mortality in CAPD patients. However, the study patients received standard therapy without adjustments for renal function and most of the variation in Kt/V was due to differences in renal function. Therefore, the CANUSA study may be demonstrating only a link between renal function at the start of treatment and mortality. When the CANUSA data was re-examined for renal GFR measured at the end of CAPD training, it was found to be a significant independent predictor of subsequent mortality. Controlling for age, diabetes, cardiovascular disease, country of treatment, and serum albumin concentration, the multivariate Cox proportional hazards model showed a relative risk of death of 0.95 for a 5 L per week greater GFR at initiation of dialysis [53].

There are many theoretical reasons why low renal clearance at the start of dialysis may result in a reduced chance of survival. They may have been referred late, when uremic complications have already developed. They may also have been referred appropriately but started dialysis late because they were malnourished and their low urea and creatinine values lead to a false sense of security. These patients may also have more aggressive form of kidney disease leading to a rapid fall-off in GFR and a more heavy reliance on CAPD in the early years of dialysis.

NUTRITIONAL STATUS

It is becoming increasingly recognized that mal-nourished patients do very badly on dialysis. Low serum albumin is the single most powerful predictor of death in dialysis patients [9]. This association between low albumin an mortality is thought to be partly due to the albumin being low in severely malnourished patients. Perhaps more convincingly, low blood urea and creatinine concentrations have also been shown to be powerful predictors of mortality [9]. These solutes are generated at a lower rate in malnutrition and low levels are markers of malnutrition in dialysis patients.

Malnutrition is common in patients with renal failure not yet on dialysis. A recent study by Ikizler et al. [10] showed that dietary protein intake (DPI) declined progressively as creatinine clearance fell below 50 mL/minute (Table 13.1)

Table 13.1. Dietary protein intake (DPI) in varying degrees of renal failure

Creatinine clearance (mL/min)	Dietary protein intake (g/kg per day)
> 50	1.01 ± 0.21
25–50	0.85 ± 0.23
10–25	0.70 ± 0.17
< 10	0.54 ± 0.16

Malnutrition may also adversely influence renal function, amplifying the decline in nutrition [11]. The nutrition status of the patient at the start of dialysis is also a powerful predictor of survival on dialysis [12, 13].

The nutritional status of dialysis patients generally improves after dialysis has started [14, 15], indicating that the malnutrition is reversed by timely dialysis.

Malnutrition is not an absolutely inevitable consequence of renal failure. Patients receiving a low-protein diet with supplementation had excellent survival [16] and good nutritional indices at the initiation of dialysis [17]. The reason for the good survival in these studies is probably the careful follow up and nutritional supervision in the pre-dialysis period. Correction of acidosis, depression, anaemia, cardiac failure and other chronic illness also has the potential for reversing the malnutrition [18].

The role of a low-protein diet in advanced renal failure is controversial. Although a low-protein diet is likely to slow the progression of renal failure, worries about its impact on an already compromised nutritional state have prevented its widespread use. The recent studies confirming the beneficial effects and demonstrating a lack of adverse effect of low-protein diets have renewed interest. However, the low protein diet is likely to be beneficial and safe only if the patient receives careful nutritional follow-up and, probably, nutritional supplementation in the pre-dialysis period.

It seems that nutrition is an important dimension of the uremic state and malnutrition has devastating consequences on the patient. Careful nutritional assessment is needed to assist in the timely initiation of dialysis and to detect or prevent malnutrition. In addition, nutritional intervention has the potential to halt or slow the progression of renal failure making it cost-effective.

ACID/BASE STATUS

One of the functions of the human kidney is to regenerate bicarbonate. Hemodialysis achieves this by including a supra-physiological concentration of bicarbonate in the dialysis fluid. During dialysis, bicarbonate diffuses into the blood across the dialyzer membrane. One of the aims of dialysis is to normalise the serum bicarbonate concentration. Optimal survival has been shown to relate to normal pre-dialysis serum bicarbonate concentration [9].

Metabolic acidosis has the potential for causing malnutrition [19]. Increasing the blood bicarbonate in hemodialysis [20] and CAPD [21] patients has been shown to increase nutritional markers. It is likely that acidosis is one of may factors inducing malnutrition although it is difficult to separate from other effects of uremia.

Metabolic acidosis also causes osteomalacia [22]. There have been few studies in the pre-dialysis period but in dialysis patients, a time-averaged serum bicarbonate of 24 mmol/L is considered to be the gold standard of optimal control [23]. Metabolic acidosis not difficult to detect and treat and so a policy to maintain the bicarbonate concentration close to this ideal is practical. In practice, metabolic acidosis is rare when dialysis is started at the current recommended level of GFR.

In my experience, patients with metabolic acidosis generally qualify for starting dialysis on other criteria and treatment with oral bicarbonate in these patients is hardly ever needed except when there is also a renal tubular bicarbonate wasting state. Similarly, by definition, an adequately dialyzed patient will not have metabolic acidosis unless there is an independent cause.

PARATHYROID AND CALCIUM

Hypocalcemia and hyperphosphatemia with secondary hyper-parathyroidism are common in chronic renal failure. In a recent study, almost 40% of patients starting dialysis had evidence of chronic hypocalcemia [24]. Calcium levels critically affect almost all cellular processes and abnormalities in calcium metabolism are likely to have a strong impact on outcome. Renal bone disease, which is mainly a disorder of calcium homeostasis is very common in dialysis patients, causes much morbidity and is difficult and expensive to treat. Secondary hyper-parathyroidism which results from chronic hypocalcemia in renal disease has been implicated in the development of left ventricular hypertrophy [25] which, in turn is a strong predictor of poor outcome [30]. Calciphylaxis [26] a more extreme manifestation of abnormal calcium metabolism is very difficult to treat and is often fatal.

The serum calcium concentrations when dialysis is started are a powerful predictor of subsequent mortality [24]. In addition to the hypocalcemia, renal bone disease is often already present when dialysis starts. In one study, 32% of 92 unselected patients with creatinine clearance < 10 mL/minute but not yet on dialysis has adynamic bone disease on bone biopsy [27].

All of these complications result from abnormal calcium metabolism over many months or years. In theory, most of the abnormalities are preventable by treatment with calcitriol and phosphate binders. But this treatment should be started long before dialysis starts. Systematic management of calcium homeostasis in the pre-dialysis period is complex and demanding. However, it is likely to prevent or reduce serious morbidity and the high cost associated with the complications of abnormal calcium metabolism.

ANEMIA

Chronic renal failure is almost invariably associated with anemia due to deficiency of erythropoition, iron or other hematinics if these are not corrected. Optimal survival and quality of life on dialysis has been shown to depend on a relatively normal hematocrit [28]. In the anemic state, reduced blood oxygen-carrying capacity must be compensated for by increasing cardiac output. This is likely to lead directly to left ventricular hypertrophy (LVH – see below) which is an important contributor to the premature death of dialysis patients [30].

Since cardiovascular problems are the commonest cause of death in dialysis patients, and LVH is often already present when dialysis starts, maintaining a normal hematocrit in the pre-dialysis period should be of supreme interest.

Treatment of renal anemia is now relatively uncontroversial and guidelines exist. Experience has shown that the use of erythropoitin in the pre-dialysis period is safe and may also slow the progression of renal failure [29].

LVH

Left ventricular hypertrophy (LVH) is known to be a powerful predictor of death in dialysis patients [30]. If it is present at the start of dialysis, it is a powerful predictor of poor survival on dialysis [31]. LVH is an adaptation to a chronically high cardiac output and is caused by hypertension, fluid overload, anemia and, possibly, vasoldilator drugs – all common factors in renal failure. The majority of deaths on dialysis, at least during the first few years, is caused by cardiac disease and LVH is thought to be a major factor in these deaths.

LVH tends to develop relatively early in the course of the renal failure [32] and is normally established when dialysis starts [30] (Table 11.2).

The LVH has been shown to be associated with high systolic, but not diastolic BP [32], high cardiac output, fluid overload, anemia [32] and high parathyroid hormone levels [33].

Fortunately, there is now plenty of evidence that treating the causes of the LVH can prevent, reverse, or at least delay the progression of LVH.

Table 13.2. Prevalence of left ventricular hypertrophy (LVH) in varying degrees of renal failure

Creatinine clearance (mL/min)	% of patients with LVH
> 30 (patients attending nephrology clinic)	16
< 30	38
At start of dialysis	70

Treatment with ACE inhibitors but not calcium antagonists has been shown to cause regression of LVH after dialysis has started, independently from hypotensive effects [34, 35]. ACE inhibition also reduced LVH in the pre-dialysis period [36]. In dialysis patients, correction of anemia by erythropoitin has resulted in a regression of LVH [37]. Treatment of hyper-parathyroidism by parathyroidectomy has also been shown to induce regression of LVH [33].

Prevention of LVH in the pre-dialysis period includes aggressive blood pressure control, use of ACE-inhibitors or angiotensin antagonists, normalization of the hematocrit and attention to fluid overload. In renal failure, hypertension is usually due to a combination of activation of the renin-angiotensin system and chronic fluid overload. Blood pressure control should logically be controlled by diuretics combined with fluid restriction and, if necessary ACE-inhibitors or angiotensin antagonists. Anti-hypertensives whose main mode of action is vasodilatory should be avoided since they will increase cardiac output and, in theory, increase LVH.

Attention to the causes of LVH in the pre-dialysis period is likely to have a dramatic impact on the survival of dialysis patients. The current prevalence of 70% of patients starting dialysis with LVH leaves no room for complacency.

PSYCHOLOGICAL AND PRACTICAL ISSUES

Professional care in the period before dialysis starts includes education, and psychological support. During this period, the patient may make a more relaxed adjustment to his impending dialysis and to make informed decisions regarding his care and type of dialysis.

In a recent study, the majority of patients offered a free choice between dialysis modalities chose self-care options including CAPD [38]. However, almost all patients who had not received nephrology care in the pre-dialysis period were treated by centre hemodialysis [39]. This suggests that nephrology care in the pre-dialysis period is important for preparing the patient to receive the most appropriate dialysis modality.

Also, patients with advanced renal failure may deny the severity of their illness and fail to comply with treatment for their renal disease. They are more likely to smoke, and to have poor compliance with blood pressure and blood sugar lowering medication. A component of the co-morbidity and mortality associated with renal failure is related to lifestyle and compliance issues.

There has been very little work to address these important issues [40]. The Vancouver pre-ESRD programs has been demonstrated to reduce urgent dialysis starts (13% vs. 35%; $p < 0.05$), increase outpatient training (76% vs. 43%; $p < 0.05$), and reduce hospital days in the first month of dialysis (6.5 days vs. 13.5 days; $p < 0.05$). Cost savings due to the program in 1993 were conservatively estimated to be $173,000 (Canadian dollars) or over $4000 per patient [41]. Also, patients who have received multidisciplinary pre-dialysis care were more likely to retain employment after dialysis starts [42].

In hemodialysis, the preferred access type is the A-V fistula [43]. This needs to be placed at least 3 weeks and preferably 3–6 months before dialysis starts [44]. The timely selection and creation of an appropriate access is clearly a quality issue in the period before dialysis starts. Morbidity and hospitalization is increased when dialysis is delivered using PTFE grafts or central venous cannulation.

BLOOD SUGAR CONTROL

Between 30–50% of patients starting dialysis have diabetic renal disease, making this the most common cause of end-stage renal failure in the US and Europe. These diabetic renal failure patients are also the most expensive and difficult to treat and have the worst outcome. As lifestyles and eating habits become "westernized" the incidence of diabetes elsewhere in the world is increasing and diabetes may soon become the most common cause of renal failure world-wide. The poorer countries who are experiencing an epidemic of diabetes are ill-equipped to cope with the resulting renal-failure.

Diabetics starting dialysis tend to be those with the worst blood sugar control, probably due to poor compliance. Intensive diabetic control started early in the course of the diabetes has been shown to almost completely eliminate the risk of developing renal failure over a 35 year period [45]. Even when diabetics with relatively advanced disease are treated with intensive blood sugar control the mortality and rate of progression of renal failure is reduced by over 40% [46]. At present, there is no conclusive evidence that diabetic renal failure can develop in well-controlled diabetics. Therefore, diabetic renal disease may be considered to be mostly or entirely preventable. Blood sugar control in the pre-dialysis period has also been shown to be a marker for subsequent mortality once dialysis starts [47].

There is now substantial evidence that ACE inhibitors can reduce the rate of progression of diabetic renal disease, independently of any hypotensive effect [48]. Furthermore, treatment with ACE inhibitors has been shown to be cost-effective, resulting in savings of over $1.5 million in a cohort of 1000 diabetic patients over a 4-year period [49].

For these reasons, strict control of blood sugar and treatment with ACE inhibitors should be one of the main aims in pre-dialysis care the diabetic. Since the families of patients with diabetic renal disease are at increased risk of developing renal failure [50], they should be encouraged to attend for screening.

The high prevalence of diabetes in patients starting dialysis should be considered as both a massive failure in past management and prevention of diabetes and also a substantial opportunity for reducing the incidence of end-stage renal failure [51].

WHEN SHOULD WE START DIALYSIS ?

A fit patient with chronic renal failure attending a clinic is likely to be far cheaper to manage than a patient who has been established on dialysis. If dialysis is started unnecessarily early then costs would increase. However, the cost-savings resulting from a delayed start to dialysis may be cancelled out by the cost of any increased morbidity or hospitalizations [52].

At present, there is no clear consensus on when dialysis should start. The confusion may be exploited by the patient who will often be in denial of the existence of his or her renal failure or unaware of its consequences and will pressurize the physician to delay the start of dialysis. In capitated or systems other than fee-for-service, hospital managers may also pressurize the physician to delay the start of dialysis for economic reasons, unaware or unconvinced of the hidden cost of delayed start.

For these reasons, it has become imperative that objective data is applied to guide the selection of the most appropriate time to start dialysis. While many of the functions of the failing kidney (e.g. hemoglobin and blood pressure homeostasis) can be supported or replaced without dialysis, the excretory and base regeneration functions cannot. Therefore, the timing of the start of dialysis must mainly be guided by measurement of clearance, acid-base and volume status. Clinical symptoms are unreliable as they are subjective and prone to bias. They also tend to occur late in the progression of renal failure and be non-specific.

Although monitoring of the patients nutritional status is necessary as part of the pre-dialysis care, it is of limited use in guiding the timing of the start of dialysis. The early signs of malnutrition are subtle and easy to miss. Patients' nutritional requirements vary and malnutrition may be caused by factors other than uremia. In my view, in realistic medical practice, unless we have very tight dietetic supervision we are likely to miss the optimal time to start dialysis if we wait for malnutrition to be detected. It is probably unrealistic to expect an objective nutritional index which will reliably detect subtle malnutrition in all patents. We need to judge the start of dialysis at that point just before the patient develops any observable adverse effect of uremia including malnutrition.

There is unlikely to be a hard threshold of renal clearance below which problems inevitably occur. However, there are already published data which quantifies risk of malnutrition and subsequent mortality according to level of renal clearance at the start of dialysis. Data from the CANUSA and other studies has suggested a normalized renal creatinine clearance of 9–14 mL/minute or a weekly SRI (Kt/V) of 2.0 as the threshold [53]. The current DOQI guidelines support this approach but accept that dialysis may be started at lower levels of renal function if nutrition is carefully monitored and shown to be adequate and if there are absolutely no adverse symptoms or signs of uremia.

The level of renal function at which dialysis should be started is a dynamic quantity. Dialysis should be started at the point at which the adverse effects of delaying dialysis further outweighs the adverse effects and disadvantages of the dialysis itself. As our ability to deliver safer, better tolerated and more powerful dialysis increases, the level of renal function at which dialysis is started will also increase. In general, this level will be close to the level considered as the minimum acceptable equivalent clearance for dialysis patients (see Appendix).

Although guided by objective measurement and analysis of the literature, the actual decision to start dialysis is the result of a subjective assessment of the impact of uremia and dialysis on the patient's life. The informed patient is best placed to make this decision.

LATE NEPHROLOGY REFERRAL.

There have been numerous studies demonstrating worse survival in patients who are referred to nephrology late in the progression of renal failure [54]. More than half of 184 consecutive nondiabetic patients starting dialysis at a centre in Brazil were referred less than one month before dialysis was started. The mortality rates during the first six months of dialysis in the late referred patients was more than 2.5 times higher than in those patients who were referred earlier [55].

Patients who are referred late generally have more co-morbidity than those who are referred earlier. This increased co morbidity may explain all of the excess mortality in this group. It is likely that some, if not all, of the co-morbidity in the late referred patients was acquired due to uremia or lack of adequate preventative care during the pre-dialysis period.

Alternatively, and more disturbingly, those patients with high co-morbidity are less likely to be referred early by the general or family physician. This may be for economic or ethical reasons. However, when these high-risk patients become moribund due to uremia, they are then referred for dialysis urgently. There is, as yet no published data quantifying this problem but, from numerous anecdotes, this practice is undoubtedly widespread. These moribund patients whose suitability for dialysis has been questioned are the most difficult and expensive to treat and have the worst outcome of all.

Although the earlier the patient is referred, the greater the opportunity for prevention, those patients who already have high co-morbidity would most benefit from early referral.

There are often economic pressures on general or family physicians to hang onto their renal failure patients as long as possible. In capitated or managed systems, these physicians have the explicit role as gatekeeper, limiting or delaying access to specialist medical services. Since these delays result in sicker patients being referred for dialysis, the costs of care of the dialysis patients are increased and their morbidity and mortality are also increased. This makes dialysis appear to be a poor value-for-money treatment and will further inhibit referral.

CONCLUSION: THE CASE FOR PRE-DIALYSIS CARE.

The aim of pre-dialysis care is to prevent or delay the progression of renal failure and its complications, and to prepare the patient so that he is able to make informed decisions regarding the treatment of his renal failure. A multi-disciplinary team with specialist expertise in treating renal failure is best able to provide better and more cost-effective care of renal anemia, renal bone disease, hypertension, and the underlying renal disease. Although pre-dialysis care is likely to result in starting dialysis at an earlier stage of declining renal function, the potential for delaying this decline means that this start may not necessarily be at an earlier point in time.

If this team also has responsibility for the patient's care after dialysis starts they will be better placed to assist in decisions regarding choice of dialysis modality and the appropriateness and timing of the start of dialysis. These decisions will be made in the context of ongoing responsibility and appreciation for the consequences and cost of these decisions after dialysis has started.

One of the biggest social challenges facing the word at present is how to provide fair and equal access to healthcare at reasonable cost. Our failure to prevent diseases which require expensive treatment such as dialysis is a major contributor to the problem. Attempts to push down the costs or limit the availability of these treatments has resulted in serious ethical and practical dilemmas. Pre-dialysis care, offers the prospect of reducing or avoiding these problems altogether. In addition to its preventative role, pre-dialysis care provides the opportunity for systematically collecting information which can be used to guide the difficult decisions which must be made when expensive treatment is inevitable.

APPENDIX

Calculation of Solute Removal Index (SRI) and Weekly Creatinine Clearance (CCr)

It is now customary to measure renal function and dialysis clearance in CAPD patients and report the result as creatinine clearance (CCr) in L/week/ 1.73 m^2 and weekly Kt/V. Both these clearance parameters have been shown to relate to survival in CAPD [8]. It seems logical to use the same methodology to measure renal clearance in the period before dialysis starts. Dialysis should be started when CCr and Kt/V fall below the minimum recommended values for CAPD regardless of the blood urea and creatinine concentrations.

In CAPD, kidney function or any continuous treatment, Kt/V is the mass of urea cleared per week divided by the mass of urea in the patient. In hemodialysis, the intermittency of the treatment results in a more complicated relationship between Kt/V and mass cleared. The more intermittent and intense the treatment (i.e. shorter or less frequent) the less mass is cleared for a given weekly Kt/V. A patient treated by hemodialysis with a Kt/V of 1.4 delivered over 4 hours three times per week will clear as much urea as a CAPD patient receiving a weekly Kt/V of 2. It has been proposed that hemodialysis dose is quantified by measuring the mass of urea removed as in CAPD or renal function. This approach leads to the solute removal index (SRI) which is the mass of urea removed per week divided by the peak mass of urea in the patient. In continuous treatments SRI is exactly equal to the weekly Kt/V. In hemodialysis, SRI can be measured using dialysate collections or from pre-and post dialysis blood urea concentrations when it is approximately equal to the urea reduction ratio (URR) multiplied by the number of treatments per week if the concept of peak toxicity is acceped.

To avoid confusion, with Kt/V in hemodialysis, I prefer to use the term SRI instead of Kt/V when quantifying renal function and CAPD. If hemodialysis is also quantified using SRI, then allowing for renal function and comparison with CAPD is greatly simplified.

In CAPD, the recent CANUSA study demonstrated a significant positive relationship between survival and total (renal plus dialytic) creatinine and urea clearance [56]. Based on the results of this study, it is now recommended that CAPD patients receive at least a Kt/V of 2 per week and a creatinine clearance of 60 L/week/1.75 m^2. In hemodialysis, the recommended minimum Kt/V of 1.4 three times per week [57] translates to a SRI of 2 per week – the same as the recommended minimum dose in CAPD. At present there is no recommended minimum creatinine clearance for hemodialysis as there is in CAPD but the same value of 60 L/week/1.73 m^2 is practically achievable and would be logical.

In this case, dialysis should be started when SRI falls below 2 and creatinine clearance below 60 L/week/1.73 m^2. These values translate to a urea clearance of 7 mL/min/1.73 m^2 and a creatinine clearance of 6 mL/min/1.73 m^2.

SRI and weekly creatinine clearance can be calculated using the equations below.

The surface area (*SA*) in m^2 and body water volume in liters (*V*) is calculated using the Watson equations from the height in cm (*H*), age in years (*A*) and body weight in Kg (*W*).

$$V = 2.447 - 0.09516 \times A + 0.1074 \qquad \text{(males)}$$
$$V = 2.097 + 0.1069 \times H + 0.2466 \times W \qquad \text{(females)}$$
$$SA = W^{0.5378} \times H^{0.3964} \times 0.024265$$

Solute removal index (SRI equivalent to weekly Kt/V for continuous treatments or renal function) is calculated from *V*, blood urea (*bU*), 24 hour urine volume in liters (*uV*) and the urea concentration in the 24 hour urine collection (*uU*)

$$SRI = \frac{uV \times uU \times 7}{V \times bU}$$

Creatinine clearance in L/week/1.73 m^2 (*CCr*) is calculated from *SA*, *uV*, blood and 24 hour urine creatinine concentrations (*bC*, *uC*).

$$CCr = \frac{uV \times uC \times 7 \times 1.73}{SA \times bC}$$

REFERENCES

1. Davies SJ, Bryan J, Phillips L and Russell GI. The predictive value of KT/V and peritoneal solute transport in CAPD patients is dependent on the type of comorbidity present. Perit Dial Int 1996; 16:S158–62.
2. Huting J and Schutterle G. Cardiovascular factors influencing survival in end-stage renal disease treated by continuous ambulatory peritoneal dialysis. Am J Cardiol 1992; 69:123–7.
3. Khan IH, Catto GR, Edward N and MacLeod AM. Death during the first 90 days of dialysis: a case control study. Am J Kidney Dis 1995; 25:276–80.
4. Balaskas EV, Yuan ZY, Gupta A, Meema HE, Blair G, Bargman J et al. Long-term continuous ambulatory peritoneal dialysis in diabetics. Clin Nephrol 1994; 42:54–62.
5. Ikizler TA, Wingard RL and Hakim RM. Interventions to treat malnutrition in dialysis patients: the role of the dose of dialysis, intradialytic parenteral nutrition, and growth hormone. Am J Kidney Dis 1995; 26:256–65.
6. Nordal KP, Dahl E, Halse J, Attramadal A and Flatmark A. Long-term low-dose calcitrol treatment in predialysis chronic renal failure: can it prevent hyperparathyroid bone disease? Nephrol Dial Transplant 1995; 10:203–6.
7. Blake PG. Adequacy of peritoneal dialysis. Curr Opin Nephrol Hypertens 1996; 5:492–6.
8. Canada-USA (CANUSA) Peritoneal Dialysis Study Group. Adequacy of dialysis and nutrition in continuous peritoneal dialysis: association with clinical outcomes. J Am Soc Nephrol 1996;7:198–207.
9. Lowrie EG and Lew NL. Death risk in hemodialysis patients: the predictive value of commonly measured vari-

ables and an evaluation of death rate differences between facilities. Am J Kidney Dis 1990; 15:458–82.

10. Ikizler TA, Greene JH, Wingard RL, Parker RA and Hakim RM. Spontaneous dietary protein intake during progression of chronic renal failure. J Am Soc Nephrol 1995; 6:1386–91.

11. Benabe JE and Martinez-Maldonado M. The impact of malnutrition on kidney function. Min Electrolyte Metab 1998; 24:20–6.

12. Avram MM, Bonomini LV, Sreedhara R and Mittman N. Predictive value of nutritional markers (albumin, creatinine, cholesterol, and hematocrit) for patients on dialysis for up to 30 years. Am J Kidney Dis 1996; 28:910–7.

13. Iseki K, Uehara H, Nishime K, Tokuyama K, Yoshihara K, Kinjo K et al. Impact on the initial levels of laboratory variables on survival in chronic dialysis patients. Am J Kidney Dis 1996; 28:541–8.

14. Edefonti A, Carcano A, Damiani B, Ghio L, Consalvo G and Picca M. Changes in body composition assessed by bioimpedance analysis in the first 6 months of chronic peritoneal dialysis. Adv Perit Dial 1997; 14:267–70.

15. Pollock CA, Ibels LS, Zhu FY, Warnant M, Caterson RJ, Waugh DA et al. Protein intake in renal disease. J Am Soc Nephrol 1997; 8:777–83.

16. Walser M. Effects of a supplemented very low protein diet in predialysis patients on the serum albumin level, proteinuria, and subsequent survival on dialysis. Min Electrolyte Metab 1998; 24:64–71.

17. Coresh J, Walser M and Hill S. Survival on dialysis among chronic renal failure patients treated with a supplemented low-protein diet before dialysis. J Am Soc Nephrol 1995; 6:1379–85.

18. Bergstrom J, Wang T and Lindholm B. Factors contributing to catabolism in end-stage renal disease patients. Min Electrolyte Metab 1998; 24:92–101.

19. Bailey JL. Metabolic acidosis and protein catabolism: mechanisms and clinical implications. Min Electrolyte Metab 1998; 24:13–9.

20. Williams AJ, Dittmer ID, McArley A and Clarke J. High bicarbonate dialysate in haemodialysis patients: effects on acidosis and nutritional status. Nephrol Dial Transplant 1997; 12:2633–7.

21. Walls J. Effect of correction of acidosis on nutritional status in dialysis patients. Min Electrolyte Metab 1997; 23:234–6.

22. Coen G, Manni M, Addari O, Ballanti P, Pasquali M, Chicca S et al. Metabolic acidosis and osteodystrophic bone disease in predialysis chronic renal failure: effect of calcitriol treatment. Min Electrolyte Metab 1995; 21:375–82.

23. Zucchelli P and Santoro A. How to achieve optimal correction of acidosis in end-stage renal failure patients. Blood Purif 1995; 13:375–84.

24. Foley RN, Parfrey PS, Harnett JD, Kent GM, Hu L, O'Dea R et al. Hypocalcemia, morbidity, and mortality in end-stage renal disease. Am J Nephrol 1996; 16:386–93.

25. Hara S, Ubara Y, Arizono K, Ikeguchi H, Katori H, Yamada A et al. Relation between parathyroid hormone and cardiac function in long-term hemodialysis patients. Min Electrolyte Metab 1995; 21:72–6.

26. Angelis M, Wong LL, Myers SA and Wong LM. Calciphylaxis in patients on hemodialysis: a prevalence study. Surgery 1997; 122:1083–9 and 1089–90.

27. Hernandez D, Concepcion MT, Lorenzo V, Martinez ME, Rodriguez A, De Bonis E et al. Adynamic bone disease with negative aluminium staining in predialysis patients: prevalence and evolution after maintenance dialysis. Nephrol Dial Transplant 1994; 9:517–23.

28. Madore F, Lowrie EG, Brugnara C, Lew NL, Lazarus JM, Bridges K et al. Anemia in hemodialysis patients: variables affecting this outcome predictor. J Am Soc Nephrol 1997; 8:1921–9.

29. Kuriyama S, Tomonari H, Yoshida H, Hashimoto T, Kawaguchi Y and Sakai O. Reversal of anemia by erythropoietin therapy retards the progression of chronic renal failure, especially in nondiabetic patients. Nephron 1997; 77:176–85.

30. Foley RN, Parfrey PS, Harnett JD, Kent GM, Martin CJ, Murray DC et al. Clinical and echocardiographic disease in patients starting end-stage renal disease therapy. Kidney Int 1995; 47:186–92.

31. Silberberg JS, Barre PE, Prichard SS and Sniderman AD. Impact of left ventricular hypertrophy on survival in end-stage renal disease. Kidney Int 1989; 36:286–90.

32. Tucker B, Fabbian F, Giles M, Thuraisingham RC, Raine AE and Baker LR. Left ventricular hypertrophy and ambulatory blood pressure monitoring in chronic renal failure. Nephrol Dial Transplant 1997; 12:724–8.

33. Hara S, Ubara Y, Arizono K, Ikeguchi H, Katori H, Yamada A et al. Relation between parathyroid hormone and cardiac function in long-term hemodialysis patients. Min Electrolyte Metab 1995; 21:72–6.

34. London GM, Pannier B, Guerin AP, Marchais SJ, Safar ME and Cuche JL. Cardiac hypertrophy, aortic compliance, peripheral resistance, and wave reflection in end-stage renal disease. Comparative effects of ACE inhibition and calcium channel blockade. Circulation 1994; 90:2786–96.

35. Cannella G, Paoletti E, Delfino R, Peloso G, Rolla D and Molinari S. Prolonged therapy with ACE inhibitors induces a regression of left ventricular hypertrophy of dialyzed uremic patients independently from hypotensive effects. Am J Kidney Dis 1997; 30:659–64.

36. Dyadyk AI, Bagriy AE, Lebed IA, Yarovaya NF, Schukina EV and Taradin GG. ACE inhibitors captopril and enalapril induce regression of left ventricular hypertrophy in hypertensive patients with chronic renal failure. Nephrol Dial Transplant 1997; 12:945–51.

37. Wizemann V, Schafer R and Kramer W. Follow-up of cardiac changes induces by anemia compensation in normotensive hemodialysis patients with left-ventricular hypertrophy. Nephron 1993; 64:202–6.

38. Prichard SS, Laemeire N, Van Biesen W, Dombros N, Dratwa M, Faller B et al. Treatment modality selection in 150 consecutive patients starting ESRD therapy. Perit Dial Int 1996; 16:69–72

39. Lameire N, Van Biesen W, Dombros N, Dratwa M, Faller B, Gahl GM et al. The referral pattern of patients with ESRD is a determinant in the choice of dialysis modality. Perit Dial Int 1997; 17:S161–S166.

40. Hayslip DM and Suttle CD. Pre-ESRD patient education: a review of the literature. Adv Ren Replace Ther 1995; 2:217–26.

41. Levin A, Lewis M, Mortiboy P, Faber S, Hare I, Porter EC et al. Multidisciplinary predialysis programs: quantification and limitations of their impact on patient outcomes in two Canadian settings. Am J Kidney Dis 1997; 29:533–40.

42. Rasgon SA, Chemleski BL, Ho S, Widrwo L, Yeoh HH, Schwankovsky L et al. Benefits of a multidisciplinary predialysis program in maintaining employment among patients on home dialysis. Adv Perit Dial 1996; 12:132–5.

43. Harland RC. Placement of permanent vascualr access devices: surgical considerations. Adv Ren Replace Ther 1994; 1:99–106.

44. NKF-DOQI Clinical Practice Guidelines for Vascular Access. Am J Kidney Dis 1997; 30:S150–S191.

45. Krolewski M, Eggers PW and Warram JH. Magnitude of end-stage renal disease in IDDM: a 35 year follow-up study. Kidney Int 1996; 50:2041–6.

46. Hellman R, Regan J and Rosen H. Effect of intensive treatment of diabetes of the risk of death or renal failure in NIDDM and IDDM. Diabetes Care 1997; 20:258–64.

47. Yu CC, Wu MS, Wu CH, Yang CW, Huang JY, Hong JJ et al. Predialysis glycemic control is an independent predictor of clinical outcome in type II diabetics on continuous ambulatory peritoneal dialysis. Perit Dial Int 1997; 17:262–8.

48. Viberti G and Chaturvedi N. Angiotensin converting enzyme inhibitors in diabetic patients with microalbuminuria or normoalbuminuria. Kidney Int 1997; 63:S32–5.

49. Hendry BM, Viberti GC, Hummel S, Bagust A and Piercy J. Modelling and costing the consequences of using an ACE inhibitor to slow the progression of renal failure in type I diabetic patients. QJM 1997; 90:277–82.

50. Freedman BI, Soucie JM and McClellan WM. Family history of end-stage renal disease among incident dialysis patients. J Am Soc Nephrol 1997; 8:1942–5.

51. Brancati FL, Whelton PK, Randall BL, Neaton JD, Stamler J and Klag MJ. Risk of end-stage renal disease in diabetes mellitus: a prospective cohort study of men screened for MRFIT. Multiple risk factor intervention trial. J Am Med Assoc 1997; 278:2069–74.

52. Jungers P, Zingraff J, Albouze G, Chauveau P, Page B, Hannedouche T et al. Late referral to maintenance dialysis: detrimental consequences. Nephrol Dial Transplant 1993; 8:1089–93.

53. Churchill DN. An evidence-based approach to earlier initiation of dialysis. Am J Kidney Dis 1997; 30:899–906.

54. Innes A, Rowe PA, Burden RP and Morgan AG. Early deaths on renal replacement therapy: the need for early nephrological referral. Nephrol Dial Transplant 1992; 7:467–71.

55. Sesso R and Belasco AG. Late diagnosis of chronic renal failure and mortality on maintenance dialysis. Nephrol Dial Transplant 1996; 11:2417–20.

56. Canada-USA (CANUSA) Peritoneal Dialysis Study Group. Adequacy of dialysis and nutrition in continuous peritoneal dialysis: association with clinical outcomes. J Am Soc Nephrol 1996; 7:198–207.

57. Held PJ, Port FK, Wolfe RA, Stannard DC, Carroll CE, Daugirdas JT et al. The dose of hemodialysis and patient mortality. Kidney Int 1996; 50:550–6.

14. Quality of life assurance in hemodialysis

ROBERT LINDSAY

INTRODUCTION

To physicians who are concerned with the impact that end-stage renal disease and hemodialysis have on the day-to-day life and psychological well-being of patients and their families, a major part of the "quality" in quality assurance consists of patient quality of life.

The patient with end-stage renal disease faces a debilitating and disruptive chronic illness, and a treatment regimen that is itself a complex, demanding and incessant intrusion into one's personal and social life. Dialysis patients are required, at the very least, to stoically endure pain, discomfort, fatigue and deprivation on a daily basis, year after year. And most dialysis patients heroically struggle to continue to fulfil their roles as spouses, parents, friends, workers and community members even as they are nudged by the healthy around them into a twilight world of the "... marginal person – here today, gone tomorrow" [1]. Thus it is not surprising to find that aspects of quality of life, often referred to as 'psychosocial factors', have been of concern in nephrology for many years.[1]

The measurement of quality of life has become an integral part of clinical research in many areas. As technological and pharmacological advances have increased the efficacy of modern medicine, concomitant research efforts have gone beyond the assessment of mortality and morbidity to include the dimensions of physiological, psychological and social functioning. Likewise, as a growing proportion of the health care system is involved with the management of long-term chronic diseases and conditions, the focus of research has widened to include the patient's physical comfort, psychological health, social and vocational activity, and the impact on the patient's family. In short, the extent to which medical treatment is consciously directed to help patients live comfortable, productive and satisfying lives is the extent to which clinical research into that treatment has included measures of patient quality of life.

In addition, there is a growing awareness among medical practitioners that knowledge of, and sensitivity to, quality of life issues can contribute to successful treatment outcome. For example, minimizing and ameliorating negative iatrogenic treatment effects promotes patient compliance with difficult therapeutic regimens that require sacrifice and commitment. Likewise, in chronic treatments such as dialysis, a downturn in some aspect of a patient's quality of life may signal the beginning of a coping problem which, if identified early enough, can be defused with a minor strategically-focused intervention before it escalates into a major problem requiring a significant investment of professional time and resources.

Apart from its practical importance, our growing understanding of the dynamics of patient quality of life within the context of disease and treatment is also contributing to our theoretical knowledge of the interaction between the mind, body and social environment. Consideration of patient quality of life leads into a holistic conceptual framework where medical treatments per se are seen as interwoven into the web of the patient's entire life. Changes in any single area of life have repercussions in many other areas; thus medical decisions will be made not in isolation, but with an ecological view as to how they will affect other aspects of the patient's life, and how they will be impacted in turn by psychological factors and social forces.

The promotion of quality assurance with respect

143

L.W. Henderson and R.S. Thuma (eds.), Quality Assurance in Dialysis, 2nd Edition, 143–154.
© 1999 *Kluwer Academic Publishers. Printed in Great Britain*

to patient quality of life, then, is called forth by the humanistic ethic of the helping professions, and is justified by its practical contribution to treatment efficacy and its potential contribution to scientific knowledge.

ACHIEVING QUALITY OF LIFE ASSURANCE IN DIALYSIS

It may be helpful to briefly sketch the outlines of how the issue of quality assurance, from the point of view of patient quality of life, could be addressed in a pragmatic way within a busy dialysis unit. The foundation would be the ongoing collection of psychosocial data from patients in a regular and systematic fashion, in much the same way that medical and physiological data is routinely collected today. In order to minimize the burden on medical staff, the bulk of this information could be collected through patient-completed questionnaires. In center dialysis units, for example, most questionnaires could be filled out before or during dialysis sessions. The role of unit staff would be limited, in most cases, to the distribution and collection of questionnaires with a quick check of completion rates. In order to minimize the burden on the patients, questionnaires need to be short, clear, and easy to read and answer. Data collection could occur relatively infrequently, perhaps quarterly, with the option of larger-scale assessments on an even less frequent cycle. Scheduling would likely be done on an individual patient basis, keyed to the date of admission to the unit. In order to maximize the utility of the information gathered, the measures chosen should meet high standards of validity and reliability; as enumerated later, a substantial number of accredited quality of life instruments are, in fact, currently available.

The routine collection of quality of life information will generate a data base with several valuable applications. The individual dialysis unit will instantly have an empirical snapshot of their caseload, a descriptive cross-section captured in the range of scores, typical values, characteristics of particular subgroups, and values associated with individual patients of interest. By matching measurements from questionnaires with personal knowledge of individuals, unit staff will immedi-ately begin to make the rather esoteric numbers derived from the quality of life scales more meaningful, with certain types of problems, for example, becoming associated with specific ranges of values on particular scales. In addition, through relatively simple statistics the inter-relationships between the different aspects of quality of life, and the relationships between quality of life and other characteristics, can be investigated at the local level, in response to local interests and concerns.

Once a series of measurements have been taken, it becomes possible to track individuals, subgroups, and the caseload as a whole over time. With experience, the emergence of individual problems can be followed and even anticipated through changes in a patient's scale scores, thus facilitating early preventative interventions. Likewise the effects of therapeutic interventions over time can be assessed. As long-term data builds up, it will be possible to trace the course of psychosocial adaptation to treatment from initial adjustments onwards, and to relate individual or subgroup patterns to other characteristics, therapeutic milestones, and events in the unit. In this way, high-calibre quality of life data, collected systematically and regularly over time, could provide valuable supplemental information useful in diagnostic and therapeutic decision-making in the dialysis unit.

When many dialysis units are routinely collecting quality of life data, their utility is further enhanced. Individual units can compare patient and performance data on a regional, national and international basis. Data on patients with rare conditions or problems can be combined for more powerful analyses. Comparisons between different types of units – rural versus urban, short-hours versus long hours, reusers versus single use units, for example – become possible on an ad hoc basis, facilitating answers to questions that today can only be addressed through expensive "extracurricular" research projects.

All of these potential benefits from quality of life assurance, however, assume that patient quality of life can be assessed in meaningful, valid, reliable and efficient ways. It is to these points that we now turn, beginning with matters of conceptual definition, followed by measurement issues.

CONCEPTUAL DEFINITIONS

Quality of Life

The term "quality of life" strikes a chord of familiarity; we all have an intuitive sense of what is implied in terms of the expectations, satisfactions and frustrations in our own personal lives. The generality and all-inclusiveness of the concept, however, means that each individual will define the quality of their own life in a unique way, with different priorities and different weights differentially assigned to the various aspects of personal existence. In order for the concept to have utility in scientific research and clinical practice, this multiplicity of personal meanings must be transcended through conceptual and operational definitions which have universal applicability[2] at the same time as they accommodate the richness of individual variation.

The first step in delimiting the concept is to note that we are concerned here with patient quality of life, as distinguished from the quality of life of a general population. The latter notion comes from within the tradition of the general social survey in the field of sociology, and is concerned with the broad assessment of the nature and grading of life along such dimensions as attitudes towards self and others, racial and ethnic groups, women, family life, work, social and leisure activities, personal economic outlook, national economic outlook, and various political issues [2–4]. While the notion of patient quality of life takes a more functional orientation within a narrower focus, a great deal of theory and methodology is imported directly from these large scale social surveys.

The concept of patient quality of life can be derived almost directly from the World Health Organization's definition of health as "[a] state of complete physical, mental and social well-being and not merely the absence of disease or infirmity" [5]. When we consider the quality of life of a dialysis patient, by definition disease is present. The central focus is thus the level of physical, mental and social functioning of the individual in the presence of kidney disease. Patient quality of life "... represents the functional effect of an illness and its consequent therapy upon a patient, as perceived by the patient" [6].

Domains and Components of Quality of Life

The main dimensions of patient quality of life are embedded in the WHO definition of health: physical functioning, social functioning and psychological functioning. While specific components of these dimensions may be chosen to fit particular research questions or clinical concerns, there are several aspects of functioning that are of primary interest and importance with dialysis patients (see Figure 14.1).

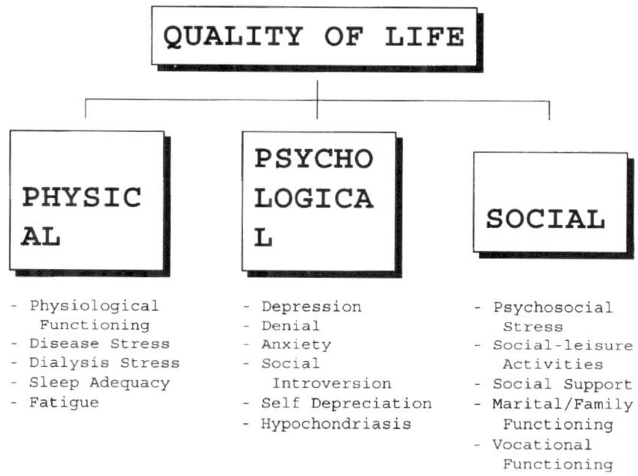

Fig. 14.1. Quality of life, dimensions and components.

PHYSICAL FUNCTIONING

The physical health, well-being and level of functioning of patients constitutes the traditional purview of medicine, and a great deal of physiological and treatment-related data is generally available to the physician in the patient's chart and dialysis records. However, there are several items that bear directly on quality of life; some of which is found in traditional medical data, and some of which is unique to the quality of life perspective. Of primary importance is a measure of physiological functioning that can provide, through a single index number, a sense of the overall health of the patient. In addition, depending on the severity and chronicity of the ESRD and accompanying conditions, an assessment of functional capacity may be helpful. This is particularly so with respect to such factors as mobility and visual acuity which are directly relevant to the self-care and home-care settings. Disease-related stress and dialysis-related distress are concerned with the impact of ESRD and its concomitant therapy on the life of the patient. The former emphasizes the incidence and severity of uremic and other symptoms, while the latter concentrates on the occurrence of physical problems and the concomitant level of discomfort during the dialysis procedure. Other aspects of treatment regimen stress, such as dietary and fluid restrictions, may also be of interest. Finally, systematic assessment of the adequacy of sleep, and the level of fatigue experienced by the patient round out the picture of the physical domain of quality of life.

PSYCHOLOGICAL FUNCTIONING

The psychological dimension of patient quality of life reflects the individual's inner experience of the illness and treatment. This will include the direct impact of the physical symptoms on subjective well-being, the meaning and significance to the person's self-concept and self-esteem of the many losses entailed in a debilitating chronic disease, adjustments to the increased immanence of the possibility of death, and the mobilization of defense and coping mechanisms. Psychological functioning is thus both influenced by, and simultaneously exerts an influence over, physiological functioning and health.

Depression is widely recognized as one potential psychological outcome of uremia and dialysis. Likewise, the importance of denial as a coping mechanism of dialysis patients is generally acknowledged. Anxiety, particularly when related to treatment issues, is also an aspect of psychological functioning with practical significance. Finally, social introversion and self-depreciation may provide important links between physical and social functioning.

SOCIAL FUNCTIONING

The strength and pervasiveness of uremic symptomatology, and the commitment of time and energy demanded by dialysis and other treatment con-

siderations, means that virtually every aspect of a patient's lifestyle changes after kidney failure. Continuing crises in the roles of marriage partner and parent will precipitate shifts in family responsibility and decision-making. Many patients must change jobs, work reduced hours, or leave their employment altogether, placing further burdens on spouse and family. And there are further changes to patterns of housework, diet, recreation and social activities.

On the other hand, social support from family and friends is one of the key resources that the dialysis patient can draw on for help in coping with the demands and disruptions of ESRD and its treatment. To the extent that the patient's social network can be protected, nurtured and strengthened, the individual can be buffered from the more extreme exigencies of their situation.

One of the important aspects of social functioning will be psychosocial stress, the stress experienced in day-to-day personal and family life related to the symptoms of kidney disease and the demands of dialysis. The level of marital and family functioning, including cohesion, conflict, communication, affection, organization and control, is both a primary resource for the patient and is itself vulnerable to disruption as a result of illness and treatment. General social support, the patient's perceptions of the degree to which he/she is loved, valued and nurtured by his/her overall social network, gives an indication of the availability of this resource. A reduction in the quality and/or quantity of social-leisure activities can signal the emergence of a deeper problem in the patient's life, as can a significant reduction in the patient's level of vocational functioning.

While the dimensions and components of quality of life outlined above are certainly not exhaustive, they do define the boundaries of the concept and give an idea of the depth of material that is relevant. As the interest in quality of life assurance spreads to more and more dialysis units, it will be important to build a consensus around the choice of components to be targeted for measurement so that a meaningful sharing and comparing of data will be possible. Equally important will be a consensus on measurement strategies.

MEASUREMENT ISSUES

Measurement Approach

There are two basic, complementary approaches to the measurement of patient quality of life: global and disease-specific. Global assessments tend to rate levels of overall functioning and/or satisfaction in general, abstract dimensions. In contrast, disease-specific assessment tools focus on concrete symptoms, stressors, dysfunctions and discomfort related to a particular disease and its treatment [7].

Within the global approach there are both "utility measures" and "health profiles". Utility measurements provide a single number representing a measure of overall quality of life. For example, the QL-Index [8] scores five items (activity; living; health; support; outlook on life) via 3-point scales (range 0–2) for an overall APGAR-type rating of from 0 to 10. Likewise the time trade-off approach generates a single number measure of quality of life by dividing the patient's current life expectancy in years into the shortest life expectancy for which the patient would settle in return for full health [9]. As health profiles, global instruments may also be long and detailed, such as the Sickness Impact Profile [10] and the Psychological Adjustment to Illness Scale [11].

The global method is most useful for assessments of a large, heterogeneous population, or when comparing different illnesses. The general approach, however, is usually too insensitive to detect small but clinically significant changes and/or differences, and thus is of limited value in evaluation research. Disease-specific assessment is generally more suitable in clinical trials of alternative interventions. Since questionnaire items have been chosen specifically to fit the research questions at hand, the scales tend to be sensitive to change and able to detect subgroup differences. On the other hand, since different illnesses affect different bodily functions and tend to contribute to different physical and emotional problems, disease-specific instruments usually have a narrow range of applicability limited to the illness and treatment for which they were designed [12].

In terms of ongoing patient quality of life assurance, both the global and disease-specific approach to measurement would be valuable. Widely used global measures would provide the basis for broad comparisons with other treatment modalities or patient populations, while a selection of disease-specific scales are required to facilitate preventative interventions, treatment evaluations, and other projects narrowly focused on issues in hemodialysis.

Disease-Specific Instrumentation

The authors have developed and/or employed a number of disease-specific instruments over the past 15 years. These have been utilized in various research projects, including a study of adaptation to home dialysis in the province of Ontario [13–18], a clinical evaluation of short-hours dialysis with the polyacrilonile membrane [19–20], and an investigation into the effects of rHuEPO and dialyser geometry on dialysis efficacy and patient quality of life [21, 22]. A selection of these instruments are briefly described below to give the reader an idea of the kinds of tools that are available. With the exception of the Physiological Index, which is compiled by medical staff using unit records, the questionnaires are all completed by patients.

1. *Physiological index*: The physiological index was developed from the "Standardized List of Somatic Criteria" of M.R. Strauch et al. and consists of 18 weighted biochemical measures selected for their relevance to an ESRD population: hepatitis; renal osteodystrophy; urine volume; serum urea, creatinine, blood pressure; hematocrit; weight increment between dialysis; potassium; diabetes; myocardial infarct; fundi; congestive heart failure; angina pectoris; pericarditis; GI ulcers; anephric. Original items and weights were validated through feedback from nephrologists from 100 West German dialysis centers [23]. Physiological Index scores range from 7 to 94, with higher values indicating poorer physiological functioning.

2. *Psychosocial stress scale*: This nine item index measures the amount of stress experienced in day-to- day personal and family life related to the symptoms of ESRD and the demands of dialysis: financial problems; marriage strain; dependency; altered sexuality; interference with

vacations, vocation, childcare and social life; and loss of family role. The scale yields a stressor count (range 0 to 9) of the number of individual stressors experienced, and a total stress score (0 to 81). An "average per-item" stress score can also be computed by dividing the total stress by the number of stressors.

3. *Disease stress scale*: A 14-item scale of distress experienced due to the symptoms of chronic uremia and ESRD: being weak and tired; shortness of breath; blood pressure problems; up/down health; headaches; being physically ill; fluid retention; cramps; itch; fear of death; inability to sleep; dizziness; sexual problems; and nausea. Additional items can be included for individual research projects. For example, in a clinical trial involving erythropoietin, three extra questions were appended: easily feel cold or chilly; inability to perspire; aching in arms/legs. The stressor count (0 to 14) indicates the number of items affecting the person, and the total stress score (0 to 126) represents the sum total of disease related stress from all 14 sources. Average per-item stress can also be computed.

4. *Sleep adequacy*: The sleep questionnaire contains 4 subscales, computed by summing the component items: Interference with Sleep (range 0 to 27), sleep disruptions (range 0 to 27), fatigue upon awakening (range 0 to 24), and fatigue during the day (range 0 to 30).

5. *Dialysis somatic symptoms distress scale*: This is an index of 11 physical symptoms that commonly occur during hemodialysis: nausea; vomiting; headache; muscle cramps; dizziness; tingling of extremities; itching; shivering; back pain; chest pain; and hypotension. Four additional items were included for the EPO project: dyspnea; wheezing; perspiration; hives, rash. Patients are scored via a symptom count (0 to 11) of the number of incidents that occurred during the dialysis session, and via a total discomfort score (0 to 99) equalling the sum total of distress reported from all items. Average per-item stress can also be computed.

6. *Fatigue rating scale*: This scale measures the mean level of fatigue experienced by patients in the time period between dialysis sessions. Scores can range from 0 to 9.00.

7. *Basic personality inventory*: The full basic personality inventory is a psychological profile composed of 12 scales, each consisting of 20 true–false items, with a corresponding score range of from 0 to 20 [24]. While the orientation of the inventory as a whole is towards the measurement of psychopathology, we have found six of the scales to be appropriate for use with populations that are psychologically normal: depression, denial, anxiety, social introversion, self-depreciation and hypochondriasis.

The Somatic Symptoms Distress Scale is included as Figure 14.2 in order to illustrate some of the characteristics of these instruments. The most efficient format is the self-completed questionnaire: data can be gathered with minimal additional work by clinical staff. In order to maximize the return rates and completion rates it is important to word the instructions and questions in simple, concrete terms, and to utilize a layout that patients with mild visual impairments find easy to read and respond to. As can be seen in the SSDS, we prefer to separate questions on the occurrence of symptoms/stressors from questions on the level of discomfort/stress, as this seems to minimize missing data. The 9-point response scale which we use for level of discomfort or stress allows for a wide range of variability within and between patients, and facilitates the sensitivity of the instrument to treatment differences and change over time.

It has been our experience that when patients report a reduction, for example, in the overall level of dialysis-related discomfort, this may be due to the fact that they are affected by a fewer number of symptoms, or due to a lessening of the level of discomfort for certain symptoms, or to some combination of the two. Hence scoring the SSDS involves taking a symptom count (the number of Yes's), computing a total discomfort score (by summing the level of discomfort for individual items with No-symptom not present weighted 0), and calculating an intensity score by dividing total discomfort by symptom count. Subsequent analysis will involve an assessment of change/difference

```
        Circle NO if you did not experience the symptom while
dialysing.


        Circle YES if you did experience the symptom and indicate the
level of
        discomfort.
```

```
+-----------------------------------------------------------------+
|                        DISCOMFORT SCALE                         |
|                                                                 |
|      very                                                       |
|                                 very                            |
|      low                        low              moderate       |
|         high                    high                            |
+-----------------------------------------------------------------+
```

```
                        Symptom          Level of
Symptom                 Level of
                          Present        Discomfort
Present                 Discomfort

   Nausea               No    Yes     [      ]    Itching        No    Yes
[      ]

   Vomiting             No    Yes     [      ]    Shivering      No    Yes
[      ]

   Headache             No    Yes     [      ]    Back Pain      No    Yes
[      ]

   Muscle Cramps        No    Yes     [      ]    Chest Pain     No    Yes
[      ]

   Dizziness            No    Yes     [      ]    Hypotension    No    Yes

[      ]
                                                  (Low blood pressure)
   Tingling of          No    Yes     [      ]
   extremities                                    Other (specify): _______
[      ]
                                                  __________________________
```

Fig. 14.2. Somatic Symptoms Distress Scale (SSDS).

in these three scale scores, as well as an examination of each individual item to locate the individual aspects of dialysis affected.

Reliability and Validity

The reliability of a scale refers to its consistency internally and its stability over time. In a scale with high internal consistency, all component items are tapping slightly different aspects of the same underlying phenomenon and are thus highly inter-correlated. Internal consistency reliability is generally expressed by Cronbach's Alpha, a conservative measure that ranges from 0 to +1. A value of 0.60 is taken by convention as the minimum level for research purposes, while a value of 0.90 may be required for diagnostic applications. Stability over time is evaluated by test-retest reliability using the correlation between scores obtained over a short period during which the measured phenomenon is assumed not to have changed [25–29]. In a recent assessment of the instruments listed earlier [22], all scales except the Physiological Index (an inventory of largely unrelated items), attained Cronbach's alphas between 0.60 and 0.88, while test-retest coefficients ranged between 0.38 and 0.92.

Validity centers on the question of whether a scale actually measures the concept it is intended to measure. Validity assessment tends to be a continuous process as new data and experience are accumulated under different conditions. The validity of a scale is usually determined relative to the specific use(s) for which it is intended; hence different types of validity assessments correspond to different research applications. The concept "quality of life", when used in clinical research, often takes the role of a secondary treatment outcome supplemental to morbidity and mortality [30]. The validity assessment of a quality of life instrument is thus normally concerned with construct validity: the adequacy with which the scale represents the underlying theoretical concept, namely a specific domain of quality of life. Generally this is demonstrated by showing that the scale scores correlate in logical directions with other variables. Again, the instruments listed above have been shown to be correlated in expected directions with related variables, and have successfully discriminated between treatment groups, at statistically significant levels [22].

It should be noted that the use of quality of life measures to assess quality assurance in dialysis units represents a new application for these instruments, for purposes other than those typically associated with clinical research. Hence the validity and reliability of the scales in the ongoing monitoring of patients' coping with ESRD and dialysis, for establishing local, regional, national and even international norms of patient functioning, and for providing supplemental input into diagnostic and treatment decisions, remains to be established through actual clinical applications.

"Subjectivity" in Quality of Life Measurement

The measurement of patient quality of life is often criticized as being "unscientific" on the grounds that it is subjective. The subjective component, present in both global and disease-specific assessment, consists of having the patient report his/her perception of the degree of discomfort, stress, palliation, interference, etc. that he/she is experiencing. The concern is that because different individuals will make this judgement on the basis of different thresholds of discomfort and stress, and different expectations regarding palliation and interference, the exact same external stimulus will prompt a variety of different ratings. This, in turn, introduces a degree of random variation into the data which reduces the reliability and consistency of the measurements.

On the other hand, it is this subjective perception which is at the root of the individual's quality of life. A person who perceives him/herself as suffering will experience their treatment and make compliance-related decisions accordingly, regardless of any objective, external determination. Thus, while the variability of individual self-ratings is an important consideration during research design, the subjective element is the target of measurement in quality of life assessment, and not something to be avoided. By focusing analyses on gain scores, ie. the amount of change within individuals over time, we can reduce the interference due to variability between individuals while preserving the essential subjective nature of the target concept.

PRELIMINARY POPULATION NORMS

This section provides descriptive statistics on several of the disease-specific scales described earlier, in order to illustrate the format of the actual hard data, and to make an initial contribution to the development of population norms. The data are drawn from two separate research studies19–22 involving a total of 300 hemodialysis patients from 27 dialysis centers in 8 countries in Europe and North America (see Table 14.1). The 173 males and 127 females ranged in age from 18 through 84 years, with a mean of 55.1, a median of 58, and a standard deviation of 14.9 years. Glomerulonephritis was the most common primary renal disease (31.3%), followed by pyelonephritis (12.7%), hypertensive nephrosclerosis (12.0%), polycystic kidneys (10.7%); and diabetic nephropathy (5.7%). Time on dialysis ranged from one month to over 21 years, with a mean of 42.9 months, a median of 22 months, and a standard deviation of 48.2. One hundred and thirteen patients (37.7%) were medically high-risk, including 88 with cardiovascular problems, 23 insulin-dependent diabetics, and 31 patients with other systemic conditions. The data reported below comes from the initial baseline assessments of patients as they entered their particular study, prior to any experimental treatment.

Table 14.1. Country of origin

	Patients	
	(n)	%
Canada	69	23.0
Denmark	5	1.7
England	30	10.0
France	21	7.0
Germany	33	11.0
Italy	72	24.0
Sweden	26	8.7
U.S.A.	44	14.7
Total	300	100.0

Table 14.2 reveals that interference due to disease and the demands of dialysis with work and housework (vocation) and vacations, are the most common complaints affecting 39% of respondents. Interference with social life, and financial and sexuality problems are also relatively common. The mean stress for an item is a measure of the seriousness of the complaint. Interference with vacation, sexuality issues, vocational interference, social interference, financial problems and child-care interference all generated average levels of stress, for those affected by the item, at levels towards the high end of the scale. Data on the scale scores indicates that 78.4% of these patients were affected by at least one item of the scale, with a sample-wide average of 2.37 items; the mean total stress level of 12.32 in a possible range of 0 through 81.

Table 14.2. Psychosocial stress

Items	Affected (%)	Mean stress	Std dev
Financial problems	29.3	5.12	2.01
Marriage strain	12.3	4.50	2.33
Dependency	28.9	4.95	1.96
Sexuality	27.5	5.55	2.48
Vacation interference	39.4	5.58	2.33
Vocation interference	39.4	5.25	2.17
Loss of family role	14.3	4.80	2.26
Childcare interference	12.2	5.06	2.57
Social interference	34.1	5.13	2.00
Scales			
Stressor count	78.4	2.37	2.08
Total stress	,,	12.32	12.26
Per-item stress	,,	3.94	2.57

The primary disease-related stressor is feeling weak and tired, which affects three quarters of the sample, although the actual amount of stress this causes is moderate (Table 14.3). The general health items (up and down health, being physically ill) affect half the sample, with itch, blood pressure problems, fluid retention and sleep disturbance also relatively common. For those affected, the worst stressor is the impairment of sexual functioning; the mean stress level for sleep problems, being weak and tired, fear of death, fluid retention and up/down health also fall towards the high end of the response scale. Almost every patient (97%) reports at least one disease-related stressor, with the average being 6 symptoms; the overall mean total stress is approximately 30 in a range of 0 to 126.

Table 14.3. Disease related stress

	Affected (%)	Mean stress	Std dev
Weak and tired	75.4	5.34	2.01
Shortness of breath	37.4	4.86	1.94
Blood pressure problems	42.6	4.96	2.02
Up and down health	50.2	5.14	1.84
Headache	28.8	4.02	2.22
Being physically ill	50.0	4.76	2.17
Fluid retention	42.8	5.16	1.92
Cramps	40.9	4.18	2.18
Itchiness	47.0	4.85	2.48
Fear of death	25.6	5.21	2.30
Sleep problems	43.5	5.37	2.35
Dizziness	22.4	3.67	1.98
Sexual functioning	25.0	6.28	2.19
Nausea	19.6	4.29	2.53
Scales			
Stressor count	96.9	6.05	3.24
Total stress	,,	29.97	20.80
Per-item stress	,,	4.60	1.69

Table 14.4. Basic personality inventory

	Range	Mean	Median	Std dev
Depression	0–18	6.41	5	4.58
Denial	1–18	10.25	11	3.21
Anxiety	0–20	6.99	6	4.10
Social introversion	0–18	5.96	5	3.96
Self depreciation	0–15	3.62	3	2.94
Hypochondriasis	0–18	7.89	8	3.92

Table 14.5. Somatic symptoms distress

Items	Affected	Mean	Std dev
Nausea	21.3	2.27	1.73
Vomiting	13.9	2.03	1.61
Headache	34.4	2.72	1.94
Muscle cramps	44.0	3.06	2.08
Dizziness	23.1	2.30	1.87
Tingling extremities	19.9	2.48	2.07
Itching	45.7	3.37	2.18
Shivering	14.6	1.83	1.50
Back pain	23.4	3.32	2.05
Chest pain	11.7	1.88	1.44
Hypotension	44.7	2.87	2.01
Symptom count	90.4	2.04	1.77
Total distress		8.15	8.71
Per-item distress	,,	3.80	1.60

Meaningful Interpretation of BPI scores reqires some standards from known groups. Several population norms are presented in the scale manual 24. In general, dialysis patients tend to score higher than the population at large on denial (a constructive defense mechanism), depression and hypochondriasis, and close to the general population on the other measures (Table 14.4).

The most commonly reported symptoms during dialysis are itch, hypotension and muscle cramps, while itch and back pain cause the most severe discomfort; however, the mean level of stress for all items are towards the low end of the response scale (Table 14.5). Ninety percent of patients experience at least one physical symptom during dialysis, with an average of 2 symptoms causing a mean total stress of 8.15 within a potential range of 0–99.

It is interesting to compare the three stress/distress scales via the mean per-item score for the scale as a whole: disease stress seems to be the most severe intrusion into patients lives (4.60) followed by psychosocial stress (3.94) and dialysis distress (3.80). It should also be noted that the standard deviations in the quality of life scales tend to be large, an indication of the high degree of individual variation.

These examples demonstrate first of all that it is possible to meaningfully quantify different aspects of patient quality of life, and secondly that a variety of comparative analyses can be undertaken to furnish the clinician with helpful information. Comparisons of an individual with other patients, comparisons of an individual's values with values at other points in time, comparisons among groups of patients, and comparisons of a unit's average values with those from other units or the region/country are all possible when quality of life data is routinely collected. Potentially, such analyses can inform diagnostic decisions, provide data for hypothesis testing, and facilitate the evaluation of new equipment and alternative therapies.

CONCLUSION

The chronic nature of end-stage renal disease, the extensive symptomatology of uremia, and the invasive character of the hemodialysis treatment regimen constitute an enormous obstacle to the maintenance of a high quality of life for renal patients. The challenge of quality of life assurance in dialysis is to overcome this obstacle. The course of action we propose is to take our already considerable skill and expertise at research, which is usually cloistered in the specialized world of clinical trials, and to integrate it with ongoing clinical practice in a synergistic methodology.

Step one involves identifying a selection of global and disease-specific measures of patient quality of life that meet high standards of efficiency, reliability and validity; many proven tools exist today, some may have to be developed. Step two is the systematic collection of quality of life data on a regular basis. This data collection is not part of an external research project, but is added to the routine record keeping of the dialysis unit. Step three consists of integrating the analysis of quality of life data into the flow of therapeutic decision making within the unit – the screening of patients into appropriate treatment modalities, the identification and diagnosis of psychosocial problems, the choice of intervention, and the deployment of preventative measures. The sharing of data between centers constitutes step four. Through this interchange, individual units can compare caseload characteristics and experiences at an empirical level. Of even greater potential is the creation of a growing quality of life database that can facilitate the investigation of unusual problems and special populations, and can support general research into the interrelationship between physical, psychological and social functioning, and the determinants of high quality of life for dialysis patients.

Quality assurance in dialysis represents the consolidation of ethical, practical and scientific goals in a unified perspective. The promise of quality of life assurance is this: through the careful and systematic attention to dialysis as delivered and dialysis as received, medical practitioners have a significant contribution to make not only to the quantity of years remaining for the renal patient, but also to the quality of that time.

NOTES

[1] The earliest paper known to the authors is: Schreiner GE. Mental and personality changes in the uremic syndrome. Med Ann DC 1959; 28:316–23, 362.

[2] Universally applicable in the sense of generally meaningful within the bounds of western industrial culture; the term assumes a shared world-view and basic commonality of values that would not be transferrable between major cultures.

REFERENCES

1. Calland CH. Iatrogenic problems in end-stage renal failure. N Engl J Med 1972; 287:334.
2. Campbell A, Converse PE and Rodgers WL. The quality of American life: perceptions, evaluations, and satisfactions. New York, Russell Sage Foundation, 1976.
3. Converse PE, Dotson JD, Hoag WJ and McGee WH III. American social attitudes data sourcebook, 1947–1978. Cambridge, Mass., Harvard University Press, 1980.
4. Campbell A. The sense of well-being in America: recent patterns and trends. New York, McGraw-Hill, 1981.
5. Fries JF andSpitz PW. The hierarchy of patient outcomes. In Spilker B, editor. Quality of life assessments in clinical trials. New York, Raven Press, Ltd., 1990; 25–35.
6. Schipper H, Clinch J and Powell V. Definitions and conceptual issues. In Spilker B, editor. Quality of life assessments in clinical trials. New York, Raven Press, Ltd., 1990; 11–24.
7. Guyatt GH, Bombardier C and Tugwell PX. Measuring disease-specific quality of life in clinical trials. CMAJ 1986; 134:889–95.
8. Spitzer WO, Dobson AJ, Hall J et al. The QL-Index. J Chronic Dis 1981; 34:585–97.
9. Churchill DN, Torrance D, Taylor DW, Barnes CC, Ludwin D, Shimizu A et al. Measurement of quality of life in end-stage renal disease: the time trade-off approach. Clin Invest Med 1987; 10:14–20.
10. Bergner M, Bobbit RA, Carter WB et al. The sickness impact profile. Med Care 1981; 19:787–805.
11. Morrow GR, Chiarello RJ and Derogatis LR. A new scale for assessing patients' adjustment to medical illness. Psychol Med 1978; 8:605–10.
12. Guyatt GH and Jaeschke R. Measurements in clinical trials: choosing the appropriate approach. In Spilker B, editor. Quality of life assessments in clinical trials. New York, Raven Press, Ltd., 1990; 37–46.
13. Lindsay RM. A comparison of CAPD and haemodialysis in adaptation to home dialysis. In Moncreith J and Popovich R, editors. CAPD ipdate – continuous ambulatory peritoneal dialysis. Masson, NY, Modern Problems in Kidney Disease, 1981; 171–9.
14. Lindsay RM, Oreopoulos D, Burton H, Conley J, Richmond J and Wells G. The effect of treatment modality (CAPD vs. haemodialysis) in adaptation to home dialysis. In Atkins RC, Thomson NM and Farrell PC, editors. Proceedings of the Pan Pacific conference on peritoneal dialysis. Edinburgh, Churchill Livingstone, 1981; 385–94.

15. Lindsay RM, Richmond J Burton H, Conley J, Clark WF and Linton AL. Is home dialysis too stressful? Controv Nephrol 1981; 3:395–405.

16. Wai L, Richmond J, Burton HJ and Lindsay RM. The influence of psychosocial factors on survival of home dialysis patients. Lancet 1981; 2;1155–6.

17. Richmond JM, Linday RM, Burton HJ, Conley J and Wai L. Psychological and physiological factors predicting the outcome on home haemodialysis. In Cluthe R, editor. Clinical nephrology. Frieburg, Germany, 1982; 109–13.

18. Burton HJ, Kline SA, Lindsay RM and Heidenheim AP. The relationship of depression to survival in chronic renal failure. Psychosom Med 1986; 48:261–9

19. Lindsay RM. Comparison of patient quality of life in short dialysis and conventional dialysis. In: Man NK, Mion C and Henderson LW, editors. Blood purification in perspective: new insights and future trends. ISAIO Press, 1987; 203–4.

20. Lindsay RM, Heidenheim AP, Spanner E, Burton HJ, Lindsay S and LeFebvre JMJ. A multi-centre study of short hours (SH) dialysis using AN69S: preliminary results. ASAIO Transactions 1991; 37:M465–7.

21. Heidenheim AP and Lindsay RM. The impact of erythropoietin and dialyzer geometry on patient quality of life. Unpublished data.

22. Lindsay RM and Heidenheim AP. Measurement of quality of life in international trials involving dialysis patients and the use of recombinant human erythropoietin. In Bauer C, Koch K, Scigalla P and Wieczorek L, editors. Clinical applications of erythropoietin. New York, Marcel Dekker Inc., 1993;81–921.

23. Strauch MR, Lipke R, Schafheutle R, Nachbauer B and Stauch-Rahaüser G. A standardized list of somatic criteria for comparative assessment of regular dialysis therapy patients. Artif Organs 1978; 2:370–2.

24. Jackson DJ. The basic personality inventory. Port Huron, Michigan, Research Psychologists Press, 1976.

25. Nunally JC. Psychometric theory, 2nd edn. New York, McGraw-Hill, 1978.

26. Carmines EG and Zeller RA. Reliability and validity assessment. Beverly Hills, Sage Publications, 1979.

27. Selltiz C, Wrightsman LS and Cook SW. Research methods in social relations, 3rd edn. New York, Holt, Rinehart, Winston, 1976.

28. Helmstadter GC. Principles of psychological measurements. New York, Appleton-Century-Crofts, 1964.

29. Lemke E and Wiersma W. Principles of psychological measurement. Chicago, Rand McNally, 1976.

30. Spilker B. Introduction. Quality of life assessments in clinical trials. Spilker B, editor. New York, Raven Press, 1990; 3.

15. Hemodialysis in the home and its impact on quality of life

CHRISTOPHER R. BLAGG

INTRODUCTION

Home hemodialysis was first developed in 1963 in the United States and Great Britain to reduce the cost of long-term dialysis for chronic renal failure in order that the limited financial and other resources available could be used to treat more patients [1–3]. Home intermittent peritoneal dialysis (IPD) was developed shortly thereafter [4], followed by continuous ambulatory peritoneal dialysis (CAPD) in 1976 [5] and then by various forms of continuous cycling peritoneal dialysis (CCPD) [6]. Today, CAPD and CCPD are the most frequently used forms of home dialysis and less than 1% of U.S. dialysis patients are treated by home hemodialysis.

Since the Medicare End-Stage Renal Disease (ESRD) Program began in 1973, almost all United States residents who develop ESRD are eligible for financial support from the federal government. This covers much of the costs of treatment by both dialysis and kidney transplantation. Of the 214,103 dialysis patients covered by the Medicare ESRD Program as of the end of 1996, 183,022 (85.5%) were on hemodialysis and 31,081 (14.5%) were on some form of peritoneal dialysis [7]. Recent years have seen a continuing annual increase in the number of patients treated by peritoneal dialysis in the home, and the percentage of all dialysis patients treated by peritoneal dialysis also gradually increased until this was 17.1% at the end of 1994. Since then, this percentage has begun to decline, and was down to 14.5% by the end of 1996. The other recent change that has occurred has been a steady increase in the percentage of peritoneal dialysis patients treated by CCPD, from 14.7% at the end of 1990 to 36.9% at the end of 1996.

Over the same period of time, the number of patients treated by home hemodialysis has continued to decline slowly. At the end of 1990, there were 2,483 patients on home hemodialysis (2.7% of all hemodialysis patients, and 1.9% of all dialysis patients), and by the end of 1996 this had fallen to 1,897 patients (1.0% and 0.9% respectively). Despite the increase in the number of patients treated by peritoneal dialysis from 20,774 at the end of 1990 to 31,081 at the end of 1996, the percentage of all patients dialyzing at home during this time declined from 16.0 to 15.2.

Of the 32,570 patients dialyzing at home at the end of 1996, 1,897 were on home hemodialysis (5.8% of all home dialysis patients), 19,184 were on CAPD (58.9%), 11,376 were on CCPD (34.9%), and 113 (0.3%) were listed as on intermittent peritoneal dialysis. Between 1990 and 1994, the annual increase in the number of dialysis patients treated by CAPD fell from 11.3% to 5.0%. However, between the end of 1994 and the end of 1995 there was a decrease of 9.9%, and between 1995 and 1996 the decrease was 10.2%. For CCPD, the average annual increase between 1990 and 1996 was 25.3%. These figures compare with an average annual increase of 8.7% in the total dialysis population between 1990 and 1996, and an annual average decline of 4.2% in the home hemodialysis population. The average annual increase for all modalities of in-center dialysis was 9.2%, while that for all modalities of home dialysis was 6.4%.

Beginning in the late 1980s, there has been concern that the mortality of United States dialysis patients is significantly higher than that of patients in Canada, Europe, Japan, and other developed countries [8, 9]. A number of possible explanations have been suggested for this, including the acceptance of older and sicker patients for treatment in the United States and possible incomplete reporting by patient registries elsewhere in the world.

L.W. Henderson and R.S. Thuma (eds.), Quality Assurance in Dialysis, 2nd Edition, 155–162.
© 1999 *Kluwer Academic Publishers. Printed in Great Britain*

Nevertheless, at least in the past, this also appears to have been related to widespread use of inadequate dialysis in the United States, and perhaps also to failure to meet the nutritional needs of patients. For example, in 1986–1987, hemodialysis patients reported to the European Dialysis and Transplant Association (EDTA) registry on average received 30% more dialysis than did patients in the United States [10]. This resulted from the common use of both shorter dialysis times and smaller less efficient dialyzers in the United States.

Because of this concern, and because of a growing interest in the evaluation and monitoring of health care, the Congress, the Health Care Financing Administration (HCFA), the Renal Physicians Association (RPA) and most recently the National Kidney Foundation (NKF), have become actively involved in looking at means to assess quality of care in dialysis and transplant patients. These efforts have resulted in HCFA's Core Indicators Project [11]; the RPA's Clinical Practice Guideline on Adequacy of Hemodialysis [12], and, most recently, the NKF's Dialysis Outcomes Quality Initiative [13]. The latter included a detailed and critical review of all the relevant literature by committees of experts, and resulted in development of clinical practice guidelines for hemodialysis adequacy, peritoneal dialysis adequacy, vascular access, and the treatment of the anemia of renal failure. However, there was little or no specific mention of how quality of care or quality of life can best be addressed in patients treated by home hemodialysis.

PATIENT SURVIVAL WITH HOME DIALYSIS

Although the benefits to patients associated with hemodialysis at home were recognized in the 1960s, it was some time before reports began to appear showing that survival with home hemodialysis is better than that with other modalities of dialysis. The first papers reporting this finding were from England [14] and Canada [15], and this has been confirmed by a number of subsequent studies [16–21]. However, apart from a report from the European Dialysis and Transplant Association [18], all these reports were from single programs and the degree of adjustment for the comorbid and other factors that might affect

survival was very varied. It is now well recognized that survival on dialysis is related to many factors, including age, sex, race, the primary cause of the renal disease, and the presence or absence of comorbid conditions. These must be taken into account in any comparisons of survival between different modalities of dialysis.

Recently, the staff at the USRDS have undertaken several different analyses using a national random sample from patients starting dialysis in 1986 and 1987 to examine survival and other results with the different modalities of dialysis. A Cox proportional hazards model was used, adjusting for age, race, sex, diabetes as the cause of renal disease, and comorbid factors present before the onset of ESRD. One of these studies confirmed the better survival with home hemodialysis, and when adjusted the relative risk (RR) of death for home hemodialysis patients was 0.58 ($p=0.03$), compared with the survival of patients on outpatient hemodialysis [22].

At the same time, concern also has been increasing about whether peritoneal dialysis as practiced until recently provides adequate dialysis for many patients [23]. The same USRDS database, adjusted for age, sex and race, in nondiabetic and in diabetic patients has been used to compare one-year survival in patients treated by outpatient hemodialysis or CAPD. The hospitalization rate for the peritoneal dialysis patients was 14% higher than for center hemodialysis patients, even after adjusting for comorbid conditions [24], and the relative risk of death, after adjusting for age, race, sex, diabetic status and duration of dialysis, was higher in peritoneal dialysis patients than in outpatient hemodialysis patients ($RR=1.19$; $p<0.001$). This risk was greater in older patients than in younger patients, and was increased in diabetic patients compared with nondiabetic patients ($RR=1.38$ vs. 1.11; both $p<0.001$) and in females compared with males ($RR=1.30$ vs. 1.11; both $p=0.001$) [25]. In addition, after adjustment for demographic factors, deaths due to infections, myocardial infarction, withdrawal from dialysis, cerebrovascular disease, other cardiac causes and "other causes" were significantly more frequent in peritoneal dialysis patients compared with outpatient hemodialysis patients [26].

QUALITY OF LIFE WITH HOME HEMODIALYSIS

One of the aims of treatment of patients with end stage renal disease is to provide them with the best possible quality of life, taking into account the effects of their disease and its treatment. Quality of life is a broad concept, and includes not only the patient's general health and their medical problems, but also the quality of their environment, their freedom to carry out the activities of daily living, and their income [27]. Unfortunately at this time the best means of estimating quality of life in patients with chronic disease remains uncertain. Part of the problem is that different quality of life measures may assess very different aspects of experience [28]. A number of instruments have been developed specifically to measure health-related quality of life in dialysis patients, although these vary widely in their ease of use and their reliability [29–32]. Typically, the measures used include some estimate of the patient's physical health and functional ability, their mental health, including depression and the effects of illness, their social health including social support, life satisfaction and adjustment to environment, vocational and sexual activities, and their general health including the severity of their illness. Measurement of these various dimensions is important in patient assessment, and quality of life can be improved by such measures as treatment of depression, improvement in social support and, where appropriate, vocational training or retraining. Some of the various measures available are discussed elsewhere in this book.

One of the important issues in comparing quality of life between different dialysis modalities is the effect of patient selection. Selection of modality is related to other factors in addition to medical ones, and the use of different modalities varies significantly in different regions of the same country and between different countries. In the United States, home hemodialysis is not readily available everywhere, and peritoneal dialysis has become increasingly popular over the last fifteen years or so, although at first it was less commonly used by for-profit dialysis facilities. In part, the growth of peritoneal dialysis reflects the demands of some patients for more independence, and in part it also reflects very successful marketing. Nevertheless,

modality selection usually is very influenced by the views of the patient's physician [33, 34], and frequently also by other financial and psychosocial considerations [35]. A study of more than 73,000 ESRD patients treated by freestanding dialysis facilities in 1993 found that home hemodialysis was most frequently used in males, native Americans, patients with polycystic kidney disease, and patients with a higher median household income, and was used less frequently in those with ESRD due to diabetes or hypertension. It was also used more frequently in patients living in areas with fewer dialysis facilities per square mile, and used less frequently in patients treated by the large dialysis chains and at for-profit units generally [36].

It has been recognized for many years that both patients and their families commonly have problems in adjusting to the effects of end stage renal disease and the burdens imposed by its treatments. Anxiety and depression are common [37, 38], physical abilities are reduced [39] and sexual dysfunction is frequent [40]. As a result, the patient and family face significant social restrictions. Patients' satisfaction with their quality of life often relates to their psychiatric status and their social circumstances. The latter is more related to various environmental factors, while psychiatric status is usually a reflection of their adjustment to these and other factors [41]. However, physical functioning appears to be the most important factor affecting patients' assessments of their global quality of life [42]. In general, patients with a functioning kidney transplant have an overall better quality of life than do patients treated by dialysis. However, those patients who have returned to dialysis following a failed transplant often have a much poorer quality of life than the average dialysis patient does [43, 44].

A number of studies have examined quality of life in dialysis and transplant patients, but only a few of these have looked specifically at patients treated by home hemodialysis. In the United States, two in particular have looked at this in relatively large patient populations treated through a number of different dialysis centers.

The largest study, by Evans and coworkers, looked at quality of life and rehabilitation in 859 dialysis and transplanted patients randomly selected from 11 dialysis and transplant centers situated across the U.S.A., and included 287 home hemodialysis patients [44]. The study examined objective and subjective indicators of quality of life, and adjusted for case-mix differences using sociodemographic and medical variables. Functional status was assessed from objective variables, the Karnofsky Index, and the patients' judgment of their ability to work. Subjective indicators reflected emotional status, and included estimates of life satisfaction, well-being and general affect.

Almost 80% of the patients with a functioning transplant were able to function at nearly normal levels, and almost 75% judged themselves to be able to work. Their quality of life, as judged in terms of life satisfaction, physical well being and psychological affect, was generally better than that of dialysis patients. Among the latter, the home hemodialysis patients fared best, having the least functional impairment, and almost 60% of home hemodialysis patients judged themselves able to work as compared with 37% of the patients treated by outpatient hemodialysis. In terms of subjective indicators of quality of life, the home hemodialysis patients scored better than patients on outpatient hemodialysis did, but not as well as the transplanted patients. Patients treated by CAPD generally scored less well than those on home hemodialysis did, but better than those on outpatient hemodialysis. These results were statistically significant, even when adjusted for case mix and other demographic differences.

Actual labor force participation among all patients was much less than that seen in the general population, although prior to the onset of ESRD treatment this was comparable. In terms of subjective indicators of quality of life, only the transplanted patients appeared similar to the general population. Even so, ESRD patients in general had scores for well being, psychological affect and life satisfaction that indicated a perception of quality of life that was only slightly lower than that of the general population. This suggests they are generally able to adapt relatively well to their adverse circumstances. Significantly, successful rehabilitation was seen primarily in the transplanted patients and some of the home hemodialysis patients, and these patients had nearly normal levels of activity and expressed general satisfaction with their lives.

The second study used a self-administered questionnaire to assess both objective and subjective quality of life in 489 patients from 59 dialysis facilities in one northeastern geographic area [45]. Forty-seven home hemodialysis patients were included in the study. Demographic and medical indicators were similar to those used in the first study. Subjective quality of life measures looked at affect, life satisfaction and well being. Quality of life was reported as similar for patients with a successful transplant and for those on home hemodialysis, and in both cases was significantly better than that of patients treated by CAPD or outpatient hemodialysis. A comparison with the study by Evans and coworkers showed very little differences in the results, the corresponding treatment groups being strikingly similar, as was the ranking of the groups. Both studies found that the patients reporting the poorest quality of life were those with a failed kidney transplant who were back on dialysis.

A study from Emory University in Atlanta assessed quality of life at two eighteen-month follow-up intervals in 97 ESRD patients, comparing transplanted patients with both home hemodialysis patients and patients treated by outpatient hemodialysis. The effects on home hemodialysis patients of receiving a kidney transplant or of transferring to CAPD were also examined [46]. In this study, the home hemodialysis patients showed the highest quality of life and the lowest hospitalization rates over time. The transplanted patients had a higher employment rate and perceived health status, but the subjective quality of life and frequency of hospitalization were not very different from those of patients on outpatient hemodialysis. Also, those home hemodialysis patients who were transplanted assessed the improvement of their quality of life as being better than did those who transferred to CAPD.

These three studies clearly show some of the major advantages of home hemodialysis with regard to quality of life, including the better opportunity for rehabilitation and ability to undertake employment or education, and the increased opportunity for patients to take greater responsibility for their own care [47]. These advantages result from the greater sense of independence, the potential for increased exercise tolerance, and the greater self-esteem seen in home hemodialysis patients compared with those on CAPD or outpatient hemodialysis in a center [44, 45].

A study from North Carolina looked at social support and health-related quality of life in 256 dialysis patients, of whom 131 were black and 125 were white [48]. This study was particularly concerned with the effects of race and the availability of social support, because black dialysis patients live significantly longer than white patients, but it did include a small number of home hemodialysis patients. Health-related quality of life, employment history, education, marital status, living arrangements, weight history, and Karnofsky's Physical Functioning Scale were evaluated, and a questionnaire was used to look at their social support and social network. Mean social support scores were not significantly different between patients on the various modalities of treatment. However, after covariate adjustment for age, sex, race and number of years on dialysis, the differences in scores between home hemodialysis (22.2), peritoneal dialysis (21.5) and outpatient hemodialysis (20.7) were statistically significant ($p=0.044$ and 0.022 respectively). In general, the health-related quality of life scores were better in the black patients, and this could not be explained by any of the other variables measured. In addition to the effect of race, this study showed a significant and positive relationship between the level of social support and health-related quality of life, suggesting that a patient's social environment influences the experience and course of their disease and also the level of functioning and their quality of life. Unfortunately, this study did not include an objective measure of health, and health status itself may be either a predictor or a component of quality of life.

Studies in other countries have produced similar findings. In Newcastle, Australia, a study was undertaken to compare quality of life in 138 dialysis patients and transplant recipients [49]. Again, the results showed that patients with a successful transplant rated highest in various aspects of quality of life, but that the home hemodialysis patients were nearly equivalent. Similarly, patients treated with CAPD ranked third, and clearly had a better quality of life than those patients treated by outpatient hemodialysis, even though their demographic characteristics were very similar. Contrary to expectations, the prevalence of clinical psychological distress among the patients was between 21% and 33%, and did not differ significantly between the four treatment groups. This rate is similar to that found in the general population of patients with other chronic illnesses. Similarly, there was no clear difference between the groups in terms of a past history of treatment for "nervous" problems. This suggests that successful adjustment to ESRD is more dependent on psychological adjustment than on the treatment modality selected, and that attention to the social and psychological adjustment of patients could be helpful in enhancing outcomes.

In terms of correlations, the strongest association found was between the general health questionnaire score and the total life satisfaction score. There were also correlations with current or past psychological distress, frequency of hospitalizations, and the feeling of control over life circumstances. In addition, for the patients treated by outpatient hemodialysis there was a significant negative association between duration of treatment and life satisfaction.

A study from Wellington, New Zealand, examined the quality of life of 108 dialysis patients, of whom 58 were on home hemodialysis [50]. Quality of life scores reported by nurses were significantly higher for the home hemodialysis patients than for those treated by outpatient hemodialysis or by CAPD ($p<0.05$ in both cases). 83% of the home hemodialysis patients were reported as working or studying normally, compared with 54% of the CAPD patients and 39% of the patients treated by outpatient hemodialysis. Similarly, the home hemodialysis patients scored significantly higher on daily living, support, and health and outlook scores.

The last several years' interest in rehabilitation and quality of life in dialysis patients has led to an increased use of exercise programs and more widespread provision of vocational assistance to help patients return to employment [51]. However, rehabilitation is much wider than just return to work or school, and a more encompassing definition is the restoration of meaningful existence in the patient's life. Better rehabilitation may also have other benefits for society, as there seems to be the possibility that rehabilitation, whether this results in return to work or not, it may also be associated with a lower hospitalization rate and a reduction in the need for nursing home care for elderly dialysis patients [52].

Patient perceptions are also important in terms

of quality of life. A number of different patient satisfaction surveys have been used over the years, but most of those in current use relate to more global aspects of dialysis care from the viewpoint of the dialysis unit. Patient surveys are not yet a standard part of the evaluation of ESRD treatment, nor are the instruments for this standardized. Recently the Agency for Health Care Policy and Research has funded a patient outcome study of dialysis care, the CHOICE (Choices for Healthy Outcomes in Caring for ESRD) study that examines the specifics of all aspects of patient care [53]. An early report from this study evaluates patients' views of dialysis care using a survey based on comments from focus groups that included both hemodialysis and peritoneal dialysis patients. These resulted in identification of the twenty-five highest rated aspects of dialysis care in terms of importance, and the twenty-five lowest rated aspects of care. From this, the authors developed a brief questionnaire for the CHOICE study that may be suitable for general use in a dialysis program. Unfortunately, home hemodialysis patients were not included in this preliminary study, but their perceptions as to what aspects of their care are most important should also be assessed and could help in comparing quality of life in patients treated by different modalities.

Finally, the last three years has seen increased attention to home hemodialysis as evidenced by sessions on this at the four most recent Annual Conferences on Peritoneal Dialysis and at other national and local meetings. This reflects the continuing interest of some patients, physicians and programs in what is seen as the best treatment for an appreciable number of patients. Most importantly, this interest is also being generated by the news about the development of new equipment designed specifically for home hemodialysis by Aksys Ltd. of Lincolnshire, Illinois [54] and others. Many years ago, Scribner in Seattle voiced the opinion that what is needed to make home hemodialysis more widely acceptable is the availability of what he called a "one-button machine". This would be so computerized, automated and fail-safe that the patient would have only have to press a button to initiate dialysis and there would not be the need for a family member or other dialysis aide to monitor the treatment. At the end of dialysis, the machine would automatically rinse, disinfect and store itself, the tubing set and the dialyzer in situ. At the appropriate time, the machine would then automatically prepare the equipment immediately prior to the time for the next dialysis. It is hoped the Aksys machine will be ready for initial clinical testing in the latter half of 1998.

At the same time, there has been a renewal of interest in more frequent hemodialysis in order to provide more adequate treatment. Over the years there have been a number of reports describing the benefits of hemodialysis carried out more often than three times weekly, and many of these have been summarized by Twardowski in a recent article that also discusses the requirements for equipment for home hemodialysis [55]. Most striking are the results of the nightly home hemodialysis program initiated by the late Robert Uldall in Toronto, Canada, and continued by Andreas Pierratos [56]. In the first two years of this, eleven patients were trained to dialyze at home for eight to ten hours overnight, six or seven times weekly, using modified standard hemodialysis equipment, a small polysulfone dialyzer and a permanently implanted Cook internal jugular catheter. Their average cumulative weekly Kt/V was 7.3 and phosphate removal was doubled. β_2-Microglobulin clearance was some five times that found with conventional dialysis, and serum β_2-microglobulin levels slowly but progressively decreased. Patients reported improvement in well-being, appetite and sleep pattern, the latter including correction of sleep apnea. They gained weight, fluid intake could be liberalized, they no longer required phosphate binders, and in some cases phosphate replacement was required. Nutritional intervention was necessary for management of the hypophosphatemia and new onset hyperlipidemia. With reuse of the dialyzers, the cost of this treatment was similar to that for CAPD [57–61]. The main remaining concern is with the blood access. Will there be problems with more frequent fistula or graft puncture and can a jugular venous catheter be used successfully long term?

This development of equipment specifically designed to make home hemodialysis simpler and less onerous, together with increased emphasis on the benefits of more frequent dialysis, whether overnight or using short high efficiency dialysis, will ultimately lead to increased acceptance and use of home hemodialysis.

CONCLUSIONS

Because of its advantages, home hemodialysis is an important option that should be available to all suitable patients. Unfortunately, this is not the case at the present time. It is just as important there be active assessment of the quality of the care provided in the home as it is for patients treated in a dialysis unit. Equally importantly, there needs to be ongoing assessment of health care-related quality of life, and the rehabilitation of home hemodialysis patients, together with the provision of all the necessary supporting services. The problems of providing these assessments and services are increased by the logistical problems associated with dialysis remote from the center.

All the studies suggest that the overall results of treatment with home hemodialysis are at least as good and probably better than those with either peritoneal dialysis or outpatient hemodialysis. Careful monitoring of quality of care and quality of life should help to maintain and expand this record. This is important as we move into what Relman has called the "Era of Assessment and Accountability" in medical care [54].

REFERENCES

1. Merrill JP, Schupak E, Cameron E, and Hampers CL. Hemodialysis in the home. JAMA 1964; 190:468–70.
2. Baillod RA, Comty C, Ilahi M, Konotey-Ahulu FID, Sevitt L and Shaldon S. Overnight haemodialysis in the home. Proc Eur Dial Transpl Assoc 1965; 2:99–103.
3. Curtis FK, Cole JJ, Fellows BJ, Tyler LL and Scribner BH. Hemodialysis in the home. Trans Am Soc Artif Intern Organs 1965; 11:7–10.
4. Tenckhoff H, Shilipetar G, vanPaasschen WJ, and Swanson E. A home peritoneal dialysate delivery system. Trans ASAIO 1969; 15:103–7.
5. Popovich RP, Moncrieff JW, Dechard JB, Bomar JB and Pyle WK. The definition of a novel portable/wearable equilibrium peritoneal dialysis technique. Abstracts, ASAIO 1976; 5:65.
6. Diaz-Buxo JA. Continuous cyclic peritoneal dialysis. In Nolph KB, editor. Peritoneal Dialysis, 3rd edition. Dordrecht, The Netherlands, Kluwer Academic Publishers; 1989:169–73.
7. Health Care Financing Administration. Research Report: End Stage Renal Disease Program Highlights 1996. Department of Health and Human Services, Health Care Financing Administration, Office of Clinical Standards and Quality. Data from the Program Management and Medical Information System, 1990–96, Baltimore, MD, August 31, 1997.
8. Hull AR and Parker TF. Introduction and summary: Proceedings from the morbidity, mortality and prescription of dialysis symposium, Dallas, TX, September 15 to 17, 1989. Am J Kidney Dis 1989; 15:375–83.
9. Held PJ, Brunner F, Odaka M, Garcia JR, Port FK and Gaylin DS. Five-year survival for end-stage renal disease patients in the United States, Europe, and Japan, 1982 to 1987. Am J Kidney Dis 1990; 15:451–7.
10. Held PJ, Blagg CR, Liska DW, Port FK, Hakim R and Levin N. The dose of hemodialysis according to dialysis prescription in Europe and the U.S., 1986–87. Kidney Int 1992; 42:S16–S21.
11. ESRD Core indicators project for hemodialysis patients. Health Care Financing Administration. Baltimore, MD, 1995, 1996, and 1997.
12. Renal physicians association working committee on clinical practice guidelines. Clinical Practice Guideline on Adequacy of Hemodialysis. Clinical practice guideline, no. 1. Washington, DC. December 1993.
13. National Kidney Foundation DOQITM Clinical Practice Guidelines. New York, NY, National Kidney Foundation; 1997.
14. Moorhead JF, Baillod RA, Hopewell JP et al. Survival rates of patients treated by home and hospital dialysis and cadaveric renal transplantation. Br Med J 1970; 4:83–5.
15. Price JDE, Ashby K and Reeve CE. Result of 12 years' treatment of chronic renal failure by dialysis and transplantation. Can Med Assoc J 1978; 118:263–6.
16. Baillod RA and Moorhead JF. Review of ten years' home dialysis. Proc Eur Dial Transpl Assoc 1974; 11:68–75.
17. Williams GW, Weller JM, Ferguson CW, Forsythe SB and Shu-Chen W. Survival of end-stage renal disease patients: Age-adjusted differences in treatment outcomes. Kidney Int 1983; 24:691–3.
18. Wing AJ. Survival on integrated therapies What assumptions shall we make? Am J Kidney Dis 1984; 4:224–32.
19. Prowant B, Nolph KD, Dutton S et al. Actuarial analysis of patient survival and dropout with various end-stage renal disease therapies. Am J Kidney Dis 1983; 3:27–31.
20. Rubin J, Hsu H, Bower J. Survival on dialysis therapy: One center's experience. J Med Sci 1989; 297:80–90.
21. Mailloux LU, Kapikian N, Napolitano B et al. Home hemodialysis: patient outcomes during a 24-year period of time from 1970 through 1993. Adv Renal Repl Ther 1996; 3:112–19
22. Woods JD, Port FK, Stannard D, Blagg CR and Held PJ. Comparison of mortality with home hemodialysis: a national study. Kidney Int 1996; 49:1464–70.
23. Teehan BP and Hakim R. CAPD Quo Vadis? J Am Soc Nephrol 1995; 6:139–43.
24. Habach G, Bloembergen W, Mauger E and Port FK. Hospitalization among United States dialysis patients: hemodialysis versus peritoneal dialysis. J Am Soc Nephrol 1995; 5:1940–8.
25. Bloembergen WE, Port FK, Mauger EA and Wolfe RA. A comparison of mortality between patients treated with hemodialysis and peritoneal dialysis. J Am Soc Nephrol 1995; 6:177–83.

26. Bloembergen WE, Port FK, Mauger EA and Wolfe RA. A comparison of cause of death between patients treated with hemodialysis and peritoneal dialysis. J Am Soc Nephrol 1995; 6:184–91.

27. Guyatt GH, Feeney DH and Patrick DL. Measuring health-related quality of life. An Intern Med 1993; 118:622–9.

28. Kimmel PL, Peterson RA, Weihs KL et al. Aspects of quality of life in hemodialysis patients. J Am Soc Nephrol 1995; 6:1418–26.

29. Gill TM and Feinstein AR. A critical appraisal of the quality of quality-of-life measurements. JAMA 1994; 272:619–26.

30. Nissenson AR. Measuring, managing, and improving quality in end-stage renal disease treatment setting: peritoneal dialysis. Am J Kidney Dis 1994; 24:368–75.

31. Kurtin P and Nissenson AR. Variation in end-stage renal disease patient outcomes: what we know, what should we know, and how do we find out? J Am Soc Nephrol 1993; 3:1738–47

32. Edgell ET, Coons SJ, Carter WB et al. A review of health-related quality-of-life measures used in end-stage renal disease. Clin Ther 1996; 18:887–938.

33. Dunham C, Mattern WD and McGaghie WC. Preferences of nephrologists among end-stage renal disease treatment options. Am J Nephrol 1985; 5:470–5.

34. Mattern WD, McGaghie WC, Rigby RJ, Nissenson AR, Dunham CB, Khayrallah MA. Selection of ESRD treatment: an international study. Am J Kidney Dis 1989; 13:457–64.

35. Nissenson AR, Prichard SS, Cheng IKP et al. Non-medical factors that impact on ESRD modality selection. Kidney Int 1993; 43:S120–S127.

36. Kendix M. Dialysis modality selection among patients attending freestanding dialysis facilities. Health Care Financing Rev 1997; 18:3–21.

37. Kutner NG, Fair PL and Kutner MH. Assessing depression and anxiety in chronic dialysis patients. J Psychsom Res 1985; 29:23–31.

38. Kaplan DeNour A. Prediction of adjustment to chronic hemodialysis. In Levy NG, editor. Psychonephrology: Psychological Factors in Hemodialysis and Transplantation, vol 1. New York, Plenum; 1981:117–32.

39. Gutman RA, Stead WW and Robinson RR. Physical activity and employment status of patients on maintenance dialysis. N Engl J Med 1981; 304:309–13.

40. Abram HS, Hester LR, Sheridan WF and Epstein GM. Sexual functioning in patients with chronic renal failure. J Nerv Ment Dis 1975; 160:220–6.

41. Kalman TP, Wilson PG and Kalman CM. Psychiatric morbidity in long-term renal transplant recipients and patients undergoing hemodialysis. JAMA 1983; 250:55–8.

42. Churchill DN, Torrance GW, Taylor DW et al. Measurement of quality of life in end-stage renal disease: The time trade-off approach. Clin Invest Med 1987; 10:14–20.

43. Julius M, Hawthorne VM, Carpienter-Alting P, Kniesley J, Wolfe RA and Port FK. Independence in activities of daily living for end-stage renal disease patients: Biomedical and demographic correlates. Am J Kidney Dis 1989; 13:61–9.

44. Evans RW, Manninen DL, Garrison LP et al. The quality of life of patients with end-stage renal disease. N Engl J Med 1985; 312:553–9.

45. Bremer BA, McCauley CR, Rona RM and Johnson JP. Quality of life in end-stage renal disease: a reexamination. Am J Kidney Dis 1989; 13:200–9.

46. Kutner NG, Brogan D and Kutner MH. End-stage renal disease treatment modality and patients' quality of life. Longitudinal assessment. Am J Nephrol 1986; 6:396–402.

47. Oberley ET and Schatell DR. Home hemodialysis: Survival, quality of life, and rehabilitation. Adv Ren Replace Ther 1996; 3:147–53.

48. Tell GS, Mittelmark MB, Hylander B, Shumaker SA, Russell G and Burkart JM. Social support and health-related quality of life in black and white dialysis patients. ANNA J 1995; 22:301–8.

49. Morris PLP and Jones B. Life satisfaction across treatment methods for patients with end-stage renal failure. Med J Aust 1989; 150:428–32.

50. Fox E, Peace K, Neale TJ, Morrison RBI, Hatfield PJ and Mellsop G. "Quality of life" for patients with end-stage renal failure. Renal Failure 1991; 13: 31–5.

51. Thornton TA and Hakim RM. Meaningful rehabilitation of the end-stage renal disease patient. Sem Nephrol 1997; 17:246–52.

52. Blagg CR. The socioeconomic impact of rehabilitation. Am J Kidney Dis 1994; 24:S17–S21.

53. Rubin HR, Jenckes M, Fink NE et al. Patient's view of dialysis care: development of a taxonomy and rating of importance of different aspects of care. Am J Kidney Dis 1997; 30:793–801.

54. Kenley RS. Tearing down the barriers to daily home hemodialysis and achieving the highest value renal therapy through holistic product design. Adv Renal Replace Ther 1996; 3:137-46.

55. Twardowski ZJ. Daily home hemodialysis: A hybrid of hemodialysis and peritoneal dialysis. Adv Renal Replace Ther 1996; 3:124–32.

56. Uldall R, Ouwendyk M, Francoeur R et al. Slow nocturnal home hemodialysis at the Wellesley Hospital. Adv Renal Replace Ther 1996; 3:133–6.

57. Pierratos A, Uldall R, Ouwendyk M, Francoeur R and Vas S. Two years experience with slow nocturnal hemodialysis (SNHD). (Abstract). J Am Soc Nephrol 1996; 7:1417.

58. Raj D, Ouwendyk M, Francoeur R, Vas S, Uldall R and Pierratos A. B2 microglobulin removal by slow nocturnal hemodialysis. A promise for prevention of dialysis related amyloidosis (Abstract). J Am Soc Nephrol 1996; 7:1495..

59. Langos V, Ecclestone A, Lum D et al. Slow nocturnal hemodialysis: Nutritional aspects. (Abstract). J Am Soc Nephrol 1996; 7:1518

60. Pierratos A, Thornely K, Ouwendyk M, Francoeur R and Hanly P. Nocturnal hemodialysis improves sleep quality in patients with chronic renal failure (Abstract). J Am Soc Nephrol 1997; 8:169

61. Dominic SC, Raj M, Ouwendyk R, Francoeur R et al. Amino acid profile in nocturnal hemodialysis (Abstract). J Am Soc Nephrol 1997; 8:170.

62. Relman AS. Assessment and accountability: the third revolution. N Engl J Med 1988; 319:1220–2.

16. Selection of adequacy criteria models for hemodialysis

WILLIAM R. CLARK

INTRODUCTION

For the past several years, the topic of hemodia-lysis (HD) adequacy has been one of the most widely discussed and investigated subjects in all of ESRD therapy. However, considerable disagree-ment on several fundamental issues in HD ade-quacy, including the defining criteria, persist. Although this topic has been reviewed extensively in the literature [1–5], this vitally important aspect of the care of the chronic HD patient has not been critically assessed from a quality assurance per-spective. The purpose of this chapter is first to provide a clinical overview, including a brief review of landmark studies that provide the basis for current HD adequacy recommendations. The remainder of the chapter deals with implementa-tion of these current recommendations and the quality assurance issues the chronic dialysis unit must consider.

RATIONALE FOR THE USE OF UREA AS A UREMIC SURROGATE

The low-molecular weight nitrogenous waste pro-ducts ("small solutes") collectively represent the class of uremic solutes that has been most exhaus-tively studied and employed for quantification (such as urea kinetic modeling: UKM) [6–8]. As a class, these solutes have certain distinct character-istics. First, neither urea nor creatinine, the solutes in this class employed clinically for quantification, is a uremic "toxin" per se. Instead, these com-pounds are felt to be surrogates for a broad class of uremic toxins whose biochemical and kinetic characteristics are similar to those of urea and creatinine. Second, as the name implies, they have

relatively low molecular weights, generally less than 200 daltons. As such, their transmembrane removal during hemodialysis is mediated primar-ily by diffusion since the rate at which this latter process occurs is inversely proportional to solute size [9]. Third, the rate at which these compounds are generated is related to protein metabolism. For example, the rate at which urea is generated is directly proportional to the rate at which net catabolism of body protein occurs. This stoichio-metric relationship is exploited clinically in UKM [10]. For patients in "steady state" with regard to protein metabolism (i.e. net anabolism = net cata-bolism), the net protein catabolic rate (PCR), which can be estimated from the UKM-derived urea generation rate, provides an estimate of diet-ary protein intake. The rate of creatinine genera-tion is also tied to protein metabolism. Creatinine is a by-product of muscle protein metabolism and the rate at which it is generated is proportional to muscle mass (lean body mass) [11]. Therefore, by use of a recently described technique called creati-nine kinetic modeling [12, 13], additional useful nutritional information can be derived.

An ongoing controversy in HD adequacy relates to the specific choice of surrogate solute used for quantifying treatment. Among nephrologists that believe therapy quantification is necessary, the majority believe the uremic state is most strongly influenced by the extent to which low-molecular weight nitrogenous waste products are removed by a dialytic therapy. Early proponents of this view-point used several studies performed in the 1970s and early 1980s [8, 14, 15] as supportive evidence. The investigation which has been most frequently cited as supportive of the mediating role of small solute retention in uremia is the National Coop-erative Dialysis Study (NCDS) [8]. In this study, a

163

L.W. Henderson and R.S. Thuma (eds.), Quality Assurance in Dialysis, 2nd Edition, 163–172.
© 1999 *Kluwer Academic Publishers. Printed in Great Britain*

total of 152 patients were randomly assigned to receive one of four possible HD regimens in which two parameters, the time-averaged concentration of urea (TAC_{urea}) and treatment time, were varied. Both TAC_{urea}, assumed to be a surrogate for small solute removal, and time, assumed to be a surrogate for middle molecule removal, were varied at two different target levels in a 2×2 study design. (The basis for using time as a middle molecule surrogate is the relative importance of time vs. blood and dialysate flow rates in the removal of slowly diffusing solutes in this size range [16].) The results of the study, in which morbidity (withdrawal from the study due to medical reasons) was followed for up to 48 weeks, were interpreted as indicating outcome in chronic HD patients is more closely related to small solute effects than to middle molecule effects. Specifically, patients in the two arms of the study in which the target TAC_{urea} was low (50 mg/dL) had significantly less morbidity than patients in the high target TAC_{urea} (90 mg/dL) groups. A statistically significant effect of time was observed only in patients having high target TAC_{urea} values. In addition, in the one year period immediately following the study's completion, significantly more deaths occurred in the high TAC_{urea} groups than in the low TAC_{urea} groups.

In a subsequent "mechanistic" analysis of the NCDS data by Gotch and Sargent [17], morbidity in the study (withdrawal from the study or "percent failure") was found to vary inversely with delivered Kt/V. Gotch and Sargent chose to characterize the relationship between percent failure and Kt/V with a step function rather than an exponentially decreasing function. Therefore, percent failure for Kt/V values of 0.8 and less was expressed at a high constant value (approximately 55%) while that for Kt/V values of 0.9 and greater was expressed at a low constant value (approximately 10%). For patients dialyzed thrice weekly, Gotch and Sargent concluded adequate dialysis was defined by a delivered Kt/V of 1.0 per treatment and a normalized PCR (dietary protein intake) of 1.0 g/kg/day. These investigators also concluded that delivery of HD at a Kt/V level of greater than 1.0 per treatment was "of no apparent clinical value with the cellulosic dialyzers in current use".

However, in a reappraisal of the NCDS data base, Keshaviah [18] provided a vastly different interpretation of the study. For this evaluation, edited data that had been mistakenly recorded or entered in the original assessment of the study results were available. Of particular interest was the reappraisal of patient outcome (percent failure) as a function of Kt/V. In contrast to the step function to which Gotch and Sargent [17] fit the unedited data, the edited data were fit more appropriately to an exponential function in the reappraisal. Therefore, as opposed to the original mechanistic analysis, this re-analysis suggested Kt/V values of greater than 1.0 per treatment indeed did afford additional clinical benefit.

INADEQUATE HD IN THE UNITED STATES: SCOPE OF THE PROBLEM

Although the Gotch and Sargent mechanistic analysis was widely disseminated and debated, its impact on HD prescription in the United States was questionable. Multiple reports [19–21] in the early 1990s suggested a large percentage of US HD patients did not even receive prescribed doses that attained the Kt/V value of 1.0 considered adequate delivered therapy by Gotch and Sargent [17]. This observation was attributed to several factors, including cost containment and patient preferences.

The possible causative role of inadequate HD prescription and delivery in the relatively high American mortality rates was addressed in a 1989 conference in Dallas [22]. In this symposium, the gross mortality of American HD patients was reported to the highest of all the reporting registries. However, emphasis was placed on the need for co-morbidity adjustment when comparing data from the various registries [23]. No information regarding delivered dialysis was presented. However, data from the large National Medical Care (NMC) data base demonstrated mortality was inversely proportional to treatment time [24], an important component of dialysis dose. This observation was confirmed by Held et al. [25] in a separate analysis.

The Dallas meeting alerted the American dialysis community to the pervasive problem of underdialysis. One response to this meeting has been the development by oversight agencies of minimal criteria defining adequate HD [26, 27]. Recent longitudinal data [28] suggest the dissemination of these recommendations have produced a gradual but measurable increase delivered dialysis dose over the past few years. These recommendations have also resulted in two other clinical devlopments. First, there has been a proliferation of HD quantification techniques available for use by clinicians. The other development has been the recent publication of a number of studies demonstrating a correlation between HD dose and outcome. The important aspects of these two developments are reviewed below.

RECENT STUDIES DEFINING RELATIONSHIP BETWEEN HD DOSE AND OUTCOME

In 1993, Owen et al. [29] published outcome data for a large cohort of patients (approximately 13,000) in whom the urea reduction ratio (URR) was employed to quantify dialysis dose. These patients were assessed over a six month period in 1990 and 1991. In this study, URR (mean $\pm$ SD: $59 \pm 9\%$) was found to be correlated inversely with death risk, although serum albumin (S_{alb}) was an even more powerful predictor of death. However, based on the assumption that S_{alb} is a nutritional index, these data failed to demonstrate a direct relationship between nutritional status and small solute removal.

Based on their experience at the Regional Kidney Disease Program (RKDP), Collins et al. [30] reported on the outcome of approximately 1,800 patients who commenced HD between 1976 and 1989. For both nondiabetic patients with comorbid risk factors and diabetics, Kt/V (less than 1.2) and S_{alb} (less than 3.5 g/dL) were both inversely related to death risk. The authors concluded that optimal survival was defined by a single-pool Kt/V of 1.2–1.4 in nondiabetics and by a Kt/V $\geqslant$ 1.4 (mean, 1.6) in diabetics.

Hakim et al. [31] described their experience at Vanderbilt University with an urban, largely African-American patient population over the years 1988–1991. From 1988 to 1991, substantial mean increases in both treatment time (195 vs. 212 minutes) and in vivo blood urea clearance (170 vs. 220 mL/minutes). These changes translated into an augmentation in mean delivered Kt/V from

0.8 ± 0.32 to 1.18 ± 0.41 and concomitant improvements in both mortality and morbidity, the latter of which was assessed by hospitalization rate.

The final recent study demonstrating a clear relationship between delivered HD dose and outcome was conducted by Parker et al. [32] of Dallas Nephrology Associates (DNA). From 1989 to 1992, the mean delivered single-pool Kt/V increased from 1.18 ± 0.28 to 1.46 ± 0.30 while the URR increased from 61.3% to 69.6% over the same time period. These changes were sufficient to yield standardized mortality rates [33] that were significantly below the mortality rates of the US reference population in the final two years of the study. These investigators concluded that both single-pool Kt/V and URR are appropriate tools in the quantification of delivered HD dose. Their recommendation was that the minimum single-pool (delivered) Kt/V should be 1.4, or an equivalent URR.

All four of these studies concluded that survival in American chronic HD patients was directly related to the dose of therapy over the dose ranges investigated. However, the manner in which HD dose was measured differed greatly among the four studies. One study used the URR while the other studies employed the Kt/V as the primary tool for measuring delivered dose. In addition, among these latter studies, one accounted for post-HD rebound while the post-HD BUN was drawn immediately after treatment in the other two. These disparities among the studies make dose comparisons difficult. However, largely in response to these four studies, a consensus statement defining minimally adequate HD as a delivered single-pool Kt/V of 1.2 was issued in 1994 [34].

COMMONLY USED SINGLE-POOL QUANTIFICATION METHODS

Urea Reduction Ratio

The URR, proposed by Lowrie and Lew [35] in 1991, is a single-pool, two-point (pre-dialysis and post-dialysis BUN) method described by the following equation:

$$ URR = 100\% \cdot (1 - R) \qquad (1) $$

where R=immediate post-dialysis BUN/pre-dialysis BUN. It is a single-pool methodology that accounts for neither intradialytic urea generation nor ultrafiltration. Although widely used, several studies [36–38] have shown that the URR is a rather insensitive method to measure changes in dialysis dose, especially at relatively high values of Kt/V. Sherman et al. [39] recently have demonstrated that substantial variability in Kt/V can be observed for a given URR, an effect which increases with increasing HD dose (Figure 16.1). These investigators showed that, for a given URR value, the single-pool Kt/V may vary by $\geqslant 0.2$ around the median value, depending on the intradialytic urea generation rate and the extent of ultrafiltration. The authors concluded that, although the URR may be a useful standardized method to assess dialysis dose in large groups of patients (i.e. data bases), it lacked sufficient accuracy for use in monitoring individual patients.

VVSP Model

This model involves application of mass balance principles to urea nitrogen during both the intradialytic and interdialytic periods and requires three successive BUN samples (pre/post/pre-dialysis) to be obtained [8, 10]. Similar to other single-pool quantification techniques, urea is assumed to be distributed in one body compartment (total body water), even during dialysis. The major output parameters are Kt/V and PCR. A problem with this technique is the requirement for an accurate estimate of in vivo dialyzer urea clearance. Dialyzer clearance determination by the classical method, which involves drawing simultaneous arterial and venous line BUN samples, is not widely applicable in clinical practice. An alternative approach is the use of dialyzer manufacturer's in vitro data to estimate in vivo clearance [37]. However, this latter approach has not been validated in a large-scale trial. Therefore, the requirement for an accurate estimate of dialyzer urea clearance is a major drawback of the VVSP model.

Daugirdas Equation

The Daugirdas second-generation equation [40] is a two-point kinetic method having a greater level

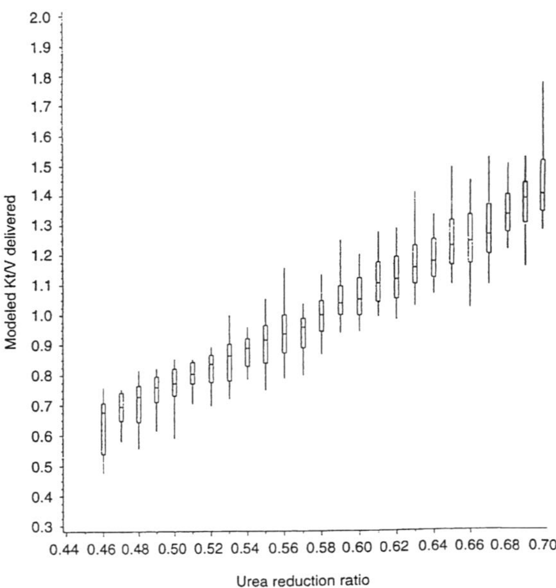

Fig. 16.1. Kt/V versus urea reduction ratio (URR). The boxes represent 50% and the whiskers represent 90% intervals. Reproduced with permission from Sherman et al [39].

of sophistication than the URR. This technique employs a logarithmic equation relating delivered Kt/V to R, the post-/pre-dialysis BUN ratio, and additional parameters:

$$Kt/V = -\ln(R - 0.008 \cdot t) + (4 - 3.5 \cdot R) \cdot (UF/W) \qquad (2)$$

In this equation, UF represents intradialytic ultrafiltration (liters) and W is post-dialysis weight (kg). The second term on the right-hand side of the equation accounts for intradialytic urea generation while the third term represents the effect of ultrafiltration. This equation was clinically validated in a group of 374 HD patients in whom the Kt/V predicted by this equation and that determined by the VVSP model were found to be highly correlated.

DRAWBACKS OF SINGLE-POOL METHODS

The increasing use of high-efficiency therapies has highlighted the general inability of single-pool methodologies to describe urea's kinetic behavior during HD adequately. A model consisting of two compartments (pools) more accurately represents urea kinetics. Urea's two-pool behavior typically results in a significant rebound in the immediate post-dialysis period [41, 42] that has three components [4] (Figure 16.2). The initial component, which is dissipated within 20 seconds, is related to access recirculation. Cardiopulmonary recirculation [43] which contributes to urea rebound for up to 2 minutes post-HD, is the second component. As described by Depner [4], cardiopulmonary recirculation, which is found only in patients with peripheral arteriovenous vascular accesses, is a disequilibrium that exists between one blood circuit comprised of the heart, lungs, and dialyzer and another circuit involving the remainder of the circulation and the dialyzer. In the heart-lung circuit, blood flow to and from the dialyzer is relatively rapid, resulting in efficient urea removal in this circuit. However, urea delivery to the dialyzer from the peripheral circulation is impaired due to the repeated delivery of already well-dialyzed blood from the heart-lung compartment to the dialyzer, which effectively limits the delivery of blood from the peripheral compartments.

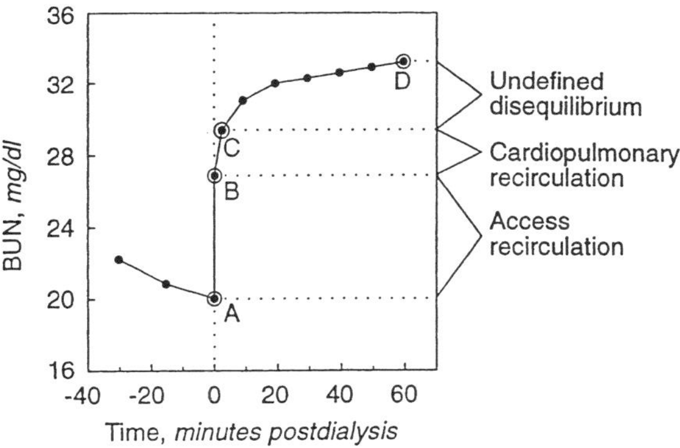

Fig. 16.2. Components of post-hemodialysis rebound. Reproduced with permission from Depner [4].

The third and most prominent component of urea rebound is related to actual compartmental differences in urea concentrations that develop during the intradialytic period and persist following treatment. One explanation for this rebound is the continued transfer of urea from the intracellular to the extracellular space, which occurs at a slower rate than dialytic removal of urea from the extracellular space [44, 45]. A second potential explanation can be found in the regional blood flow model, proposed by Daugirdas and Schneditz [46]. In this model, post-HD rebound is correlated with the degree of mismatch between blood supply and urea content in different body compartments. The failure of single-pool models to account for post-HD urea rebound may result in a substantial overestimation of the amount of dialysis actually delivered [47], which may lead to the prescription of insufficient therapy. Based on the above concern, kinetic models accounting for the two-pool behavior of urea during rapid dialysis have been proposed and these are described below.

DOUBLE-POOL QUANTIFICATION METHODS

Daugirdas Rate Equation

In this equation [46], a factor proportional to the efficiency (rate) of dialysis is used to account for the double-pool behavior of urea:

$$\Delta Kt/V = -0.6 \cdot (K/V) + 0.03 \tag{3}$$

In this equation, the rate of dialysis (K/V) is defined as the ratio of the dialyzer urea clearance to the distribution volume and $\Delta Kt/V$ is the estimated difference between the single-pool Kt/V and the double-pool Kt/V that would be determined from an equilibrated (30 minutes post-HD) BUN sample. Therefore, this estimation of delivered Kt/V incorporates the effect of post-HD urea rebound without the need for drawing a true equilbrated BUN sample. To estimate K/V, the delivered Kt/V derived from equation (1) is divided by dialysis time [K/V=(Kt/V)/t].

Dialysate-Side Therapy Quantification

Dialysate-side quantification of HD, a second double-pool methodology, was first described by Malchesky et al. in 1982 [48]. Similar to UKM, this method involves application of a urea nitrogen mass balance during the intradialytic and interdialytic periods, permitting the measurement of actual dialytic urea removal. However, no measurement of dialyzer urea clearance is required. A collection of the entire volume of spent dialysate along with BUN samples before and after dialysis are required. Although the logistics of this methodology preclude its widespread clinical use, it is generally regarded as the gold-standard quantification technique and, therefore, serves as a reference point for methods.

Advances in clinical chemistry methodologies and computer microprocessor technology have enabled the development of devices capable of accurately measuring effluent dialysate urea nitrogen concentrations. A number of on-line dialysate urea sensors recently have undergone clinical evaluations [49–52] and several of these have been cleared for human use by regulatory agencies around the world. However, only one (BioStat 1000; Baxter Healthcare Co., McGaw Park, Illinois, USA) [50] of these devices has been cleared by the FDA for use in the United States as of this writing. This device samples the effluent dialysate to produce a dialysate urea nitrogen vs. time profile. A typical profile, shown in Figure 16.3, is best fit with a double-exponential function, consistent with double-pool urea kinetics. The double-pool Kt/V is determined from the slopes of the individual exponential curves while total urea nitrogen removal is quantified by a graphical integration technique.

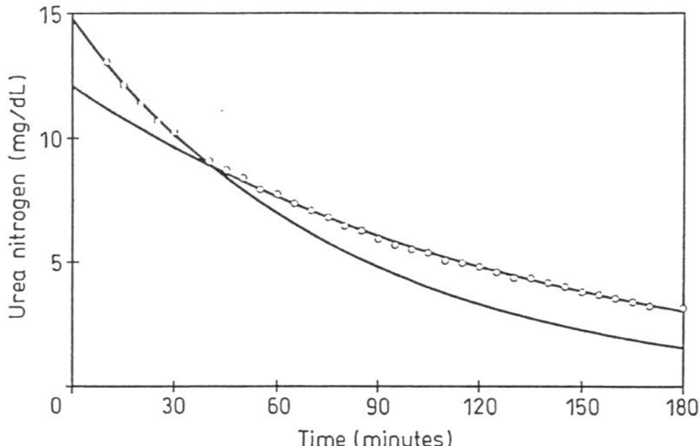

Fig. 16.3. Effluent dialysate urea nitrogen concentration, measured by a urea sensor, versus time during a typical patient treatment. The characteristic double-exponential profile is shown. Reproduced with permission from Keshaviah et al [49].

CURRENT RECOMMENDATIONS FOR THE DELIVERY OF ADEQUATE HD: THE NKF DIALYSIS OUTCOMES QUALITY INITIATIVE (DOQI)

The National Kidney Foundation (NKF) recently convened a working group whose goal was to develop HD adequacy guidelines for American patients. This group performed an exhaustive review of the literature and has recently published its recommendations [53]. For ESRD patients receiving thrice-weekly treatment, some of these guidelines are: 1) the delivered dose of HD should be measured using formal UKM, employing the single-pool, variable-volume model; 2) the minimum delivered dose of dialysis should be a Kt/V of 1.2 or a URR of 65% per treatment; 3) the prescribed dose of dialysis should be a Kt/V of 1.3; 4) the delivered dose of HD should be measured at least once a month; 5) post-dialysis BUN samples should be drawn using the Slow Flow/Stop Pump technique that prevents sample dilution with recirculated blood and minimizes the confounding effects of urea rebound (vide infra); and 6) the BUN sampling method used for a given patient should remain consistent.

Although the working group acknowledged that compartment effects can reduce the accuracy of single-pool urea kinetic calculations, they did not advocate the use of double-pool methodologies for the following reasons: 1) two-pool methods that require drawing a 30 minutes post-HD BUN sample are impractical in the outpatient HD setting; 2) studies demonstrating a relationship between HD dose and survival have employed single-pool methods; and 3) at present, there are no prospective outcome studies based on two-pool models. However, the working group acknowledged the need both for prospective studies employing blood-based double-pool models, such as the ongoing NIH HEMO Study [54], and further evaluation of on-line, dialysate-based quantification methodologies.

One of the most important issues addressed by the DOQI work group is the post-HD sample, as small differences in its timing can have a large impact on the measured HD dose. The work group recommended that this sample be drawn between 15 and 30 seconds after the blood pump has been turned down either to 50 mL/minute or off. This timing minimizes the component of rebound related to access recirculation (Figure 16.2).

DIFFERENCES BETWEEN THE PRESCRIBED AND DELIVERED DOSE OF HD: ASSESSMENT OF CAUSES

In many HD treatments, the actual (delivered) dose of therapy may be significantly less than the amount prescribed [20]. As detailed in Table 16.1, a large discrepancy between prescribed and delivered therapy has numerous possible causes. Both access recirculation and low access blood flow rate may limit delivered HD therapy. At present, considerable controversy regarding the most appropriate manner to diagnose access recirculation exists, as methodologies that employ BUN determinations [55], access pressure [56], and ultrasound [57] are all currently used. Devices designed to quantify access flow also have been developed recently [58].

Dialyzer dysfunction is another common cause of inadequate delivered HD and is usually related to membrane surface area loss secondary to clotting or the effects of reprocessing. Gotch originally demonstrated that maintaining total cell volume in reprocessed low-flux cellulosic hollow fiber dialyzers at greater than 80% of the baseline value preserves urea clearance at greater than 90% of the baseline value [59]. Although this original observation has generally been corroborated in subsequent studies [60], there are exceptions in the literature [61, 62]. These latter data suggest that additional investigation of the relationship between total cell volume and urea clearance during dialyzer reprocessing is warranted. As shown in Table 16.1, numerous other factors may account for large discrepancies between prescribed and delivered HD doses, including blood/dialysate pump miscalibrations, patient compliance issues (tardiness or early sign-off), and laboratory or blood sampling errors.

Recently, algorithms designed to assist the clinician in troubleshooting the cause of a less than expected delivered HD dose have been developed [63, 64]. As shown in Figure 16.4, the first step in assessing an unexpected decrease in delivered HD dose is dictated by the number of patients involved. If the problem involves multiple patients

Table 16.1. Causes of shortfalls in hemodialysis delivery [adapted from Reference 53]

Reduction in dialyzer urea clearance
- Access recirculation
- Inadequate access blood flow
- Reliance on manufacturer's in vitro clearance data for prescription
- Loss of membrane surface area secondary to reprocessing
- Dialyzer clotting
- Blood/dialysate pump miscalibration

Reduction in treatment time
- Patient tardiness
- Patient premature sign-off
- Miscalculated effective treatment time (failure to account for interruptions)

Laboratory or blood sampling errors (see text)

in the unit, it may be related to recent changes in equipment or policy. The major equipment-related problems include pump miscalibration and dialyzer dysfunction, both reuse-related and non-reuse-related. An example of a policy change would be a liberalization of the manner in which patients arriving late and signing off early are handled. If the shortfall in dialysis delivery occurs for an individual patient in whom the prescription was attained, the vascular access is implicated. If recirculation (determined by the BUN method) is greater than 10–15% and needle placement is correct, these investigators recommend a fistulogram. On the other hand, a recirculation value less than 10% would lead to an empiric increase in the HD dose in the hands of these investigators.

SUMMARY

In conclusion, considerable progress has been made in the past several years in defining the relationship between delivered HD dose and outcome. However, the most appropriate methodology for quantifying HD remains controversial, particularly with regard to single-pool vs. double-pool techniques. Current recommendations (e.g. National Kidney Foundation DOQI) for adequate delivery of chronic HD are based on single-pool methodologies. However, the growing interest in double-pool quantification techniques, and specifically, on-line dialysate-based methodologies will probably lead to their routine use in the future.

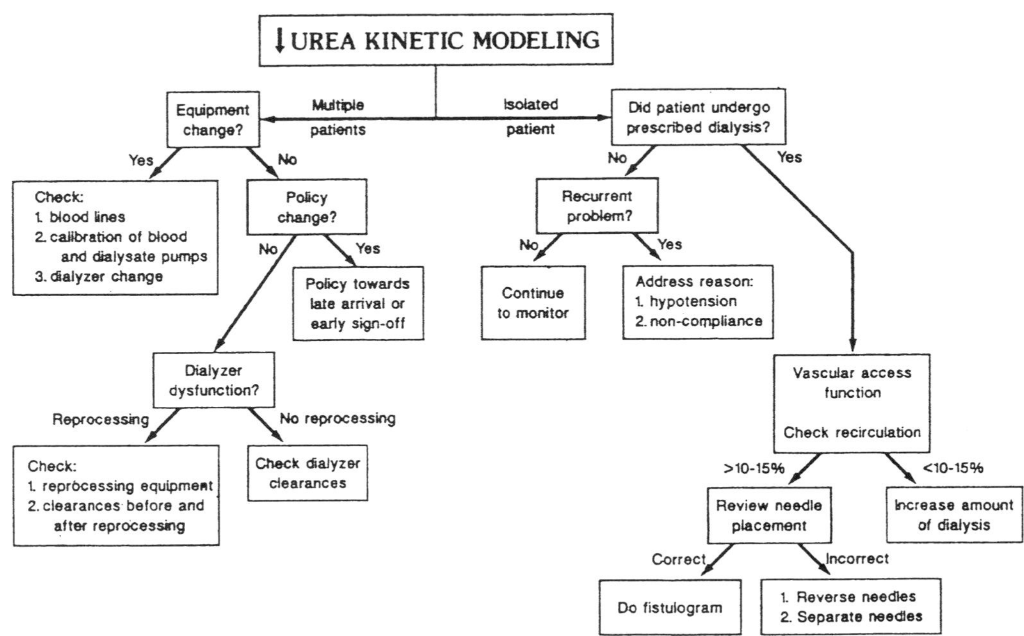

Fig. 16.4. An algorithm for an approach to evaluating patients with unexpected differences between prescribed and delivered hemodialysis dose. Reproduced with permission from Delmez and Windus [63].

REFERENCES

1. Levine J and Bernard D. The role of urea kinetic modeling, TAC_{urea}, and Kt/V in achieving optimal dialysis: a critical reappraisal. Am J Kidney Dis 1990; 15:285–301.
2. Hakim R, Depner T and Parker T. Adequacy of hemodialysis. Am J Kidney Dis 1992; 20:107–13.
3. Vanholder R and Ringoir S. Adequacy of dialysis: a critical analysis. Kidney Int 1992; 42:540–58.
4. Depner T. Assessing adequacy of hemodialysis: urea modeling. Kidney Int 1994; 45:1522–35.
5. Clark W, Rocco M and Collins A. Quantification of hemodialysis: analysis of methods and the relevance to patient outcome. Blood Purif 1997; 15:92–111.
6. Sargent J and Gotch F. The study of uremia by manipulation of blood concentrations using combinations of hollow fiber devices. Trans Am Soc Artif Intern Organs 1974; 20:395–401.
7. Sargent J and Gotch F. Mathematical modeling of dialysis therapy. Kidney Int 1980; 18:S2–10.
8. Sargent J. Control of dialysis by single-pool urea model: the National Cooperative Dialysis Study. Kidney Int 1983; 23:S19–25.
9. Henderson L. Of time, TAC_{urea}, and treatment schedules. Kidney Int 1988; 33:S105–6.
10. Gotch F. Kinetic modeling in hemodialysis. In Nissenson A, Fine R and Gentile D, editors. Clinical dialysis, 3rd edition. Norwalk: Appleton and Lange, 1995; 156–88.
11. Forbes G and Bruining G. Urinary creatinine excretion and lean body mass. Am J Clin Nutr 1976; 29:1359–66.
12. Keshaviah P, Nolph K, Moore H, Prowant B, Emerson P, Meyer M et al. Lean body mass estimation by creatinine kinetics. J Am Soc Nephrol 1994; 4:1475–85.
13. Canaud B, Garred L, Argiles A, Flavier J, Bouloux C and Mion C. Creatinine kinetic modelling: a simple and reliable tool for the assessment of protein nutritional status in haemodialysis patients. Nephrol Dial Transplant 1995; 10:1405–10.
14. Teschan P, Ginn H, Bourne J and Ward J. Neurobehavioral probes for adequacy of dialysis. Trans Am Soc Artif Intern Organs 1977; 23:556–60.
15. Lowrie E, Laird N, Parker T and Sargent J. Effect of the hemodialysis prescription on patient morbidity. Report from the National Cooperative Dialysis Study. N Engl J Med 1981; 305:1176–81.
16. Babb A, Popovich R, Christopher T and Scribner B. The genesis of the square meter-hour hypothesis. Trans Am Soc Artif Intern Organs 1971; 17:81–91.
17. Gotch F and Sargent J. A mechanistic analysis of the National Cooperative Dialysis Study. Kidney Int 1985; 28:526–34.

18. Keshaviah P. Urea kinetic and middle molecule approaches to assessing the adequacy of hemodialysis and CAPD. Kidney Int 1993; 43:S28–S38.

19. Gotch F, Yarian S and Keen M. A kinetic survey of US hemodialysis prescriptions. Am J Kidney Dis 1990; 15:511–15.

20. Delmez J and Windus D. Hemodialysis prescription and delivery in a metropolitan community. Kidney Int 1992; 41:1023–8.

21. Held P, Port F, Garcia J, Gaylin D, Levin N and Agodoa L. Hemodialysis prescription and delivery in the US: results from the USRDS case mix study (abs). J Am Soc Nephrol 1991; 2:328.

22. Hull A and Parker T. Proceedings from the morbidity, mortality, and prescription of dialysis symposium, Dallas, Texas, September 15 to 17, 1989. Am J Kidney Dis 1990; 15:375–83.

23. Collins A, Hanson G, Umen A, Kjellstrand C and Keshaviah P: Changing risk factor demographics in end-stage renal disease patients entering hemodialysis and the impact on long-term mortality. Am K Kidney Dis 1990; 15:422–32.

24. Lowrie E and Lew N. Death risk in hemodialysis patients: the predictive values of commonly measured variables and an evaluation of death rate differences between facilities. Am J Kidney Dis 1990; 15:458–82.

25. Held P, Levin N, Bovbierg R, Pauly M and Diamond L. Mortality and duration of hemodialysis. J Am Med Assoc 1991; 265:871–5.

26. Health care financing adminstration end-stage renal disease network scope of work 1991–1993.

27. Renal Physicians Association Working Committee on Clinical Practice Guidelines. Clinical practice guidelines on adequacy of hemodialysis. Clinical practice guideline, no. 1, Washington, 1993.

28. Helgerson S, McClellan W, Frederick P, Beaver S, Frankenfield D and McMullan M. Improvement in adequacy of delivered dialysis for adult in-center hemodialysis patients in the United States, 1993–1995. Am J Kidney Dis 1997; 29:851–61.

29. Owen W, Lew N, Liu Y, Lowrie E and Lazarus JM. The urea reduction ratio and serum albumin as predictors of mortality in patients undergoing hemodialysis. N Engl J Med 1993; 329:1001–6.

30. Collins A, Ma J, Umen A and Keshaviah P. Urea index and other predictors of long-term outcome in hemodialysis patient survival. Am J Kidney Dis 1994; 23:272–82.

31. Hakim R, Breyer J, Ismail N and Schulman G. Effects of dose of dialysis on morbidity and mortality. Am J Kidney Dis 1994; 23:661–9.

32. Parker T, Husni L, Huang W, Lew N and Lowrie E. Survival of hemodialysis patients in the United States is improved with a greater quantity of dialysis. Am J Kidney Dis 1994; 23:670–80.

33. Wolfe R, Gaylin D, Port F, Held P, and Wood C. Using USRDS generated mortality tables to compare local ESRD mortality rates to national rates. Kidney Int 1992; 42:991–6.

34. Morbidity and mortality of renal dialysis. An NIH consensus conference statement. Ann Intern Med 1994; 121:62–70.

35. Lowrie E and Lew N. The urea reduction ratio (URR): a simple method for evaluating hemodialysis treatment. Contemp Dial Nephrol 1991; 12:11–20.

36. Depner T. Estimation of Kt/V from the urea reduction ratio for varying levels of dialytic weight loss. Semin Dial 1993; 6:242.

37. Daugirdas J and Depner T. A nomogram approach to hemodialysis urea modeling. Am J Kidney Dis 1994; 23:33–40.

38. DeOreo P and Hamburger R. Urea reduction ratio is not a consistent predictor of Kt/V (abs). J Am Soc Nephrol 1995; 6:597.

39. Sherman R, Cody R, Rogers M and Solanchick J. Accuracy of the urea reduction ratio in predicting dialysis delivery. Kidney Int 1995; 47:319–21.

40. Daugirdas J. Second generation logarithmic estimates of single-pool variable volume Kt/V: an analysis of error. JASN 1993; 4:1205–13.

41. Pedrini L, Zereik S and Rasmy S. Causes, kinetics, and clinical implications of post-hemodialysis urea rebound. Kidney Int 1988; 34:817–24.

42. Phlederer B, Torrey C, Priester-Coary A, Lau A and Daugirdas J. Estimating equilibrated Kt/V from an intradialytic sample: effects of access and cardiopulmonary recirculation. Kidney Int 1995; 48:832–7.

43. Schneditz D, Kauffman A, Polaschegg H, Levin N and Daugirdas J. Cardiopulmonary recirculation during hemodialysis. Kidney Int 1992; 42:1450–6.

44. Heineken F, Evans M, Keen M and Gotch F. Intercompartmental fluid shifts in hemodialysis patients. Biotech Prog 1987; 3:69–73.

45. Pastan S and Colton C. Transcellular urea gradients cause minimal depletion of extracellular volume during hemodialysis. Trans Am Soc Artif Intern Organs 1989; 35:247–50.

46. Daugirdas J and Schneditz D. Overestimation of hemodialysis dose depends on dialysis efficiency by regional blood flow but not by conventional two pool urea kinetic analysis. ASAIO J 1995; 41:M719–24.

47. Bankhead M, Toto R and Star R. Accuracy of urea removal estimated by kinetic methods. Kidney Int 1995; 48:785–93.

48. Malchesky P, Ellis P, Nosse C, Magnusson M, Lankhorst B and Nakamoto S. Direct quantification of dialysis. Dial Transplant 1982; 11:42–4.

49. Keshaviah P, Ebben J and Emerson P. On-line monitoring of the delivery of the hemodialysis prescription. Ped Nephrol 1995; 9:S2–8.

50. Depner T, Keshaviah P, Ebben J, Emerson P, Collins A, Jindal K et al. Multi-center clinical validation of an on-line monitor of dialysis adequacy. J Am Soc Nephrol 1996; 7:464–71.

51. Garred L, St. Amour N, McCready W and Canaud B. Urea kinetic modeling with a prototype urea sensor in the spent dialysate stream. ASAIOJ 1993; 39:M337—41.

52. Ronco C, Brendolan A, Crepaldi C, Frische P, Ghiotto F, Zamboni S et al. On-line urea monitoring: A further step towards adequate dialysis prescription and delivery. Int J Artif Organs 1995; 18:534–43.

53. NKF-DOQI Hemodialysis Work Group. NKF-DOQI clinical practice guidelines for hemodialysis adequacy. Am J Kidney Dis 1997; 30:S12–64.

54. Eknoyan G, Levey A, Beck G, Agodoa L, Daugirdas J, Kusek J et al. Hemodialysis (HEMO) study: rationale for selection of interventions. Semin Dial 1996; 9:24–33.

55. Windus D, Audrain J, Vanderson R, Jendrisak M, Picus D and Delmez J. Optimization of high-efficiency dialysis by detection and correction of vascular access dysfunction. Kidney Int 1990; 38:337–41.

56. Besarab A, Al-Saghir F, Al-Nabhan N, Lubkowski T and Frinak S. Simplified measurement of intra-access pressure. ASAIO J 1996; 42:106–16.

57. Depner T, Krivitski N and MacGibbon D. Hemodialysis access recirculation measured by ultrasound dilution. ASAIO J 1995; 41:M749–53.

58. Krivitski N. Theory and validation of access flow measurement by ultrasound dilution technique during hemodialysis. Kidney Int 1995; 48:244–50.

59. Gotch F. Mass transport in reused dialyzers. Proc Dial Transplant Forum 1980; 10:81–5.

60. Ouseph R, Smith B and Ward R. Maintaining blood compartment volume in dialyzers reprocessed with peracetic acid maintains Kt/V but not $\beta 2$-microglobulin removal. Am J Kidney Dis 1997; 30:501–6.

61. Murthy B, Sundaram S, Jaber B, Perrella C, Meyer K and Pereira B. Effect of formaldehyde/bleach reprocessing on *in vivo* performances of high-efficiency cellulose and high-flux polysulfone dialyzers. J Am Soc Nephrol (in press).

62. Delmez J, Weerts C, Hasamear P and Windus D. Severe dialyzer dysfunction undetectable by reprocessing validation tests. Kidney Int 1989; 36:478–84.

63. Delmez J and Windus D. Impaired delivery of dialysis: diagnosis and correction. Am J Nephrol 1996; 16:29–34.

64. Coyne D, Delmez J, Spence G and Windus D. Impaired delivery of hemodialysis prescriptions: an analysis of causes and an approach to evaluation. J Am Soc Nephrol 1997; 8:1315–18.

17. Water treatment for hemodialysis

P. KESHAVIAH

INTRODUCTION

According to an Italian proverb "Aqua torbido non lava" i.e. "Dirty water does not wash clean". This can be most aptly applied to the water used for hemodialysis. If the water used for hemodialysis is "dirty", the blood of the hemodialysis patient will not be "washed clean". The hemodialysis patient is exposed to more water in one year than the normal population in 20 years. Further, the hemodialysis patient's blood is exposed to this large quantity of water across a thin non-selective membrane that has none of the "wisdom" of the gastrointestinal tract of a normal individual. Also, the hemodialysis patient's ability to excrete harmful toxins from such exposure is limited by compromised renal function. The combination of large volume of exposure, non-selective transport across the dialyzer membrane, and compromised renal function make for a situation that is potentially hazardous to the health and well-being of the patient on hemodialysis. Unless the water used for hemodialysis is analyzed periodically and subjected to appropriate treatment processes whose efficacy is monitored regularly, there may be serious risks to patient well-being that have been well documented in the dialysis literature.

CONTAMINANTS WITH DOCUMENTED TOXICITY IN HEMODIALYSIS

The risks and hazards associated with inadequately treated water are summarized in Table 17.1 along with the lowest contaminant levels at which toxicity has been observed. It should be noted that many of the contaminants associated with toxicity in the hemodialysis setting are not regulated by the Safe Drinking Water Act of 1974 [1]. Also, even for contaminants that are regulated by the Safe Drinking Water Act, the levels at which toxicity is observed in hemodialysis are lower than the safe limits established for drinking water.

Aluminium. Aluminium may not be naturally occurring in the source water but may be added to the water by the municipal supplier as alum (aluminium sulphate) to treat water with a high content of suspended colloids. Exposure of the hemodialysis patient to aluminium levels greater than 0.06 mg/L has been associated with a progressive syndrome of neurological deterioration and encephalopathy [2–5]. This syndrome, called dialysis dementia, is often fatal and is characterized by personality changes, reduced short term memory, speech disturbances, muscle spasms, seizures, and dementia. Bone diseases such as osteomalacia and osteodystrophy have also been associated with a prolonged exposure to high levels of aluminium [6, 7]. A type of anemia called microcytic hypochromic anemia may also result from

Table 17.1. Water contaminants associated with toxicity in the hemodialysis setting

Contaminants	Lowest concentration associated with toxicity (mg/L)
Aluminium	0.06
Copper	0.49
Zinc	0.2
Calcium/magnesium	88 (Ca^{++})
Sodium	300
Fluoride	1.0
Nitrate	21 (as N)
Sulphate	200
Chloramines	0.25
Microbiological contaminants	–

L.W. Henderson and R.S. Thuma (eds.), Quality Assurance in Dialysis, 2nd Edition, 173–187.
© 1999 *Kluwer Academic Publishers. Printed in Great Britain*

aluminium exposure [8, 9]. Patients on hemodialysis may be exposed to aluminium from two sources – for water used for preparing dialysate and from ingestion of aluminium-containing phosphate binders. Water as the source of exposure has been well established by epidemiological studies [10].

Copper. Copper may be leached from the water distributing system or from the dialysate delivery system, by acidic water causing chills, nausea and headache, liver damage, and fatal hemolysis [11–13]. Water may become acidic if a dual bed deionizer is in use with exhaustion of the anionic resin bed.

Zinc. Zinc may be leached into the water from galvanized iron components used in the water distribution system or the dialysate delivery system. The toxic effects of zinc exposure include nausea, vomiting, fever, and anemia [14].

Calcium or magnesium. Calcium or magnesium levels are elevated in water supplies that are hard. If the water is not softened, exposure to high levels of calcium or magnesium may result in a syndrome characterized by nausea, vomiting, muscular weakness, skin flushing, and hypertension or hypotension [15–17].

Sodium. Sodium levels may be naturally elevated in the water supply or may be the result of softening extremely hard water. Also, softener malfunction may result in high sodium levels [18]. Hypernatremia, increased thirst, and excessive water intake are consequences of a high sodium level in the water supply.

Fluoride. Fluoride is often added to the municipal water supply to prevent dental caries. Even at the Safe Drinking Water level of 1 mg/L, prolonged hemodialysis exposure may result in bone diseases such as osteomalacia and osteoporosis [19, 20]. Accidental over-fluoridation of the water by the supplier has been associated with adverse symptoms and one fatality [21].

Nitrate. Contamination of the water supply by fertilizers or excessive bacterial contaminants may result in high nitrate levels with consequences of methemoglobinemia, cyanosis, hypotension, and nausea [22, 23]. Very high nitrate levels may also cause hemolysis [23].

Sulphate. High sulphate levels in dialysis water have been associated with nausea, vomiting, and metabolic acidosis [24].

Chloramines. Chloramines are commonly used bactericidal agents in municipal water treatment. Because they are powerful oxidants, inadequate removal of chloramines may result in hemolysis, hemolytic anemia (characterized by Heinz body formation) and methemoglobinemia [25–29].

Microbiological contaminants. There have been documented clusters of pyrogen reactions associated with high levels of Gram-negative bacteria in the water supply [30–35]. Symptoms noted include shaking chills, fever, hypotension, headaches, myalgia, nausea and vomiting.

WATER QUALITY AT THE SOURCE

The various sources of water may be broadly classified into two major categories – ground waters and surface waters. In both cases, the water is derived from the natural water cycle, water evaporating from oceans, rivers, and other reservoirs into the atmosphere, the vapor condensing and returning to earth as rain, snow, or hail. Some of this water flows on the earth's surface as streams and rivers and collects in closed bodies of water such as lakes and ponds. Precipitated water may also seep into the earth, collecting in underground reservoirs and aquifers, being classified as ground water.

The quality of surface water depends on the location. In agricultural locations, surface water may be contaminated by fertilizers and pesticides. In urban locations, surface water may be contaminated by industrial wastes and sewage. Unless surface water is appropriately treated for hemodialysis use, it may pose a grave risk to the well-being of the hemodialysis patient.

Ground water percolates through various layers of soil and its quality may depend on the geology of that area. Organic contaminants are usually removed by the percolation of water through the various soil layers. However, inorganic contaminant levels may increase. Ground water percolated through limestome is usually hard containing high levels of calcium and magnesium compared to water percolated through granite.

In 1974, landmark legislation was passed by Congress called the Safe Drinking Water Act [1] which mandated the surveillance of drinking water supplies by federal and state governments with the EPA assigned the responsibility of enforcing these regulations. However, these regulations only apply to public water systems defined as "any system, publicly or privately owned, that serves an average of 25 persons daily or has at least 15 service connections for at least 60 days of the year" [34]. Even with public water systems that are subject to EPA regulations, the level of compliance is of the order of 90% so that approximately 10% of public water systems may be supplying unsafe water. It should not be assumed, a priori, that the water supply for a hemodialysis unit meets the EPA standards. It is essential that contact be established between the staff of the dialysis unit and the municipal water supplier regarding water quality and treatment practices. There should also be an on-going dialogue to ensure that changes in water treatment procedures by the supplier are communicated to the dialysis unit. This communication is particularly important with water supplies that are fluoridated, situations where large amounts of aluminium may be used to flocculate organic contaminants, and with the use of chlorine and chloramines for disinfection of the water. Also, if the supply source (ground/surface) changes during the year or the mix of these sources varies, there may be large seasonal variations. Appropriate plans need to be implemented at the dialysis unit to ensure appropriate quality of product water used for dialysis despite large seasonal variations.

The National Interim Primary Drinking Water Regulations [35] established by the EPA set maximum contaminant levels for inorganic and organic contaminants in drinking water. These maximum levels are summarized in Table 17.2. While water meeting these levels is safe for drinking and for cooking purposes, it is not, as previously noted, safe for dialysis because of the larger volume of exposure, exposure to blood across a thin non-selective membrane, and compromised renal function. More stringent limits

Table 17.2. National interim primary drinking water standards

Chemical	Maximum level (mg/L)
Inorganic	
Arsenic	0.05
Barium	1.00
Cadmium	0.01
Chromium	0.05
Lead	0.05
Mercury	0.002
Nitrate (as N)	10.0
Selenium	0.01
Silver	0.05
Fluoride*	1.4–2.4
Organic	
Endrin	0.0002
Lindane	0.004
Methoxychlor	0.1
Toxaphene	0.005
2, 4-D	0.1
2, 4, 5 – TP (Sivex)	0.01

*Varies according to annual average air temperature

than the EPA standards must be met, and these have been established by the Association for the Advancement of Medical Instrumentation [36].

AAMI WATER QUALITY STANDARDS

The contaminants occurring in municipal water supplies may be categorized into inorganic, organic, radioactive, and microbiological contaminants. The water quality standard in hemodialysis established by AAMI addresses inorganic and microbiological contaminants. Organic and radioactive contaminants are addressed by the Safe Drinking Water Act and no further limits have been set by AAMI, as the potential toxicity of organic and radioactive contaminants in the hemodialysis setting is not well established.

The AAMI Water Quality Standards for hemodialysis were established in 1982 and were based in part on recommendations made in an FDA sponsored study of the risks and hazards of hemodialysis [37]. The AAMI standards have been adopted by the American National Standards Institute. The AAMI standard is summarized in Table 17.3.

To understand the rationale underlying the

Table 17.3. AAMI water quality standard

Category	Chemical	Maximum level (mg/L)
Normal constituents of dialysate	Calcium	2 (0.1 mEq/L)
	Magnesium	4 (0.3 mEq/L)
	Potassium	8 (0.2 mEq/L)
	Sodium	70 (3.0 mEq/L)
Toxic contaminants regulated	Arsenic	0.005
by national interim primary	Barium	0.01
drinking water standards	Cadmium	0.001
	Chromium	0.014
	Lead	0.005
	Mercury	0.0002
	Selenium	0.09
	Silver	0.005
Other contaminants with documented	Aluminium	0.01
toxicity in hemodialysis	Chloramines	0.10
	Free chlorine	0.5
	Copper	0.10
	Fluoride	0.20
	Nitrate (as N)	2.0
	Sulphate	100
	Zinc	0.10

AAMI standard, it is convenient to divide the inorganic contaminants into three categories: normal constituents of dialysate, toxic contaminants regulated by National Interim Primary Drinking Water Standards, and other contaminants with documented toxicity in hemodialysis.

The maximum acceptable level for substances normally included in dialysate was established based on clinically acceptable variations of these substances in dialysate. As an example, the AAMI has set a maximum level of 2 mg/L (0.1 mEq/L) for calcium. Variations of this magnitude in the calcium content on dialysate (typically 2.5–4.0 mEq/L) are both hard to measure and unlikely to have adverse patient consequences. For contaminants regulated by the Drinking Water Standards, a maximum level was chosem that was one-tenth of the drinking water level, unless the limits of detection or the no-transfer level for that contaminant were higher than the one-tenth level. The no-transfer level is the contaminant level in dialysate at which no diffusive transfer occurs from dialysate to blood. For contaminants with documented treatment in hemodialysis, the AAMI level was set at the lowest level at which treatment had been documented.

The AAMI standard of 200 cfu/mL for bacterial contamination was based on studies conducted by the Centers for Disease Control [38, 39] which showed that at levels higher than 200 cfu/mL, there would be amplification of bacterial contamination in dialysate with the potential for pyrogenic reactions. In addition to the 200 cfu/mL level for water used to prepare dialysate, AAMI has also set limits of 2000 cfu/mL for final dialysate and 1 ng/mL (Limulus amebocyte lysate (LAL) assay) for the bacterial lipopolysaccharide level in water used for the reprocessing of dialyzers for multiple use, with a requirement that this water should have a bacterial count of less than 200 cfu/mL and should be filtered through a nominal 5 μm filter.

With high flux hemodialysis, back filtration from dialysate to blood occurs in the distal section of the dialzyer. The potential for biologically active endotoxic fragments or dissociated endotoxin to cross over from dialysate to blood is enhanced in the presence of back filtration [40, 41]. According to the interleukin hypothesis [42, 43], even small amounts of endotoxin, undetected by the LAL test, may stimulate cytokine production by monocytes. These cytokines have been associated with a wide variety of adverse effects. Whether endotoxin-induced cytokine production occurs with high flux dialysis is a subject of lively debate, but there are investigators who are recommending the use of filtered endotoxin-free dialysate for high flux dialysis.

The concentration of chlorinated hydrocarbons (pesticides, chlorophenoxys), herbicides, and radioactive substances are limited by the Drinking Water Standards. However, no further reduction of levels of these contaminants for hemodialysis applications has been recommended as the potential risks from these contaminants are not known. The combined use of activated carbon and reverse osmosis to treat water for hemodialysis use provides some measure of protection against these contaminants. Activated carbon is effective in adsorbing organic contaminants in a molecular weight range of 60–300 daltons whereas reverse osmosis is capable of removing larger inorganic contaminants (>200–300 daltons). Treatment processes that are effective for non-radioactive contaminants are expected to be effective for removal of their radioactive isotopes.

ACHIEVING THE WATER QUALITY STANDARDS

A variety of water treatment technologies are available that need to be used alone or in combination, depending on the source water quality, to achieve the water quality standard for hemodialysis. These various methods are listed in Table 17.4 along with the type of contaminants that they are capable of removing. We will describe here some

Table 17.4. Water treatment processes used in hemodialysis

Process	Contaminants removed
Filtration	Particulates, bacteria, viruses, endotoxins
Activated carbon adsorption	Small organics, chlorine, chloramines
Reverse osmosis	Large organics ($\sim$300 daltons), ionic species and bacteria
Softening	Calcium and magnesium
Deionization	Ionic species (cationic and anionic)

of the commonly used treatment methodologies along with a description of the operating principles, guidelines for selecting particular treatment methods, and how these various methods can be integrated into a suitable water treatment system.

Filtration

Filters play a key role in water treatment with a variety of uses from removal of large particulates to removal of bacteria and viruses. There are basically two filtration mechanisms – depth filtration and surface filtration. Depth filtration is typically used for removal of coarse particulate material from water by allowing the water to permeate the filter matrix and by trapping the particulates mechanically in channels that are smaller than the particulate or by adsorptive capture. Some depth filters (e.g. bed filters) consists of multiple layers of filter media, each layer capable of retaining progressively smaller particles. The largest particles are removed by the first layers and the smallest in the final layers of the bed. Bed filters are suited for removing particles up to 10 μm in size. Surface filters exclude solute at the surface of the filter primarily by size exclusion, although charge and hydrophobic and hydrophilic interactions may also be involved. Surface filters are suited to removal of both dissolved and suspended solutes.

Cartridge filters typically consist of a filter medium with a central drainage core. Cartridge filters may employ both depth and surface filtration. Cartridges of cellulosic materials and synthetic polymers are available with solid, mesh, pleated, wound and woven configurations. The cartridge is contained in a filter having both inlet and outlet ports. Cartridge filters capable of removing particles as small as 1 μm are available.

Membrane filters employ surface filtration and are usually in the configuration of a thin sheet of porous material with the filter being capable of retaining solutes that are larger than the pores. Water passes freely through the membrane pores. As the pores of the filter may not all be of the same size, the size cutoff of the membrane is not sharply defined and is usually quoted as the size at which 90% retention is achieved. Cellulosic and polymeric membranes are used in water treatment applications. Membrane filters can be classified as microporous filters, ultrafiltration, and reverse osmosis filters. Microporous filters are suited to removing particulates, bacteria, and viruses up to 0.1 µm in size. Ultrafilters are capable of removing endotoxins, proteins, and solutes as small as 0.001 µm ($\sim$ 200–300 daltons). Reverse osmosis filters exclude larger organic solutes ($\sim$ 200 daltons) and ionic species as small as 0.001 µm. Reverse osmosis filters are discussed in greater detail below.

Filters may be operated in a dead end configuration or with cross flow as shown in Figure 17.1. Depth filters are usually used in the dead end configuration whereas membrane filters are commonly used with cross flow. In cross flow, the tangential flow sweeps away solutes from the surface of the membrane and reduces filter clogging.

Filters should be sized on the basis of the desired

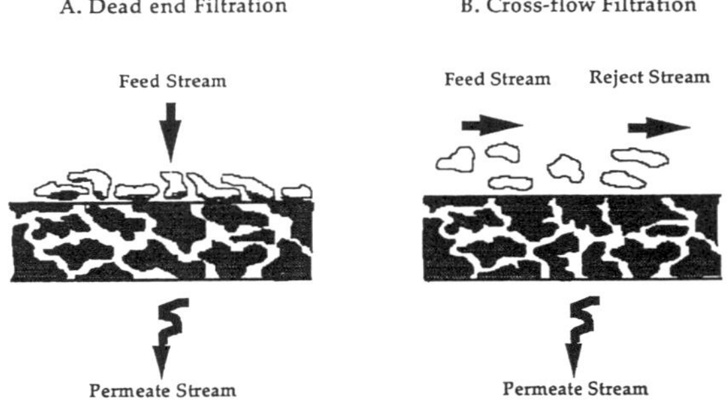

Fig. 17.1. Schematic representation of dead end and cross flow filtration.

flow rate of water through the filters. Filters have a finite capacity and need to be replaced or regenerated once this capacity is exceeded. The pressure drop across the filter is monitored and used to determine when the filtration capacity has been reached. If used beyond this capacity, pressure drops will increase, flow rates decrease, and filter performance (solute retention) will deteriorate. Depth filters may be regenerated by back washing, and the use of regenerative chemicals. Cartridge and membrane filters are usually replaced when the specified maximum pressure drop is exceeded. In a water treatment system, filters may become potential sites for bacterial colonization and proliferation. This potential should be considered in choosing a filter and determining its location in the

water treatment system. Water treatment systems may also require frequent disinfection or filter replacement to control bacterial proliferation.

Activated Carbon Adsorption

Activated carbon adsorption is suited to the removal of a wide variety of organic concentration especially of a size too small to be removed by reverse osmosis filters. Activated carbon has an extremly porous internal structure with a very high internal surface area. This porous structure is achieved by pyrolysis of materials such as coal, peat, wood, and bone in regulated atmospheres. Porous carbon granules thus produced are contained in a bed, water percolating through the granular bed, solutes being absorbed within the internal porous structure of the carbon granules. Once the adsorption capacity of the bed is exceeded, solute breakthrough occurs and the maximum acceptable outlet concentration of solute is exceeded. The carbon bed then needs to be replaced. Because of the porous structure of the granules, there is a tendency for fragmentation of the granules by mechanical attrition, and the particles or 'fines' so released need to be trapped by a suitable downstream filter to prevent them from blocking orifices and clogging equipment downstream.

In the hemodialysis application, activated carbon is used to remove contaminants such as chlorine, chloramines, hypochlorites, and chloroform. Chloramines are replacing chlorine as bactericidal agents in municipal water treatment because free chlorine has a tendency to combine with organic chemicals to form carcinogenic compounds called trihalomethanes. Trihalomethanes are not found with chloramine usage. However, chloramines are powerful oxidants and are toxic in the hemodialysis setting causing hemolysis, hemolytic anemia, and methemoglobinemia.

In hemodialysis, the breakthrough of chloramine or total chlorine (free chlorine + chloramines) should be used as a criterion for detecting exhaustion of the carbon bed. The monitoring of free chlorine alone may result in an overestimation of the remaining adsorptive capacity. The life of a carbon bed can be extended by operating at low water flow rates. Such low flow rates utilize the adsorptive capacity of the bed more completely.

Often two carbon beds in series are used in a water treatment system. When the upstream bed is exhausted, the second bed is moved upstream and a new bed added downstream. This arrangement provides an adequate marginof safety.

Because of the high surface area of carbon beds, they provide a good site for bacterial proliferation, the organics adsorbed by the carbon serving as nutrients for the colonized bacteria. Also the removal of chlorine and chloramines by the carbon exacerbates the proliferation of bacteria. Suitable water treatment equipment must be used downstream to remove bacteria and endotoxins.

Reverse Osmosis

Reverse osmosis is a membrane separation process that forces flow of solvent across a semipermeable membrane under hydrostatic pressure. As shown in Figure 17.2, when a semipermeable membrane separates a dilute solution from a concentrated solution, there is a tendency for solvent flow from the dilute solution to the concentrated solution across the osmotic gradient. In order to impede the flow of solvent across the membrane, a pressure equal to the osmotic pressure needs to be applied to the concentrated solution side of the membrane. If the pressure applied to the concentrated solution side of a membrane exceeds the osmotic pressure, there will be a reverse flow of solvent i.e. flow the the concentrated to the diluted side. This is the rationale behind the name 'reverse osmosis' for this water treatment process.

Reverse osmosis membranes are operated in a

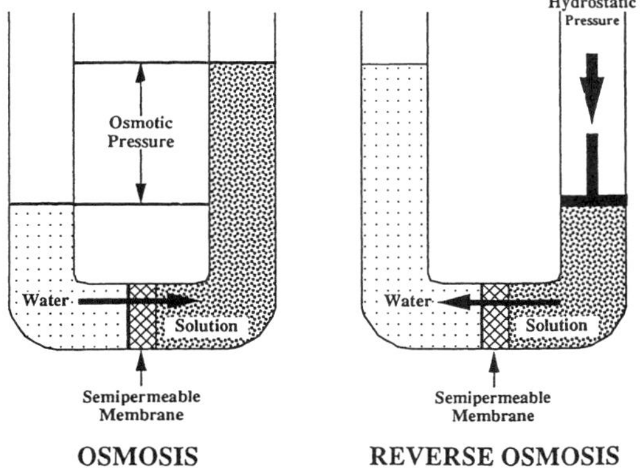

Fig. 17.2. Illustration of the principle of reverse osmosis.

cross flow configuration. The permeate is called product water and the cross flow containing the concentrated contaminants is called the reject stream. Typically the product water to feed water ratio is of the order of 25 to 50% for hemodialysis applications.

There are 3 major types of reverse osmosis membranes: cellulosic, fully aromatic polyamide, and thin film composite membranes. Reverse osmosis as a water treatment process was first demonstrated in the 1950's with cellulosic membranes (cellulose acetate). These membranes are asymmetric having a thin, dense layer that provides the solute rejection capability and a thick porous substructure that provides structural support and strength. It is because of this substructure that the membrane can withstand high hydrostatic pressures. However, under very high pressures, compaction occurs with the thin dense layer merging into the porous structure with a reduction in product water flux. Compaction is accelerated under high temperatures. Cellulose acetate membranes can only be used with a limited pH range of 4–8 because of their susceptibility to hydrolysis. They are also susceptible to bacterial degradation. Cellulose acetate membranes have a high water permeability but poor solute rejection. Aromatic polyamide membranes are also asymmetric but are resistant to hydrolysis and bacterial degradation. They can withstand higher temperatures and a wider pH range (4–11), but at the extremes of this range they are more prone to irreversible membrane degradation. They have better solute rejection characteristics than cellulosic membranes but are extremely sensitive to oxidant damage. Water containing chlorine or chloramine must be treated with activated carbon before being fed to reverse osmosis modules with polyamide membranes. Thin film composites are made by casting a thin, dense film onto a porous substrate, so that the materials and manufacturing process for the two layers can be different and can be optimized for providing the best characteristics of water flux, solute rejection, pH and temperature tolerance and compaction resistance. The supporting structure is usually polysulphone and the thin dense layer materials include aromatic polyamide, alkylarylpolymer/polyamide, and polyfurane cyanate. These membranes are more stable than the aromatic polyamide membranes to oxidant exposure, but exposure to oxidants must still be limited.

The reverse osmosis module contains the reverse osmosis membrane with provisions for access to feed, product, and reject streams. There are 2 common module configurations used in hemodialysis – spiral wound modules and hollow fiber membranes. In the spiral wound configuration, a membrane fabric sandwich is created by attaching two layers of membrane back to back to a woven fabric like nylon or dacron. This membrane-fabric sandwich is wound around a central perforated hollow tube in a jelly roll configuration with plastic mesh used to separate adjacent layers (Figure 17.3). This configuration is not unlike the coil dialyzer configuration used in the early days of dialysis. Product water flows through the membrane into the woven fabric and from the fabric into the central hollow core. The plastic mesh controls the feed stream channel height and improves mixing of the feed stream with 'quasi' turbulence. The spiral wound module is contained in a pressure vessel designed for high operating pressures. The spiral wound configuration provides a high membrane packing density and is low in manufacturing cost. However, it provides stagnation areas in the plastic mesh and in the dead spaces between the module and the pressure vessel and may be hard to clean and disinfect completely. In the hollow fiber configuration, the membrane is formed into fine hollow fibers with inside diameters of 80–250 µm. The fiber bundle is potted in a polyurethane or epoxy tube sheet and may be a straight or U-shaped bundle (Figure 17.4). The feed water stream flows on the outside of the fiber, and the product stream through the fiber lumen. The fiber bundle is contained in an appropriate pressure vessel. No supporting structures are required, making this configuration even more compact than the spiral wound configuration. However, the hollow fibers are susceptible to fouling and plugging and may be hard to clean to that appropriate pretreatment is required upstream of the hollow fiber reverse osmosis module. The water flux of the hollow fibers is lower than that of flat sheet membranes, but because of the higher packing density, more membrane surface area can be accomodated in the same volume as the spiral wound design.

Reverse osmosis membranes have a broad spectrum of solute rejection from particulates, bacteria

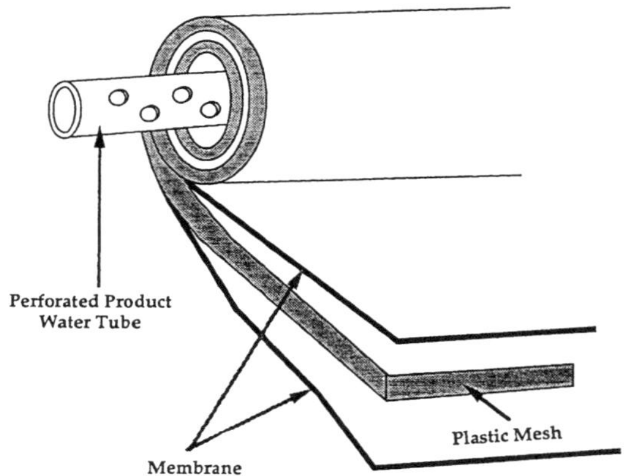

Fig. 17.3. Representation of the spiral wound reverse osmosis configuration.

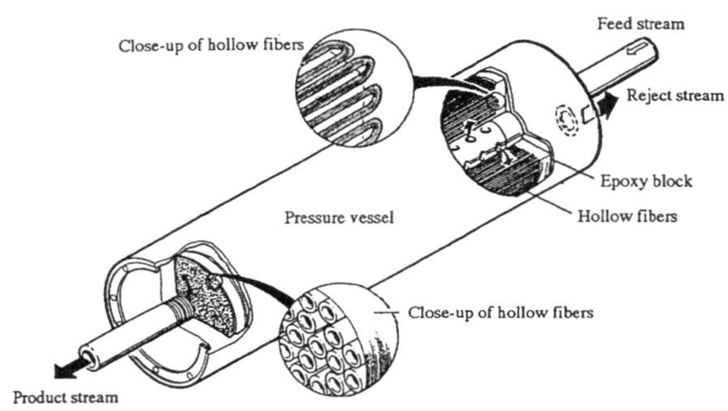

Fig. 17.4. Representation of the hollow fiber reverse osmosis configuration.

and viruses, to larger organics and small dissolved inorganic solutes. Ionic species are rejected more readily than non-charged species and the rejection increases with valence. pH may influence solute rejection. Typical rejection rate for inorganic contaminants are shown in Table 17.5. While larger organics (200–300 daltons) are readily rejected by reverse osmosis membranes, smaller, non-polar, dissolved organics like methanol, ethanol, and ethylene glycol are poorly rejected. While bacteria and viruses are rejected by most reverse osmosis membranes, because of membrane defects and minute seal leaks, reverse osmosis devices generally cannot be relied upon to produce sterile, endotoxin-free water.

Performance of reverse osmosis devices is

Table 17.5. Typical reverse osmosis membrane rejection of inorganic contaminants

	Contaminant	% Rejection*
Cations	Ca^{++}	98
	Mg^{++}	98
	Fe^{++}, Fe^{+++}	98
	Na^+	95
	K^+	95
Anions	HCO_3^-	85–95
	CL^-	95
	$SO_4^=$	98
	NO_3^-	85–90

*Cellulose acetate membrane with 1500 mg/L TDS feed water, 75% recovery, 400 psi

assessed by the rejection of ionic contaminants measured as the ratio of product water to feed water conductivity. Product water flux rates depend not only on membrane characteristics, but also on operating pressures (typically 200–400 psi), temperature ($\sim 25°C$), and feed water quality (ionic concentration). As the total dissolved solids content in the feed water increases, product water recovery (ratio of product water to feed water flow) decreases. In addition to conductivity monitoring of rejection, product water and reject stream flow meters, pressure gauges (pre and post pump as well as product and reject stream pressures) and low and high pressure switches (loss of water supply and flow path obstructions) are used to monitor the performance of the reverse osmosis unit. Means for safe cleaning and disinfection with an interlock switch to safeguard against accidental institution of these procedures contribute to good unit design. A periodic high velocity auto-flush feature for removing foulants from the membrane surface is also a convenient feature.

When water flux or solute rejection begin to diminish, it may be time to clean the reverse osmosis membrane. The module can be flushed from the feed to the reject side at a low feed pressure so as to have almost no product flow. In addition chemical cleaning with cleaning agents such as hydrochloric acid, citric acid, sodium hydroxide, sodium EDTA, and detergents may be necessary to restore membrane performance. The chemical stability of a membrane, type of foulants in the feed water and materials of construction

dictate the choice of cleaning agent. The manufacturer of the reverse osmosis device has the responsibility for providing complete instructions for cleaning and restoring membrane function. Though the capital cost of reverse osmosis modules is high, with appropriate water pretreatment, suitable operating conditions, and regular maintenance, cleaning and disinfection, a module life of several years is feasible making reverse osmosis a highly effective water treatment process from the solute rejection and cost-effectiveness points of view.

Ion Exchange

In this water treatment process, water flows through a resin bed, the resin having ion-exchange properties, i.e. able to exchange certain ions on the resin for certain ions in the feed water. Softeners and deionizers are both examples of ion exchange devices. In a softener, the resin exchanges sodium ions for calcium and magnesium ions in the hard water (Figure 17.5). Deionizers may contain cationic and anionic resins or a mixture of the two. The cationic exchange resin exchanges hydrogen ions for cationic species in the feed water. Anionic exchange resins exchange hydrogen ions for anionic species in the feed water. In a mixed bed deionizer, the hydrogen and hydroxyl ions released from the resin combine to form neutral water (Figure 17.6). Ion-exchange resins are usually in a bead configuration contained in a cylindrical column (Figure 17.7). These resins have a finite ion-exchange capacity and when exhausted, they need

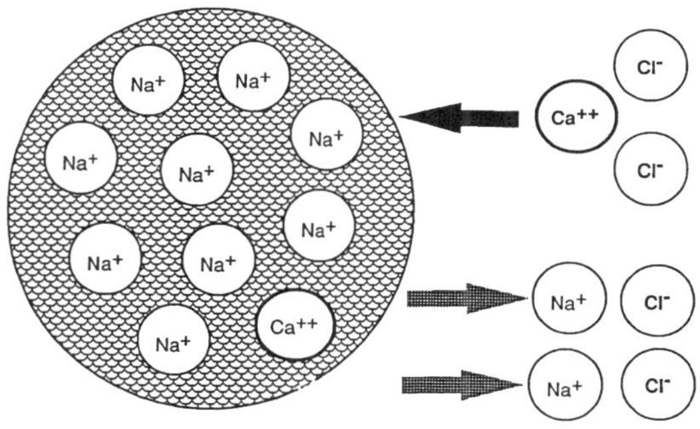

Fig. 17.5. Representation of the ion-exchange process used for softening hard water.

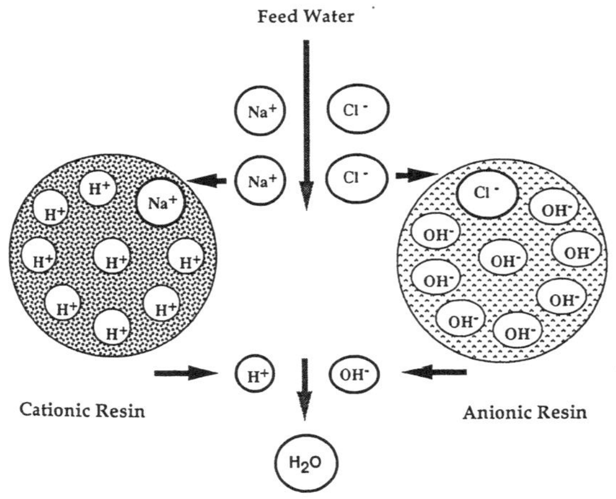

Fig. 17.6. Principle of mixed bed deionizers.

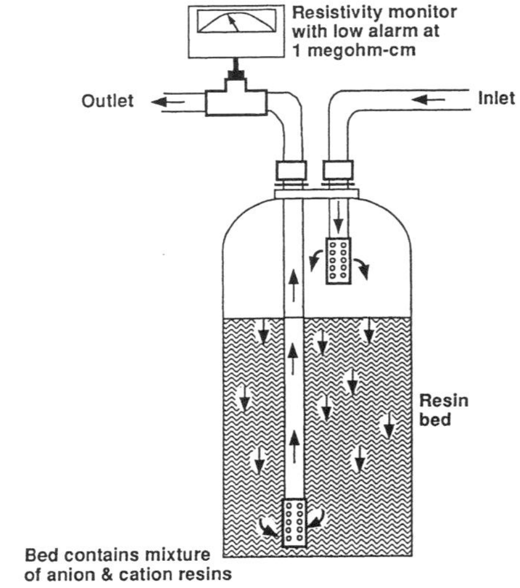

Fig. 17.7. Physical configuration of resin bed deionizer.

to be regenerated. With softener resins, regeneration is accomplished using a saturated sodium chloride solution (brine). Softener resin regeneration is usually done onsite at periodic intervals in an automated fashion under timer control. A brine tank containing sodium chloride pellets or crystals is located adjacent to the resin bed and at appropriate regeneration times, the saturated brine solutions is drawn from the brine tank by a venturi mechanism. The volume of brine drawn depends

on the regeneration frequency and exchange capacity of the resin bed. The frequency of regeneration in turn depends upon the water volume of feed water processed and the hardness of the feed water.

With deionizer resins, it is more common to have regeneration performed off-site in a central facility because caustic acids (cationic resins) and alkalis (anionic resins) are used for regeneration. The central facility will usually pick up the exhausted exchange tank, leaving a regenerated tank in its place. For hemodialysis applications, it should be ensured that the central regeneration facility uses only food-grade chemicals and does not mix resins from industrial users with hemodialysis resins. In industrial applications, deionizers may be used for recovery of heavy metals or other hazardous contaminants which may pose a serious threat to the hemodialysis patient. Similarly, for softeners, it is recommended that a purer form of sodium chloride than crude rock salt be used for regeneration.

In the hemodialysis setting, a common configuration for deionizers is to have two mixed bed deionizer tanks in service. As the first one gets exhausted, the second downstream tank is moved up and a new tank placed in its stead.

The performance of deionizers is usually monitored using a resistivity meter in units of ohm-cm. The minimum resistivity for hemodialysis water is 1 million ohm-cm or 1 meg ohm-cm. When the resistivity falls below this value, the deionizer tank needs to be regenerated. As resistivity depends on temperature, the resistivity meter needs to be temperature compensated. Instead of a meter, a monitor light may be provided.

Because of the large resin surface area and bed configuration with stagnant areas, deionizers are susceptible to bacterial colonization. Water treatment processes such as ultrafilters or ultraviolet irradiators may be required downstream to limit bacterial levels in the final water used for hemodialysis.

In situations where dual bed deionizers are used, it must be ensured that the cationic and anionic beds are appropriately sized to that they reach exhaustion together. If the anionic resin gets exhausted first, the cationic resin bed will continue to release hydrogen ions resulting in acidic product water. As stated earlier, acidic water may leach copper or other toxic materials from the water distribution system or from the dialysis equipment creating a potentially hazardous situation. Deionizer capacity is usually rated in terms of grains of total dissolved solids as calcium carbonate. This term includes all dissolved ionized species. In the case of softeners, the hardness of the water is also measured as grains of calcium carbonate and in cases where the water is extremely hard, allowance should be made for the increased sodium content of the product water following softening. For example, if reverse osmosis is used downstream, the increased sodium burden will need to be removed by an apropriately sized reverse osmosis module.

SYSTEM DESIGN

In the previous section, we have described briefly the major water treatment processes used in hemodialysis applications. A water treatment system may combine some or all of these processes depending on feed water quality, seasonal variations, product water flow rates required, and economic factors. It is beyond the scope of this chapter to get into the details of system design. However, some broad guidelines for selecting water treatment process combinations will be delineated along with some requirements for the water distribution system used to distribute the product water.

The steps involved in the design of the system area:

1. Determine product water requirements (flow rates, usage factors, application (e.g. reuse vs. dialysate water).

2. Define product water quality (e.g. AAMI standards).

3. Assess feed water quality including seasonal variations and worst case scenarios.

4. Determine the concentration reduction ratio for various contaminants for various water treatment processes based on manufacturers' specifications.

5. Select combinations of water treatment pro-

cesses taking into consideration economics, product flow rates, and impact of various combinations of pretreatment requirements and final bacteriological quality.

We will consider an illustrative case. The use of reverse osmosis will yield a concentration reduction ratio of 0.1 for most inorganic contaminants but is not as effective in removing small organics, free chlorine, and chloramines. Further, oxidants like free chlorine may damage aromatic reverse osmosis membranes. The use of activated carbon may, therefore, be a necessary pretreatment to remove free chlorine and chloramines as well as small organics. As carbon filters may release fines, a sediment filter may be necessary downstream of the carbon filter. Also carbon filters and sediment filters may promote bacterial proliferation. The reverse osmosis membrane may be quite capable of handling the bacterial burden imposed by the use of activated carbon and sediment filters. If either because of product flow requirements or economics, this approach to limiting bacterial contaminants is not feasible, an ultrafilter may also be required. Further, if the level of an inorganic contaminant like aluminium is so high as to require a concentration reduction ratio of better than 0.1, a deionizer may be necessary. From a bacteriological point of view, locating a deionizer upstream of the reverse osmosis device is preferred. However, economic reasons may dictate that using deionization to 'polish' the reverse osmosis product water is the preferred approach. In such cases, ultrafiltration may be necessary as the last step for maintaining bacteriological quality of the product water. If usage requirements are such that the reverse osmosis device is incapable of satisfying peak product water requirements, a holding tank may be necessary to meet peak flow requirements, the tank being filled during periods of lower product flow demand. In such situations, the bacteriological quality of the product water may suffer because of stagnant conditions in the holding tank and exposure to the atmosphere. The holding tank may need to be designed to reduce such exposure with a recirculation loop through an ultraviolet irradiator to limit bacteriological quality.

As the brief example demonstrates, many factors dictate the design of the total system and many of these factors may have contradictory requirements and consequences. Skill and experience with juggling these varying factors is therefore necessary in designing a safe, reliable, and cost effective system.

DISTRIBUTION SYSTEM REQUIREMENTS

The product water distribution system consists of piping and associated fittings such as valves, pressure and flow gauges, pumps, pressure regulators and seals. Care must be exercised in the choice of these various components to ensure that the product water quality does not deteriorate during distribution and that various product water locations can be served at the desired flow rates. Materials of contamination such as brass, copper, aluminium, and zinc should be avoided because they are contaminants of known toxicity in hemodialysis. The piping should be made of more inert materials such as polyvinyl chloride (PVC), non-pigmented polypropylene, stainless steel, or glass. PVC is widely available and inexpensive. However, according to some authorities PVC may not be acceptable as the surface of PVC is considered to be conducive to bacterial growth. Not only should the materials of construction be relatively inert, they should also not degenerate with exposure to commonly used disinfectants such as bleach. If PVC is used, it should be Type 1 (non-plasticized) and meet the requirements of the National Sanitation Foundation for potable water. If solvent welding is used for joints, enough curing time should be allowed before use, and vigorous flushing of the distribution system to remove residual solvent is recommended.

In designing the distribution system, care should be taken to ensure that stagnant areas are avoided because such areas promote bacterial proliferation. Also, the system should be designed to ensure that all parts of the system are exposed to cleaning agents and disinfectants where necessary. The system should be designed to promote high flow velocity, avoiding dead ends, and long, multiple branching layouts.

WATER TREATMENT AND QUALITY ASSURANCE

An obvious area of quality assurance with regard to water treatment is the monitoring of final product water quality. While we will also consider this aspect of quality assurance, it is important to point out that the role of quality assurance in water treatment begins almost as soon as the decision is made to establish a dialysis unit. At this early planning stage, it is critical that feed water quality be evaluated and communications established with the municipal water supplier regarding source of the water, seasonal variations in water quality at the source, seasonal variations in the blending of water from different sources at the municipal water treatment facility, and details of municipal water treatment practices and seasonal variations in these practices to cope with source quality fluctuations. Armed with this information, one can begin to design the appropriate water treatment system at the hemodialysis unit. While the area of system design is a specialized one requiring the appropriate knowledge and experience, the clinical staff must at least be well informed consumers who can study the proposals of various water treatment system vendors to ensure that an appropriate system is being proposed with appropriate safety margins and maintenance requirements that are within the technical abilities at the hemodialysis unit and are not so labor intensive or expensive as to adversely affect compliance with maintenance requirements. If an alternate design is available that has less stringent requirements, it may be preferred, even if initial capital costs are higher, because of the long term goal of uniform and appropriate product water quality to safeguard patient well-being. Prospective vendors should be informed that upon installation of the system, formal acceptance of the equipment is contingent upon validation of the entire system including the distribution system in terms of both product water quality and quantity. Vendors should be responsible for compliance with local plumbing and electrical codes in addition to meeting AAMI product water requirements. Complete operating manuals should be provided by the vendor including operator training requirements, monitoring requirements, recommended cleaning and maintenance schedules and procedures, and troubleshooting guidelines.

Monitoring Product Water Quality

Even if the water treatment system meets product water requirements at the time of installation, deviations from these requirements may occur as a consequence of deterioration of system performance, source water quality variations, and changes in municipal water treatment practices. It is therefore, essential that appropriate monitors of water quality be installed at appropriate locations of the water treatment system and that samples be drawn at specified intervals for more detailed laboratory analyses to ensure compliance with the AAMI Water Quality Standard. Appropriate documentation procedures should be established for long term surveillance of water quality.

In 1988, many municipal suppliers in California switched from free chlorine to chloramine. Despite all of the advance information provided regarding the change and its impact on hemodialysis facilities, failure to check product water for chloramines resulted in an outbreak of hemolytic anemia [29].

System performance may deteriorate with scaling and fouling of reverse osmosis membranes, exhaustion of components such as activated carbon or deionizer resin beds, bacterial contamination of the system, etc. Maintenance schedules and practices should be designed to prevent such deterioration of system performance. Monitoring will also alert the staff to system performance deviations from desired levels due to unforseen circumstances or will indicate that the monitoring schedules may be inappropriate and may require some tightening and fine tuning.

In describing the various water treatment processes, we have already outlined the monitoring requirements for each process. Many of these monitors are active, on-line monitors such as resistivity monitors, flow, pressure, and temperature gauges, rejection ratio indicators, etc. However, the final determinant of the adequacy of the water treatment system is the concentration of various key contaminants in the final product water. These contaminant levels should be determined at regular intervals using a certified laboratory. Also other tests such as free chlorine/chloramine levels and bacterial count may need to be performed on site within minutes or hours of drawing the appropriate samples. Dialysis unit personnel should have the appropriate training to perform these procedures and the appropriate assay tests should be available on site as needed. Standard clinical laboratory techniques available in a hospital laboratory for measuring bacterial contamination may not be appropriate for water samples. Nutrient-poor media and lower culturing temperatures may be required.

Unfortunately no specific guidelines regarding frequency of monitoring can be laid down as they vary with feed water quality and system design. The AAMI Water Quality Standard does make some recommendations regarding the frequency of monitoring certain water treatment processes and additional guidelines may be imposed by the Public Health authority in each state. For example, California requires that chloramine levels be checked before every patient shift. However, as stated by AAMI, "The monitoring of water purity levels is considered the sole responsibility of the physician in charge of hemodialysis or the medical professional designated by the physician as the person in charge".

Some general guidelines apply. Parameters such as pressures, flows, rejection ratios that are measured continuously on-line should be logged at least daily. For off-line monitors, daily monitoring may not be necessary. Initially, a conservative approach with very frequent monitoring is advisable and as time trends are established, less frequent monitoring may be suitable. Any time there is a change in system design or maintenance, a new schedule of monitoring may have to be established. Monthly testing of bacteria and endotoxin levels is recommended. A complete chemical analysis of the product water using a certified laboratory should be performed at least annually.

CONCLUDING REMARKS

Inadequate or inappropriate water treatment poses one of the gravest risks to the well-being of the dialysis patient because of the large volume of exposure across a relatively non-selective membrane. Even if the water is appropriately treated by the municipal supplier and is safe for drinking, it may be hazardous to the health of the dialysis patient. The literature is replete with many catastrophic consequences of inadequately treated water, and unless staff at dialysis units are well informed about these consequences, history may repeat itself. While water treatment technology is complex and many choices are available relative to system design and configurations, clinical staff at dialysis programs must become well informed consumers in order to deal effectively with vendors of water treatment systems. Ultimately, the responsibility for appropriate system performance, adequate water quality, and patient well-being rests with the clinical staff in charge of the dialysis program.

REFERENCES

1. The Safe Drinking Water Act of 1974. PL 523, 93rd Congress, Dec. 16, 1984.
2. Alfrey AC, Mishell JM, Burks J, Contiguglia SR, Rudolph H, Lewin E et al. Syndrome of dyspraxia and multifocal seizures associated with chronic hemodialysis. Trans Am Soc Artif Intern Organs 1972; 18:257–61.
3. Alfrey AC. Dialysis encephalopathy syndrome. Ann Rev Med 1978; 29:93–8.
4. Dunea G, Mahurkar SD, Mamdani B and Smith EC. Role of aluminium in dialysis dementia. Ann Intern Med. 1978; 88:502–4.
5. McDermott JR, Smith AI, Ward MK, Parkinson IS and Kerr DNS. Brain-aluminium concentration in dialysis encephalopathy. Lancet 1978; 1:901–3.
6. Elliot HL, Dryburgh F, Fell GS, Sabet S and MacDougall AI. Aluminium toxicity during regular haemodialysis. Br Med J. 1978; 1:1101–3.
7. Pierides AM, Edwards WG, Cullum UX, McCall JT and Ellis HA. Hemodialysis encephalopathy with osteomalacic fractures and muscle weakness. Kidney Int 1980; 18:115–24.
8. Short AI, Winney RJ and Robson JS. Reversible microcytic hypochromic anaemia in dialysis patients due to aluminium intoxication. Proc Eur Dial Transpl Assoc 1980; 17:226–33.
9. McGonigle RJS and Parsons V. Aluminium-induced anaemia in haemodialysis patients. Nephron 1985; 39:1–9.
10. Schreeder MT, Favero MS, Hughes JR, Petersen NJ, Bennett PH and Maynard JE. Dialysis encephalopathy and aluminium exposure: an epidemiological analysis. J Chronic Dis 1983; 36:581–93.
11. Matter BJ, Pederson J, Psimenos G and Lindeman RD. Lethal copper intoxication in hemodialysis. Trans Am Soc Arfif Intern Organs 1969; 15:309–15.
12. Ivanovich P, Manzler A and Drake R. Acute hemolysis following hemodialysis. Trans Am Soc Artif Intern Organs 1969; 15:316–18.
13. Manzler AD and Schreiner AW. Copper-induced hemolytic anemia. A new complication of hemodialysis. Ann Intern Med. 1970; 73:409–12.
14. Gallery EDM, Blomfield J and Dixon SR. Acute zinc toxicity in haemodialysis. Br Med J 1972; 4:331–3.
15. Freeman RM, Lawton RL and Chamberlain MA. Hard-water syndrome. N Engl J Med 1967; 276:1113–18.
16. Evans DB and Slapak M. Pancreatitis in the hard water syndrome. Br Med J 1975; 3:748.
17. Drukker W. The hard water syndrome: a potential hazard during regular dialysis treatment. Proc Eur Dial Transpl Assoc 1969;5:284–7.
18. Nickey WA, Chinitz VL, Kim KE, Onesti G and Swartz C. Hypernatremia from water softener malfunction during home dialysis (letter). J Am Med Assoc 1970; 214:915.
19. Jowsey J, Johnson WJ, Taves DR and Kelly PJ. Effects of dialysate calcium and fluoride on bone disease during regular hemodialysis. J Lab Clin Med 1972; 79:204–14.
20. Lough J, Noonan R, Gagnon R and Kaye M. Effects of fluoride on bone in calcium renal failure. Arch Pathol 1975; 99:484–7.
21. Anderson R, Beard JH and Sorley D. Fluoride intoxication in a dialysis unit – Maryland. Morbid Mortal Wkly Rep 1980; 29:134–6.
22. Carlson DJ and Shapiro FL. Methemoglobinemia from well water nitrates: a complication of home dialysis. Ann Intern Med 1970; 73:757–9.
23. Salvadori M, Martinelli F, Comparini L, Bandini S and Sodi A. Nitrate induced anemia in home dialysis patients. Proc Eur Dial Transpl Assoc 1984; 21:321–5.
24. Compty C, Luehmann D, Wathen R and Shapiro F. Prescription water for chronic hemodialysis. Trans Am Soc Artif Intern Organs 1974; 20:189–96.
25. Yawata Y, Howe R and Jacob HS. Abnormal red cell metabolism causing hemolysis in uremia. A defect potentiated by tap water hemodialysis. Ann Intern Med 1973; 79:362–7.
26. Eaton JW, Kolpin CF, Swofford HS, Kjellstrand CM and Jacob HS. Chlorinated urban water: a cause of dialysis-induced hemolytic anemia. Sciences 1973; 181:463–4.
27. Kjellstrand CM, Eaton JW, Yawata Y, Swofford H, Kolpin CF, Buselmeier TJ et al. Hemolysis in dialyzed patients caused by chloramines. Nephron 1974; 13:427–33.
28. Botella J, Traver JA, Sanz-Guajardo D, Torres MT, Sanjuan I and Zabala P. Chloramines, an aggravating factor in the anemia of patients on regular dialysis treatment. Proc Eur Dial Transpl Assoc 1977; 14:192–9.
29. Safety alert: chloramine contamination of hemodialysis water suppliers. Food and Drug Administration, Department of Health and Human Services, February 19, 1988.
30. Favero MS, Petersen NJ, Carson LA, Bond WW and Hindman SH. Gram-negative water bacteria in hemodialysis systems. Health Lab Sci 1975; 12:321–34.
31. Lauer J, Streifel A, Kjellstrand C and DeRoos R. The bacteriological quality of hemodialysis solution as related to several environmental factors. Nephron 1975; 15:87–97.
32. Blagg CR, Tenckhoff H. Microbial contamination of water used for hemodialysis. Nephron 1975; 15:81–6.
33. Robinson PJA and Rosen SM. Pyrexial reactions during haemodialysis. Br Med J 1971; 1:528–30.
34. Stacha JA and Pontius FW. An overview of water treatment practices in the United States. J Am Water Works Assoc 1984; 76:73–85.

35. Environmental Protection Agency, Office of Water Supply – National Interim Primary Drinking Water Regulations, U.S. Government Printing Office, Washington D.C., 1978.
36. American National Standard for Hemodialysis Systems. (RD-5) Association for the Advancement of Medical Instrumentation, Arlington, VA, 1982.
37. Keshaviah P, Luehmann D, Shapiro F and Comty C. Investigation of the risks and hazards associated with hemodialysis systems. (Technical Report, Contract 223-78-5046). U.S. Department of Health and Human Services, Public Health Service, Food and Drug Administration, Bureau of Medical Devices, Silver Spring, MD, June 1980.
38. Favero MS, Carson LA, Bond WW and Petersen NJ. Factors that influence microbial contamination of fluids associated with hemodialysis machines. Appl Microbiol 1974; 28:822–30.
39. Favero MS and Petersen NJ. Microbiological guidelines for hemodialysis systems. Dial Transplant 1977; 6:34.
40. Man NK, Ciancioni C, Faivre JM, Diab N, London G, Maret J et al. Dialysis-associated adverse reactions with high-flux membranes and microbial contamination of liquid bicarbonate concentrate. Contr Nephrol 1988; 62:24–34.
41. Klinkman H, Falkenhagen D and Smollich BP. Investigation of the permeability of highly permeable polysulfone membranes for pyrogens. Contr Nephrol 1985; 46:174–83, 185.
42. Dinarello C. The biology of interleukin 1 and its relevance to hemodialysis. Blood Purif 1983; 1:197–224.
43. Lonnemann G, Koch KM and Shaldon S. Induction of interleukin 1 from human monocytes adhering to hemodialysis membranes. Kidney Int 1987; 31:238.

18. Reuse of dialyzers – implications for adequacy of dialysis

B.V.R. MURTHY AND B.J.G. PEREIRA

INTRODUCTION

Reprocessing of hemodialyzers was originally introduced in the 1960s to reduce costs in coil and Kiil dialyzers [1, 2]. Reuse of dialyzers is now widely practiced in many countries to partially defray the burgeoning cost of end-stage renal disease therapy [3, 4]. Prior to 1982 (when a change in dialysis reimbursement was introduced), only 20% of units in the U.S.A. were practicing reuse [5]. Since then, the use of reprocessed dialyzers has steadily increased from 18% of dialysis centers and 18% of patients in 1976 to 75% of centers and 81% of patients in 1994 [4]. Reuse is more common in for-profit centers and free-standing units compared to hospital-based centers or not-for-profit centers [4]. Further, reuse is more common in larger centers compared to smaller centers. Among centers that reuse dialyzers, median of the average number of reuses has increased from 9 in 1986 to 14 in 1994, and the median of the maximum number of reuses obtained increased from 23 in 1986 to 30 in 1994 [4]. The prevalence of reuse in other parts of the world varies widely. In Japan, reuse is prohibited by law. Reuse penetration is modest in Western Europe where dialysis reimbursement rates are high, but is gaining in popularity in U.K. and Poland who are experiencing limitations on spending. In developing countries, reuse has facilitated the availability of dialysis where supplies are expensive and resources limited.

The germicides currently used for reprocessing of dialyzers in the U.S. include peracetic acid and hydrogen peroxide (Renalin) in 52% of centers, formaldehyde in 40% of centers, glutaraldehyde (a proprietary derivative of formaldehyde) in 7% of centers, and heat as a physical germicide in <1%

of centers [4]. In addition, many of the centers that use formaldehyde or glutaraldehyde also use sodium hypochlorite (bleach) to improve the appearance of the dialyzers and increase the number of reuses obtained. Glutaraldehyde, when used in a concentration of 0.8%, is equivalent to 4% formaldehyde, and is associated with less residual active compound compared to formaldehyde. However, reuse rates with glutaraldehyde are lower than those with formaldehyde [6].

The major advantage of reuse is the decrease in cost of dialysis. Theoretically, the amount that is saved by reuse of dialyzers would be available for further investment to increase the quality of care. However, the proliferation of for-profit dialysis chains world-wide, and the overwhelming dependence on reuse among these chains, suggests that the savings from reuse only enhance profit margins. Reprocessing of dialyzers also eliminates exposure to ethylene oxide, a potential allergen [7], thus decreasing the incidence of the "first-use" syndrome [8–10]. In addition, reprocessing of cellulose dialyzers with formaldehyde or peracetic acid is associated with decreased activation of complement system [11, 12], and may render them more biocompatible. Reprocessing of synthetic membranes, which are already more biocompatible, adds no further advantage in terms of biocompatibility. Further, the addition of cleansing agents such as bleach eliminates any potential biocompatibility advantage that reprocessing may confer [13]. The disadvantages of reuse are multiple and are listed in Table 18.1. An extensive review of the disadvantages are beyond the scope of this review and have been discussed elsewhere [14]. This review will focus on the impact of reprocessing on dialyzer performance.

L.W. Henderson and R.S. Thuma (eds.), Quality Assurance in Dialysis, 2nd Edition, 189–198.
© 1999 *Kluwer Academic Publishers. Printed in Great Britain*

Table 18.1. Reprocessing of dialyzers

Advantages
- Economic

- Increased biocompatibility?

- Protection against "First-Use Syndrome"

Disadvantages
- Inadequate dialysis due to loss of membrane surface

- Qualitative change in the dialysis membrane leading to activation of plasma or cellular elements

- Infection and pyrogen reactions
  - Infections due to improper sterilization
  - Retention of bacterial products/contaminants from reprocessing fluids
  - Increased permeability to bacterial products/contaminants from the dialysate

- Increased permeability and loss of plasma proteins into dialysate

- Sterilant-related
  - Accidental infusion of sterilant
  - Long-term risks of exposure to small doses of sterilants

CLEARANCE OF UREMIC TOXINS

Reuse of dialyzers could potentially decrease the clearance of uremic toxins and may lead to a decrease in the delivered dose of dialysis [15]. Unfortunately, limited data is available on the clearance of dialyzers in the clinical situation. Guidelines by the Association for Advancement of Medical Instrumentation (AAMI) require that urea clearance of reprocessed dialyzers should be within 10% of the urea clearance by a new dialyzer [16]. However, it is impractical to measure urea clearance before each reuse. Therefore, based on studies by Gotch showing that a decrease in total cell volume (TCV) of reprocessed hollow-fiber dialyzers by 20% decreases the urea clearance by only 10% [17], AAMI recommends that a hollow-fiber dialyzer may be reused until its TCV is 80% of the original volume [16]. However, these observations were made based on limited *in-vitro* studies with 'low-flux' dialyzers, with low blood flow rates, and these were done with very few number of dialyzers, without rigorous statistical analysis [7, 15]. Further, quality assurance of reprocessing procedures has not been investigated systematically, and could have a large impact on the incidence of complications as well as the outcomes of patients treated with these procedures [5]. Consequently, the need for evaluation of the perfor-

mance of reprocessed dialyzers that are currently used, and under clinical conditions.

SMALL MOLECULAR WEIGHT SOLUTES

Cellulose Dialyzers

Reprocessing with formaldehyde (with or without bleach) or peracetic acid does not affect small molecular weight solute (urea or creatinine) clearances of cellulose or substituted cellulose dialyzers. In the early 1980s, Kant and colleagues observed that reprocessing cellulose dialyzers with formaldehyde (without bleach) did not affect the dialysance of urea and creatinine [8]. Likewise, Hoenich and colleagues observed no significant decrease in urea and creatinine clearance with cuprophan dialyzers reprocessed with formaldehyde and bleach, up to six times [18]. Similarly, Kaye and colleagues observed that *in-vitro* and *in-vivo* urea and creatinine clearances and *in-vitro* vitamin B_{12} clearance of cuprophan dialyzers reprocessed with formaldehyde, were not significantly altered after 30 uses [19]. Finally, in a cross-over study using low-flux cellulose dialyzers, Churchill and colleagues observed no clinically or statistically significant change in predialysis urea or creatinine between single-use dialyzers and those reprocessed with formaldehyde/bleach up to five times [20].

Vanholder and colleagues observed that with formaldehyde reprocessing, urea and creatinine clearances and ultrafiltration capacity remained unaltered for the low surface area (1.0 m²) cuprophan dialyzers. However, there was a small, but significant decrease in urea and creatinine clearance for the large surface area (1.8 m²) cuprophan dialyzers [21]. Formaldehyde reuse resulted in a substantial volume loss of these large surface area dialyzers, which may have been the reason for the decrease in dialyzer clearance. In contrast, in a recent *in-vivo* study of cellulose dialyzers (T220L) reprocessed with formaldehyde and bleach, we have shown that urea or creatinine clearance did not decrease with reuse (Figure 18.1) [22].

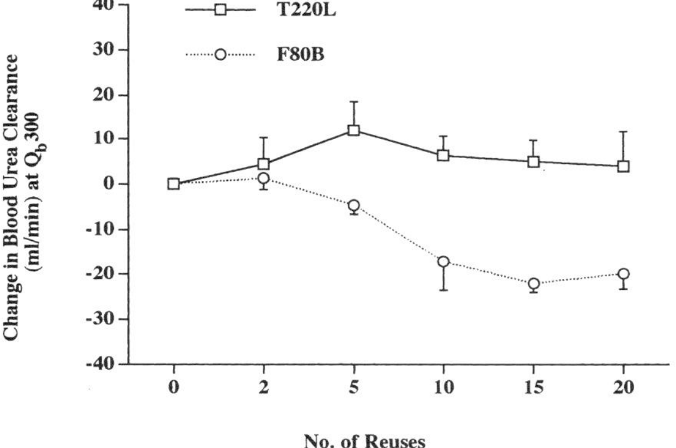

Fig. 18.1. Change in blood-side urea clearance of T220L and F80B dialyzers reprocessed with formaldehyde and bleach, at a blood flow rate (Q_b) of 300 ml/min. Using clearance of new dialyzer as baseline, urea clearance of T220L was significantly higher than that of F80B at 5th, 10th, 15th and 20th reuses ($p < 0.001$, 0.005, 0.004 and 0.006, respectively). Urea clearance of F80B decreased significantly with reuse ($p < 0.001$), while that of T220L did not ($p = 0.23$). Data is mean ± standard error of the mean, from six patients. Reproduced with permission from reference [22].

Peracetic acid reprocessing also does not affect small molecular weight solute clearance of cellulose dialyzers. Vanholder and colleagues observed that reprocessing small or large surface area cuprophan dialyzers with peracetic acid resulted in neither a loss of volume nor a loss of clearance [21]. Likewise, Leypoldt and colleagues observed

that the small molecule (urea and phosphate) clearances of low-flux cellulose (TAF175) or substituted cellulose dialyzers (CA210) reprocessed with peracetic acid did not significantly decrease between first and 15th use [23]. The reason for the volume loss of large surface area cuprophan dialyzers with formaldehyde reprocessing but not with peracetic acid reprocessing in the study by Vanholder and colleagues is not clear [21].

In summary, neither the small molecule clearances nor the ultrafiltration capacity of cellulose dialyzers are affected with reuse, irrespective of the germicide used. With large surface area cellulose dialyzers, formaldehyde reprocessing may result in volume loss, with a consequent decrease in small molecule clearance.

Synthetic Dialyzers

The small molecule clearances of synthetic dialyzers reprocessed with formaldehyde (with or without bleach) appears to decrease with reuse. Vanholder and colleagues observed a significant fall in urea and creatinine clearances and ultrafiltration capacity during the seventh use of PAN dialyzers (reprocessed with formaldehyde) compared to first use [21]. Indeed, urea clearance of PAN membrane dialyzers reprocessed with formaldehyde decreased from 117 mL/min during the first use to 91 mL/min during the seventh use, and creatinine clearance decreased from 99 mL/min during first the use to 77 mL/min during the seventh use. Likewise, the ultrafiltration capacity decreased from 1.01 mL/min/mmHg during the first use to 0.41 mL/min/mmHg during the seventh use [21]. Thus, the urea clearance of PAN membranes fell by a mean of 22% in spite of TCV remaining more than 80% of the initial volume [21]. Similarly, we have shown that urea and creatinine clearances of polysulfone dialyzers (F80B) reprocessed with formaldehyde and bleach decreased significantly from first use to 20th reuse (Figure 18.1) [22]. Urea clearance of F80B dialyzers at a blood flow rate of 300 mL/min (Q_b 300) decreased from 241 ± 2 mL/min for new dialyzers to 221 ± 5 mL/min after 20 reuses, and at a blood flow rate of 400 mL/min (Q_b 400), from 280 ± 4 mL/min for new dialyzers to 253 ± 7 mL/min after 20 reuses. Likewise, creatinine clearance of F80B dialyzers also decreased significantly with reuse [22].

Peracetic acid reprocessing does not seem to affect the clearance of small molecules of polysulfone dialyzers. Garred and colleagues did not observe a decrease in urea or creatinine clearances for up to a median of 15 reuses with high-flux polysulfone dialyzers (F60 and HF80) reprocessed with peracetic acid [24]. Two other studies of polysulfone dialyzers (F60 and F80A) reprocessed with peracetic acid observed no change in small molecular weight solute clearances after five reuses [21] and 15 reuses [23], respectively. However, peracetic acid reprocessing appears to decrease the small molecular weight clearances of other synthetic membranes. Vanholder and colleagues observed that PAN or AN69 dialyzers, reprocessed with peracetic acid, showed a significant decrease of urea and creatinine clearances with reuse, with a concomitant fall of ultrafiltration capacity [21].

Thus, with respect to small molecular weight solute clearances, polysulfone dialyzers behave differently when reprocessed with formaldehyde or peracetic acid. Formaldehyde reprocessing adversely affects the clearance of small molecular weight solutes, but peracetic acid reprocessing does not. However, the clearance of small molecular weight solutes with other synthetic dialyzers is adversely affected with reuse, whether reprocessed with formaldehyde or peracetic acid.

In view of the toxicity reported with reprocessing chemicals, innovative physical methods (using heat), and a combination of physical and relatively less toxic chemical method (using heat and citric acid) for reprocessing of dialyzers, have been recently reported. These methods have not been adequately standardized, and limited data are available on their efficacy and safety. Nonetheless, the available data suggest that these physical methods of reprocessing do not affect urea clearances of polysulfone dialyzers for up to 10–12 uses [25, 26]. One of the major drawbacks of the physical methods of reprocessing is a limited number of reuses obtained. Indeed, Kaufman and colleagues have reported that heat reprocessed polysulfone dialyzers achieved a mean of 7 uses, and only 12% of dialyzers reached the prescribed maximum number of 12 uses [27]. Of the discarded dialyzers, 44% failed a bedside integrity test, 36% failed automated fiber bundle volume or pressure holding tests and 8% were discarded due to a

blood leak. The major advantage of heat reprocessing rests in the fact that pyrogenic reactions, sepsis, and subjective symptoms are a rarity with this method of reprocessing. Although heat sterilization is a safe method of dialyzer reprocessing, further improvements in the technique to increase the number of reuses are required, and quality control of the process is essential.

MIDDLE MOLECULAR WEIGHT SOLUTES

Although 'flux' has been defined as a function of ultrafiltration coefficient (Kuf) of the membrane, high-flux dialyzers also clear middle molecular weight solutes more efficiently than 'low-flux' dialyzers. β_2Microglobulin (molecular weight 11,800 daltons) has been used as a convenient marker for assessment of the clearance of solutes in the middle molecular weight range. Hence, some study groups have adopted the clearance of β_2-microglobulin of >20 mL/min as a measure of 'high-flux' nature of the dialyzer [28]. Studies on the behavior of 'low-flux' dialyzers following reprocessing are limited. The β_2-microglobulin clearance of 'low-flux' dialyzers is consistently <5 mL/min. Indeed, we have shown that the clearance of β_2-microglobulin with formaldehyde and bleach reprocessed cellulose dialyzers (T220L) remained <5.0 mL/min across 20 reuses (Figure 18.2 and Table 18.3) [22]. Thus, reprocessing with formaldehyde and bleach does not alter the ability of these dialyzers to clear β_2-microglobulin.

The β_2-microglobulin clearance with new 'high-flux' dialyzers (cellulose or synthetic) is expected to be >20 mL/min for new dialyzers. However, β_2-microglobulin clearance with reused dialyzers varies with the germicide/ cleansing agent used and the number of reuses. Finally, within a given family of 'high-flux' dialyzers, β_2-microglobulin clearance can vary between dialyzers. This is best illustrated for 'high-flux' polysulfone dialyzers of the F80 family, which were originally manufactured as F80, but subsequently as F80A or F80B. The β_2-microglobulin clearances of new F80A and F80B dialyzers are different from each other [29].

Several investigators have demonstrated that β_2-microglobulin clearance with polysulfone dialyzers increases when reprocessed with bleach. Kaplan and colleagues observed that during clinical dialy-

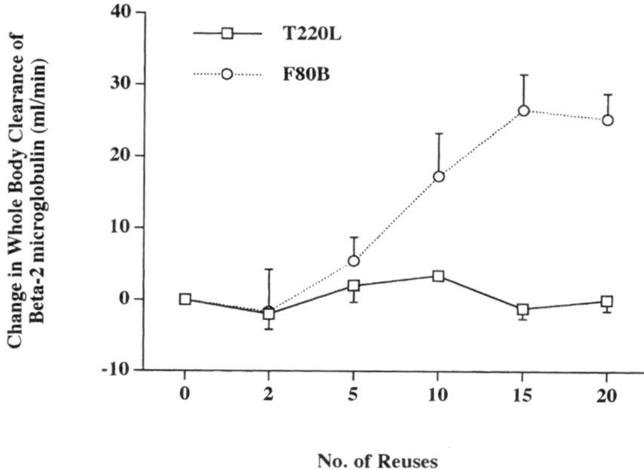

Fig. 18.2. Change in whole body clearance of β_2-microglobulin with T220L and F80B dialyzers reprocessed with formaldehyde and bleach. Using the clearance by a new dialyzer as baseline, the whole body β_2-microglobulin clearance with F80B was significantly higher than that with T220L at 5th, 10th, 15th and 20th reuses ($p = 0.02$, <0.001, <0.001 and <0.001, respectively). The whole body clearance of β_2-microglobulin with F80B increased significantly with reuse ($p < 0.001$), while that with T220L did not ($p = 0.16$). Data is mean$\pm$standard error of the mean, from six patients. Reproduced with permission from reference [22].

L) [30]. Similarly, data from the HEMO study shows that the β_2-microglobulin clearance with polysulfone dialyzers (F80A and F80B) reprocessed with bleach increased with reuse, particularly after 10–20 reuses (Table 18.2) [29]. We have also shown that the plasma β_2-microglobulin clearance of polysulfone dialyzers (F80B) reprocessed with formaldehyde and bleach, increased from a mean of 15.8 mL/min for new dialyzers to 35.8 mL/min for dialyzers reused up to 20 times (Figure 18.2 and Table 18.3) [22]. The dialyzer β_2-microglobulin clearance (as opposed to the treatment clearance stated above) of F80B dialyzers was < 5.0 mL/min for new dialyzers, but increased to 21.2 ± 5.3 mL/min at Q_b 300 after 20 reuses (Table 18.3) [22]. The ability of bleach to increase β_2-microglobulin is also related to the number of reuses of the membrane. Measurement of β_2-microglobulin removal and/or clearance of reused polysulfone dialyzers reused < 10 times, did not reveal a significant increase in the clearance with reuse, compared to the first use [31–33]. These studies indicate that the increase in β_2-microglobulin clearance of polysulfone dialyzers repro-

Table 18.2. Effect of reuse of high-flux dialyzers on plasma β_2-microglobulin clearance – results from the HEMO study[a]

Membrane type (dialyzer)	Germicide/ cleansing agent	Clearance (mL/min)[b] Use 1	Clearance (mL/min)[b] – Reuses 10–20	Clearance (mL/min)[b] – All uses
Polysulfone (F80A)	Peracetic acid	28.0 (3.3)	10.6 (3.8)	14.5 (1.4)
Cellulose (CT190G)	Peracetic acid	45.1 (2.6)	14.7 (1.1)	22.9 (0.8)
Polysulfone (F80B)	Bleach	11.5 (1.8)	45.2 (2.4)	29.4 (1.3)
Polysulfone (F80A)	Bleach	28.0 (3.3)	56.8 (3.1)	42.0 (1.9)
Cellulose (CT190G)	Bleach	45.1 (2.6)	47.9 (4.5)	47.9 (3.1)

[a]Adapted from reference 29.

[b]Values indicate mean (standard error of the mean)

sis with polysulfone dialyzers (F80) reprocessed with formaldehyde and bleach, the dialysate β_2-microglobulin concentration increased with increasing number of reuses [30]. The mean dialysate β_2-microglobulin concentration during clinical dialysis with polysulfone dialyzers (F80) reprocessed > 10 times (1.54 ± 0.15 mg/L) was significantly higher than that with new polysulfone dialyzers (1.05 ± 0.13 mg/L) or dialyzers reprocessed > 10 times without bleach (0.5 ± 0.15 mg/

cessed with bleach usually occurs after 10 reuses.

In contrast to polysulfone dialyzers, the β_2-microglobulin clearance with 'high-flux' cellulose dialyzers (CT190G) reprocessed with bleach, does not increase with reuse (Table 18.2) [29]. Thus, following bleach reprocessing, the increase in sieving coefficient that is observed with polysulfone dialyzers is not observed with 'high-flux' cellulose dialyzers.

In contrast to bleach reprocessing, the ability to

Table 18.3. β_2-Microglobulin dialyzer clearance, percent removal from plasma and whole body clearance during clinical dialysis with T220L and F80B dialyzers reprocessed with formaldehyde and bleach[a]. Adapted from reference [22] and printed with permission.

		No. of reuses						
Dialyzer	β_2-Microglobulin	0 (new)	2	5	10	15	20	p[b]
T220L	Dialyzer clearance at Q_b 300[c]	<5.0	<5.0	<5.0	<5.0	<5.0	<5.0	ns
	Percent removal from plasma[d]	13.0 ± 1.4	9.1 ± 3.2	13.8 ± 3.7	15.6 ± 1.4	11.1 ± 2.4	11.4 ± 0.7	ns
	Whole body clearance (mL/min)[e]	9.8 ± 1.0	7.8 ± 2.5	11.9 ± 2.8	13.3 ± 1.4	9.0 ± 2.1	9.1 ± 1.3	ns
F80B	Dialyzer clearance at Q_b 300[c]	<5.0	<5.0	6.4 ± 0.4	10.3 ± 0.9	24.3 ± 3.5	21.2 ± 5.2	<0.001
	Percent removal[d]	19.8 ± 3.6	16.9 ± 3.6	24.1 ± 1.9	$35.8 \pm 4,5$	41.0 ± 7.1	40.1 ± 5.5	<0.001
	Whole body clearance (mL/min)[e]	15.8 ± 3.5	13.1 ± 2.3	20.0 ± 0.7	31.6 ± 2.6	37.1 ± 4.2	35.8 ± 2.7	<0.001

[a]Values are presented as mean $\pm$ standard error of mean, from six patients

[b]Calculated using analysis of variance (ANOVA) for repeated measurements. Indicates the significance of increase across the reuses studied

[c]Blood flow rate of 300 mL/min

[d]Percent removal of β_2-microglobulin from plasma with F80B dialyzers was significantly higher than with T220L dialyzers at 5th, 10th, 15th and 20th reuses ($p = 0.03$, 0.001, 0.007 and 0.007, respectively). p-values calculated using two sample t-test

[e]Whole body clearance of β_2-microglobulin with F80B dialyzers was significantly higher than with T220L dialyzers at 5th, 10th, 15th and 20th reuses ($p = 0.02$, <0.001, <0.001 and <0.001, respectively). p-values calculated using two sample t-test

clear β_2-microglobulin decreases following reprocessing with peracetic acid both with 'high-flux' polysulfone as well as 'high-flux' cellulose dialyzers. Leypoldt and colleagues observed that the dialyzer clearances of β_2-microglobulin with high-flux cellulose (CT190G) as well as polysulfone dialyzers (F80A) reprocessed with peracetic acid decreased significantly between first and fifteenth use [23]. Likewise, results from the HEMO study show that during clinical dialysis with either 'high-flux' polysulfone (F80A) or 'high-flux' cellulose triacetate (CT190G) dialyzers reprocessed with peracetic acid, the β_2-microglobulin clearance decreased significantly with reuse (Table 18.2) [29]. Thus, although peracetic acid reprocessing does not affect small molecular weight solute clearance, it does decrease β_2-microglobulin clearance of both 'high-flux' cellulose as well as polysulfone dialyzers.

Studies on the behavior of synthetic membranes other than polysulfone, reprocessed with bleach or peracetic acid, are limited. The principal mechanism of β_2-microglobulin clearance with 'high-flux' PMMA membranes is by adsorption to the dialysis membranes [34]. The efficacy of β_2-microglobulin removal with PMMA is expected to decrease when reprocessed with peracetic acid, because

peracetic acid does not strip the membrane of the protein coat formed from an earlier exposure of the membrane to blood. However, during clinical dialysis with PMMA dialyzers, Westhuyzen and colleagues observed that serum β_2-microglobulin concentrations decreased significantly at 15, 60 and 240 minutes into dialysis compared to the predialysis values during first use, as well as 2nd and 4th uses, following peracetic acid reprocessing [35]. Interestingly, the dialysate concentrations of β_2-microglobulin significantly increased with reuse from the first to the fourth use [35]. The increased dialysate removal of β_2-microglobulin may have accounted for an increased removal of β_2-microglobulin during the 4th use of the membrane compared to its first use. The mechanisms underlying this increased clearance into the dialysate are currently unclear. It is possible that when reused beyond 4 times, the β_2-microglobulin removal by these dialyzers may decrease. Indeed, Kerr and colleagues observed a decrease in β_2-microglobulin clearance with peracetic acid reprocessed PMMA hemofilters, after the fourth use [36].

AN69 dialyzers remove β_2-microglobulin by both adsorption and filtration [34]. *In-vitro* studies observed that reprocessing of these dialyzers with peracetic acid significantly decreased their ability to clear β_2-microglobulin, but bleach reprocessing did not [34]. This observation is consistent with the fact that bleach strips the membrane of the protein coat from a previous exposure to blood, but peracetic acid does not. Data on β_2-microglobulin clearance of AN69 dialyzers are limited, and are derived from dialyzers reused only a few times. An *in-vivo* study observed that the percent removal of serum β_2-microglobulin by AN69 dialyzers reprocessed with peracetic acid showed no significant decrease up to the 4th use [35]. Whether the removal of serum β_2-microglobulin increases significantly with higher number of reuses of these dialyzers, is a matter of conjecture. In contrast to the PMMA dialyzers, the dialysate concentrations of β_2-microglobulin with AN69 dialyzers did not increase following reprocessing with peracetic acid [35].

A consistent pattern emerges from the above discussed studies. For polysulfone dialyzers, reprocessing with bleach increases and reprocessing with peracetic acid decreases β_2-microglobulin clearance. While peracetic acid reprocessing also decreases β_2-microglobulin clearance with 'high-flux' cellulose dialyzers, bleach reprocessing does not. The cause for increase in β_2-microglobulin clearance with bleach reprocessing of polysulfone dialyzers is probably an increase in sieving coefficient. The lack of removal of the protein coat on the membranes by peracetic acid may account for the decrease in clearance of β_2-microglobulin observed during reuse of 'higfh-flux' dialyzers.

PROTEIN AND/OR ALBUMIN LOSS

In 1992, with *in-vitro* experiments, by Donahue and colleagues showed that the clearance of small (molecular weight 1,400 daltons) and middle molecular weight (molecular weight 10,000 daltons) polymers by polysulfone dialyzers (F60) significantly increased following reprocessing with 1% bleach and formaldehyde [37], suggesting that reprocessing with bleach alters the membrane permeability of polysulfone dialyzers. Subsequently, Kaplan and colleagues observed that polysulfone dialyzers (F80) reprocessed with bleach, led to the loss of proteins and albumin into the dialysate, and the degree of protein and albumin loss was directly related to the number of

times the membrane was reprocessed with bleach [30]. The mean dialysate protein concentrations progressively increased from 1.5 mg/dL during the first use, to 19.9 mg/dL after 23 to 25 reuses [30]. The mean dialysate protein losses during the entire treatment for bleach reprocessed dialyzers were 1.2 g for first use, 1.8 g during the fifth use, 2.9 g during tenth reuse, 6.4 g during the twelfth through fifteenth use, 10.4 g during the sixteenth through twentieth use and 17.5 g during the twenty-third through twenty-fifth use [30]. Total dialysate albumin losses were unmeasurable from first to fifth use, increased exponentially thereafter, attaining a mean concentration in the dialysate of 14.4 mg/dL after 23 to 25 uses. In contrast, dialyzers reprocessed without bleach had significantly lower protein losses and did not reveal a relationship with reuse. The mean dialysate protein concentrations of the dialyzers with non-bleach reprocessed polysulfone dialyzers after 10 reuses (2.1 mg/dL) was not significantly different from that of the first use (dry pack) of dialyzers (1.5 mg/dL) [30]. Further, none of the dialysate samples from the non-bleach reprocessed dialyzers had detectable albumin levels across 20 reuses [30].

Kaplan and colleagues also observed that the mean serum albumin levels ranged from 3.5 to 3.6 g/dL during the six months prior to discontinuing the bleach from the reprocessing cycle compared to 3.8 to 3.9 g/dL three weeks after discontinuing bleach reprocessing of polysulfone dialyzers, in the same patients [30]. This suggests that the decrease of serum albumin among patients dialyzed with bleach reprocessed polysulfone (F80) dialyzers may be due to the massive protein and albumin leak from these dialyzers.

The leak of protein during dialysis with bleach reprocessed polysulfone dialyzers varies with the dialyzers studied. Gotch and colleagues studied the overall permeability-area product (KoA) for cytochrome C, a surrogate marker of β_2-microglobulin, and protein sieving coefficient (KsP) for polysulfone dialyzers (F80A and F80B) reprocessed with either peracetic acid, heat or bleach. After 20 reuses, heat resulted in no increase in either KoA or KsP, and bleach resulted in a small but insignificant increase in KoA and KsP [38]. Thus, the protein loss using bleach reprocessed polysulfone dialyzers in this study was negligible. Similarly, we have shown that albumin loss with bleach reprocessed F80B dialyzers was negligible for up to 20 reuses [22]. The modification in the F80 dialyzer membrane that led to the correction of albumin leak also appears to have decreased the ability of these dialyzers to clear β_2-microglobulin, such that the F80B dialyzers behaves as 'low-flux' up to 10 reuses [22, 29]. Thus, the issue of protein leak by polysulfone dialyzers reprocessed with bleach is still controversial, and clearly more studies are required to elucidate the permeability characteristics of different membranes following reprocessing with various germicides, and the long-term clinical consequences of these effects.

Protein losses with polysulfone dialyzers (F80) reprocessed with peracetic acid have been shown to be much lower compared to that of dialyzers reprocessed with formaldehyde/ bleach. Protein loss after 15 or more uses of polysulfone dialyzers (HF80R) reprocessed with peracetic acid was 3.2 ± 1.1 g, not significantly different from that with first use (dry pack) of the dialyzer [39].

REUSE AND DELIVERY OF DIALYSIS PRESCRIPTION:

The recently released Dialysis Outcomes Quality Initiative (DOQI) guidelines [40] recommend monitoring of dialysis with urea kinetic modeling (Kt/V) or urea reduction ratio (URR). The mortality risk among hemodialysis patients is lower by 7% for each 0.1 increment in delivered Kt/V, and by 11% for each 5% increase in delivered URR [41]. Whether the mortality plateaus with Kt/V values exceeding 1.3 and URR exceeding 70% is currently unknown [42]. However, in the U.S., data from the Unites States Renal data System (USRDS) shows that, between July and December 1993, the mean delivered single pool Kt/V was 1.22 and mean was URR 63.1% in a national random sample of in-center hemodialysis patients (43). These values are lower than the currently recommended Kt/V of 1.3 for routine hemodialysis patients [40]. One of the possible reasons for a decreased dialysis adequacy is a decline in dialyzer performance following re-use of dialyzers. The effect of reuse on dialysis delivery has not been adequately studied. In a multi-center study, Sherman and colleagues observed a significantly increased delivered Kt/V (urea) (1.08 vs. 1.02) in centers with low reuse of dialyzers (mean of 3.8 times) compared to centers with high reuse of dialyzers (mean of 13.8 times), suggesting a decline in performance of dialyzer with reuse [15]. In 43% of the centers using formaldehyde reprocessing, the difference in Kt/V values between low and high-reuse averaged 0.17 [15]. However, this study showed a strong center difference, probably related to practices associated with differences in reprocessing techniques. In the context of an increased mortality risk with decreased dose of dialysis, this decline in dialysis dose with reuse is a matter of concern. In contrast, in a prospective study of patients randomized to single use or reuse of cellulose dialyzers with glutaraldehyde and bleach, we did not observe a significant difference in URR between groups, over a period of three months [44]. Although most dialysis units monitor the dose of dialysis delivered by measurement of URR or urea kinetic modeling, such measurements are usually performed on a montly basis, and do not provide timely identification of sub-optimal delivered dose. The newer on-line monitoring systems (blood-side and dialysate-side monitoring of Kt/V) may help assess the efficacy of delivery of dialysis prescription during dialysis with reprocessed dialyzers.

REFERENCES

1. Shaldon SH, Silva H and Rosen SM. The technique of refrigerated coil preservation hemodialysis with femoral venous catherization. Br Med J 1964; 2:672–4.
2. Pollard TL, Barnett BMS, Eschbach JW and Scribner BH. A technique for storage and multiple reuse of Kill dialyzer and blood tubing. ASAIO Trans 1967; 13:24–8.
3. Baris E and McGregor M. The reuse of hemodialyzers: an assessment of safety and potential savings. Can Med Assoc J 1993; 148:175–83.
4. Tokars JI, Alter MJ, Miller E, Moyer LA and Favero MS. National surveillance of dialysis associated diseases in the United States – 1994. ASAIO J 1997; 43:108–19.
5. Schoenfeld PY. The technology of dialyzer reuse. Semin Nephrol 1997; 17:321–30.
6. Husni L, Kale E, Climer C, Bostwick B and Parker TF. Evaluation of a new disinfectant for dialyzer reuse. Am J Kidney Dis 1989; 14:110–8.
7. Shusterman NH, Feldman HI, Wasserstein A and Strom BL. Reprocessing of hemodialyzers: a critical appraisal. Am J Kidney Dis 1989; 2:81–91.

8. Kant KS, Pollack VE, Cathey M, Goetz D and Berlin R. Multiple use of dialyzers: safety and efficacy. Kidney Int 1981; 19:728–38.

9. Bok D and Pascual LCH. Effect of multiple use of dialyzers on intradialytic symptoms. Proc Clin Dial Transplant Forum 1980; 10:92–5.

10. Robson M, Charoenpanich R and Kant K. Effect of first and subsequent use of hemodialyzers on patient well-being. Am J Nephrol 1986; 6:101–6.

11. Hakim RM and Lowrie EG. Effect of dialyzer reuse on leukopenia, hypoxemia and total hemolytic complement system. Trans Am Soc Artif Intern Organs 1980; 26:159–64.

12. Chenoweth DE, Cheung AK, Ward DM and Henderson LW. Anaphylatoxin formation during hemodialysis: a comparison of new and re-used dialyzers. Kidney Int 1983; 24:770–4.

13. Sundaram S, King AJ and Pereira BJ. Lipopolysaccharide-binding protein and bactericidal/permeability-increasing factor during hemodialysis: clinical determinants and role of different membranes. J Am Soc Nephrol 1997; 8:463–70.

14. Miles AMV and Friedman EA. A review of hemodialyzer reuse. Semin Dialysis 1997; 10:32–7.

15. Sherman R, Cody R, Roger M and Solanchick J. The effect of dialyzer reuse on dialysis delivery. Am J Kidney Dis 1994; 24:924–6.

16. AAMI. Reuse of hemodialyzers. AAMI standards and recommended practices. Arlington, VA, Association for the Advancement of Medical Instrumentation, 1995; 3:106–7.

17. Gotch FA. Dialyzer transport properties and germicide elution. Proceedings: Seminars on reuse of hemodialyzers and automated and manual methods. New York, National Nephrology Foundation, 1984.

18. Hoenich NA, Johnston SRD, Buckley P, Harden J, Ward MK and Kerr DNS. Hemodialysis reuse: impact on function and biocompatibility. Int J Artif Organs 1983; 6:261–6.

19. Kaye M, Gagnon R, Mulhearn B and Spergel D. Prolonged dialyzer reuse. Trans Am Soc Artif Intern Organs 1984; 30:491–3.

20. Churchill DN, Taylor DW, Shimizu AG et al. Dialyzer reuse – a multiple crossover study with random allocation to order of treatment. Nephron 1988; 50:325–31.

21. Vanholder RC, Sys E, DeCubber A, Vermaercke N and Ringoir SM. Performance of cuprophane and polyacrylonitrile dialyzers during multiple use. Kidney Int 1988;24:S55–6.

22. Murthy BVR, Sundaram S, Jaber BL, Perrella C, Meyer KB and Pereira BJG. Effect of formaldehyde/bleach reprocessing on *in-vivo* performances of 'high-efficiency' cellulose and 'high-flux' polysulfone dialyzers. J Am Soc Nephrol 1998 (in press).

23. Leypoldt JK, Cheung AK and Deeter RB. Effect of Renalin R reprocessing on small and large solute clearances (K) by hemodialyzers (HD). J Am Soc Nephrol 1995; 6:A607.

24. Garred LJ, Canaud B, Flavier JL, Poux C, Polito-Bouloux C and Mion C. Effect of reuse on dialyzer efficacy. Artif Organs 1990; 14:80–4.

25. Levin NW, Parnell SL, Prince HN et al. The use of heated citric acid for dialyzer reprocessing. J Am Soc Nephrol 1995; 6:1578–85.

26. Schoenfeld P, McLaughlin MD and Mendelson M. Heat disinfection of polysulfone hemodialyzers. Kidney Int 1995; 47:638–42.

27. Kaufman AM, Frinak S, Godmere RO, Levin NW. Clinical experience with heat sterilization for reprocessing dialyzers. ASAIO J 1992; 38:M338–40.

28. The HEMO Study Group. Manual of operations, The Hemodialysis (HEMO) Study, Page 3.5: National Institutes of Health, National Institute of Diabetes and Digestive and Kidney Diseases, Bethesda, MD, 1995.

29. Leypoldt JK, Cheung AK, Clark WR et al. Characterization of low and high-flux dialyzers with reuse in the Hemo Study: interim report (Abstract). J Am Soc Nephrol 1996; 7:1518.

30. Kaplan AA, Halley SE, Lapkin RA and Graeber CW. Dialysate protein losses with bleach processed polysulfone dialyzers. Kidney Int 1995; 47:573–8.

31. Diaz RJ, Washburn S, Cauble L, Siskind MS and Van Wyck D. The effect of dialyzer reprocessing on performance and beta 2-microglobulin removal using polysulfone membranes. Am J Kidney Dis 1993; 21:405–10.

32. DiRaimondo CR and Pollak VE. Beta 2-microglobulin kinetics in maintenance hemodialysis: a comparison of conventional and high-flux dialyzers and the effects of dialyzer reuse. Am J Kidney Dis 1989; 13:390–5.

33. Petersen J, Moore R, Jr., Kaczmarek RG et al. The effects of reprocessing cuprophane and polysulfone dialyzers on beta 2-microglobulin removal from hemodialysis patients. Am J Kidney Dis 1991; 17:174–8.

34. Goldman M, Lagmiche M, Dhaene M, Amraoui Z, Thayse C and Vanherweghem JL. Adsorption of beta 2-microglobulin on dialysis membranes: comparison of different dialyzers and effects of reuse procedures. Int J Artif Organs 1989; 12:373–8.

35. Westhuyzen J, Foreman K, Battistutta D, Saltissi D and Fleming SJ. Effect of dialyzer reprocessing with Renalin on serum beta-2-microglobulin and complement activation in hemodialysis patients. Am J Nephrol 1992; 12:29–36.

36. Kerr PG, Argiles A, Canaud B, Flavier JL and Mion C. The effects of reprocessing high-flux polysulfone dialyzers with peroxyacetic acid on beta 2-microglobulin removal in hemodiafiltration. Am J Kidney Dis 1992; 19:433–8.

37. Donahue PR and Ahmad S. Dialyzer permeability alteration by reuse (Abstract). J Am Soc Nephrol 1992; 3:363.

38. Gotch F, Gentile D, Kaufman A and Levin N. Effects of reuse with peracetic acid, heat and bleach on polysulfone dialyzers (Abstract). J Am Soc Nephrol 1994; 5:A415.

39. Peterson DE, Hyver T, Yeh I and Petersen J. Reprocessing dialyzers with peracetic acid-hydrogen peroxide does not cause substantial protein losses (Abstract). J Am Soc Nephrol 1994; 5:424.

40. Anonymous. NKF-DOQI clinical practice guidelines for hemodialysis adequacy. National Kidney Foundation. Am J Kidney Dis 1997; 30:S15–66.

41. Anonymous. National Kidney Foundation report on dialyzer reuse. Am J Kidney Dis 1997; 30:859–71.

42. Held PJ, Port FK, Wolfe RA et al. The dose of hemodialysis and patient mortality. Kidney Int 1996; 50:550–6.

43. U.S. Renal Data System. The USRDS dialysis morbidity and mortality study (Wave 1). Am J Kidney Dis 1996; 28:S58–78.

44. Pereira BJG, Natov SN, Sundaram S et al. Impact of single use versus re-use of cellulose dialyzers on clinical parameters and indices of biocompatibility. J Am Soc Nephrol 1996; 7:861–70.

19. The impact of membrane selection on quality assurance in dialysis

LEE W. HENDERSON

INTRODUCTION

Broadly considered, the selection of a membrane for treatment of the patient with kidney failure determines whether transplantation (glomerular basement membrane), peritoneal dialysis or treatment with the artificial kidney occurs. I will narrow the topic by excluding kidney transplantation but will explore the various options within the latter two modes of treatment. I recognize, however, that receipt and retention of a good quality kidney graft offers the best duration and quality of life and must be considered as the gold standard against which all other modes of treatment must be judged.

There is still much that remains unknown about membrane selection in spite of a professional lifetime's worth of investigation of this topic by many researchers, myself included. The wealth of choices today, as contrasted with the early 1960s when the only choice lay between cellulosic and peritoneal membrane, is both a tribute to the skill of the membrane manufacturer and an indictment of the nephrologist for failing to understand the pathophysiology of uremia with sufficient clarity to define the requirements for an ideal treatment membrane.

In the subsequent pages I will describe reported differences in membrane properties and how they may impact on quality of care. I will try to be clear about where data ends and informed speculation begins. I will describe categories or classes of membrane and typical properties rather than specific membranes, i.e. a "generic" approach.

Quality assurance in the treatment of end stage renal disease has at least two dimensions; quantity and quality of life. Offering an "adequate" dialysis prescription is of course central to both. I will

make the case that membrane selection is the single most important primary variable in the dialysis prescription that can be selected by the dialysis unit director as it drives the decisions such as treatment time and home versus dialysis center treatment and impacts on both quantity and quality of life. What follows is a discussion aimed at illuminating that choice. The importance of this choice is underscored by government reimbursement agencies and their requirement to report presumed parameters of adequacy such as Kt/V, for urea and plasma albumen concentration, treatment time, etc.

HOW MAY WE DEFINE ADEQUATE DIALYSIS?

At present we turn to urea kinetic modeling and the results of the National Cooperative Dialysis Study (NCDS) [1] to provide a clinically qualified quantitative definition of adequate hemodialysis.[1] The derivative analysis by Gotch and Sargent [4] has provided us with the now familiar "Domain Map" (Figure 19.1) in which normalized dietary protein intake is plotted against predialysis blood urea nitrogen concentration with isopleths drawn out of the origin like spokes from the hub of a wheel that show the amount of therapy rendered in terms of the dimensionless parameter for urea of Kt/V. A patient consuming 1 gram of protein/ kilogram lean body mass with a value for Kt/V of [3] 1.2 is now widely considered to be adequately hemodialyzed [5]. K represents the diffusive dialyzer clearance (in mL/min) for urea; a value that is directly related to the overall mass transfer resistance of the membrane for urea as well as the area of the membrane employed i.e. membrane selec-

L.W. Henderson and R.S. Thuma (eds.), Quality Assurance in Dialysis, 2nd Edition, 199–213.
© 1999 *Kluwer Academic Publishers. Printed in Great Britain*

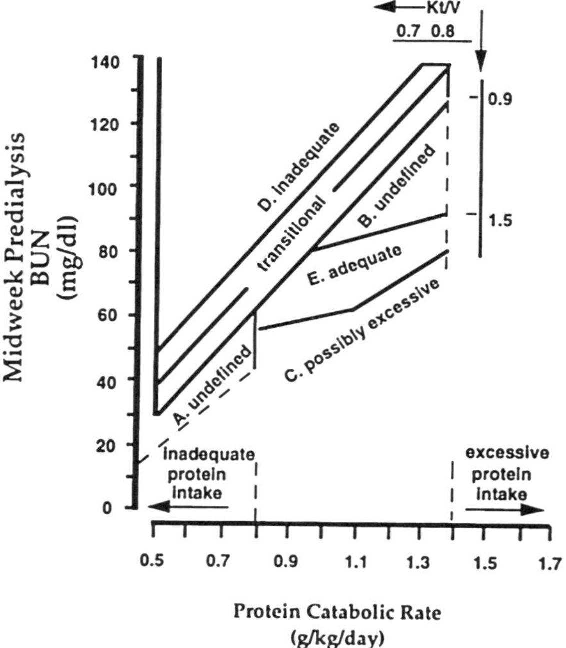

Fig. 19.1. A domain map showing the interrelationship between predialysis blood urea nitrogen concentration, protein catabolic rate and the dimensionless parameter Kt/V (modified from reference [3]).

tion; t is the length of the treatment in minutes and V, the total body water in milliliters. Before exploring the relevance of this ratio further, it will be important to understand some of the underlying assumptions of the NCDS and the limitations that they impose upon interpretation of this parameter.

The NCDS study was designed to determine whether urea kinetic modeling could predict clinical outcome with sufficient accuracy to make it a useful clinical tool for dialysis prescription. The answer by those conducting the study and for many others, myself among them, was yes. But what of the limitations? Little has been written on this subject [6, 7] and many unwarranted extrapolations exist in the literature.

CAPD adequacy parameters have now been amply clinically qualified by the CANUSA Study [8]. Weekly Kt/V urea for CAPD, while about a factor of 2 less than hemodialysis for technical reasons [6, 8], has been shown to correlate with both mortal and morbid outcome as have two

nutritionally-based parameters – plasma albumin concentration and global clinical assessment of nutritional status. While it is not the thrust of this work to provide details of how these measurements are made, it will be important to understand the strengths and limitations of urea kinetic modeling as it is the most widely employed technique for assessing adequacy for both CAPD and HD.

Urea as surrogate for uremic yoxins: It is generally conceded that urea, itself, is not the most significant uremic toxin but rather that it is surrogate for other more toxic solutes [9]. With reference to Table 19.1, all that is required of urea to achieve this surrogate status is that it maintain an "orderly" relationship over a therapeutic cycle (e.g. a week) in terms of its concentration in the plasma water with the concentration of solutes for which it is considered surrogate (Table 19.2). Comparability of molecular size, charge, space of distribution, polarity and rate of generation would

Table 19.1. The surrogate status of urea

1.	Requires an orderly relationship between the rate of: Generation Catabolism Elimination
2.	Does not require comparable molecular Size Charge Space of distribution

Table 19.2. Factors affecting surrogate status

1.	Membrane area
2.	Residual renal function
3.	Number of spaces of distribution, i.e. solute transcellular kinetics
4.	Cytokine release – Membrane – Dialysate
5.	Flow rate of blood by the membrane
6.	Membrane solute clearance profile – Degree of openness: to diffusion to convection
7.	Peak and valley chemistries vs. steady state (i.e. HD versus CAPD)
8.	Treatment time
9.	Frequency of treatment

likely assure such an orderly relationship but are by no means required. For example, a solute of larger molecular weight with a purely extracellular space of distribution could sustain a proportional change in concentration to urea during a given weekly treatment prescription in a reproducible manner that would qualify it as having an orderly relationship to urea. As will be explored subsequently, this latter surrogacy for solutes of larger size and/or differing space of distribution will be more easily perturbed by variations in the treatment prescription than would that for solutes with a molecular size and space of distribution that is comparable to urea. Note that there have been several promising candidates identified since Scribner's original postulate that middle molecules were pathophysiologically important in uremia, e.g. β_2-microglobulin [10] the polypeptide inhibitor of polymorph activity described by Hörl, et al. [11]. Inferential evidence for their presence and pathophysiologic importance is strong however [12–14].

Time as surrogate for uremic toxins: A secondary outcome measure of the NCDS that was less rigorously addressed by the study protocol and almost ignored in the published interpretation [1] is the impact of treatment time (in minutes) on adequacy as assessed by the incidence of morbid events [13]. Time enters the numerator of the parameter Kt/V. As the numerator is a clearance, time product one might simplistically assume shortening dialysis time could be completely compensated for, clinically, by an increase in the clearance of urea that holds this product constant, i.e. use of a larger or more permeable membrane. While this is perfectly correct mathematically, this is not the case clinically. For example, doubling the clearance of urea so that treatment time can be cut in half may shift the limiting mass transfer resistance area product for urea away from the dialyzer membrane and place it upon the cell membrane (averaged across the body) resulting in a significant disequilibrium between plasma water and cell water [15]. This may be quantitatively appreciated by the increase in urea rebound that occurs at the conclusion of an high efficiency treatment [16] as urea moves across the cell wall into the plasma discharging the gradient caused by the dialysis treatment, i.e. urea is not distributed in a single

pool. A clue to this event would be noting that the volume of distribution for urea calculated from the drop in plasma water urea concentration measured at the end of treatment was identifiably less than the commonly accepted value computed as 58 to 60% of the body weight in kilograms. One must now ask how the increase in clearance was obtained with high efficiency hemodialysis. This would most commonly be accomplished by using a somewhat larger membrane and increasing blood flow rate to utilize this augmented area. This, of course, is the strategy used in group III of the NCDS in which low (comparable to control) pretreatment urea concentration and short treatment time were employed. Figure 19.2, modified from Laird et al. [17], points out that this strategy is associated with a significant increase in morbid events. As previously pointed out [13], this is a surprising finding in that the increase in membrane area should have worked toward preserving the surrogate status for urea for toxins that diffuse

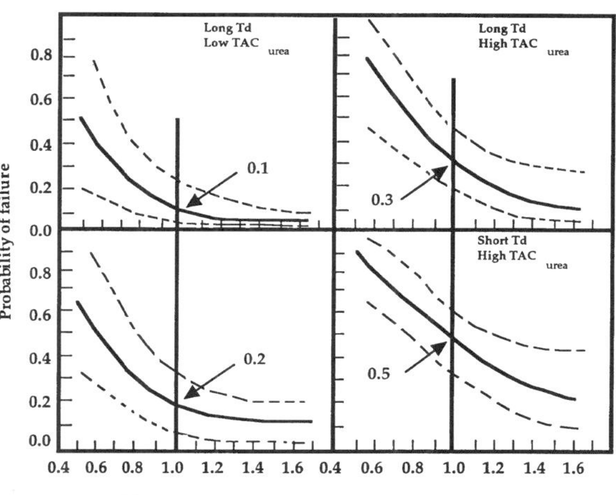

Fig. 19.2. The probability of failure is here defined as any patient who died, withdrew for medical reasons or was hospitalized prior to 24 weeks in the experimental phase of the protocol. The date of failure was the date of death, withdrawal or first hospitalization, whichever occurred first. The solid curves were calculated from NCDS data. The dashed lines represent 95% confidence limits. The impact of treatment time (Td) may be read vertically for low and high time average concentration of urea (TAC_{urea}) and horizontally for the impact of TAC_{urea} on probability of failure. The probability of failure approximately doubles when going from long treatment time to short treatment time for both low TAC_{urea} (0.1 to 0.2) or high TAC_{urea} (0.3 to 0.5).

more slowly than urea, making the therapy more nearly comparable to that offered in the control group. The increase in morbid events with this strategy supports the interpretation that the shortened time outweighs, in importance, the increase in membrane area, resulting in a build up of pathophysiologically important slowly diffusing solutes. Said another way, in this time/flux trade-off, the increased solute flux from use of the larger membrane failed to compensate for the reduction in treatment time [6].

The reports of an increase in mortality and its association with shortened treatment time (low t, no change in K) from Lowrie et al. [18] using a large database from a private dialysis chain and of Held [19, 20] using the powerful USRDS database, provide experimental support for the importance of solutes for which urea is surrogate in determining the quality of treatment provided. It is important to note that these retrospectively examined data of Lowrie and Held were not associated with any effort to sustain a satisfactory dietary protein intake, nor to provide a Kt/V^3 of 1.2. In the NCDS, of course, a major component of this prospectively conducted protocol was aimed at sustaining nutritional status with the maintenance of a dietary protein intake of 1 g/day/kg body weight. The comparability of the pretreatment blood urea nitrogen concentrations noted by Held, et al. [19] between his short and standard treatment time patient groups, points up the reduced dietary protein intake in the short treatment group. This points to the concern about malnutrition and its role in determining a satisfactory treatment outcome. It remains to be determined what the respective contributions are of those factors that cause death in association with malnutrition vs. those that do so in association with retained, slowly diffusing toxins (i.e. middle molecules) and whether these factors interrelate (See, for example, Anderstram et al. [21]).

A more recent analysis from the Japanese registry from Shinzato et al. [22], selecting patients who have been on the treatment for at least 2 years, provides the correlation between relative risk of death and the hours per treatment of the 3 times weekly schedule. A reference value of 4.0–4.5 hours/treatment thrice weekly was assigned a relative risk of 1.0. They report that values shorter than that e.g. 3.5–4.0, show an increased relative risk at 1.68 ($p < 0001$). Factoring Kt/V received per treatment by the time of treatment, i.e. Kt/V/t offers an index of efficiency for urea removal, i.e. the rate of delivery of Kt/V. This calculation shows that in this population ($n = 53,867$) shortening treatment time but maintaining high removal rates of urea by increasing membrane area and flow rates is detrimental to longevity (Maeda et al. Mannheim [23]), i.e.

$$\frac{Kt/v}{t} \propto \frac{1}{\text{longevity}}$$

The importance of treatment time as being a significant prescription variable, of course reaches back to the work of Scribner and Babb on middle molecules and the square meter hour hypothesis [24]. Treatment time may be taken as surrogate for middle molecule clearance, i.e. clearance of molecular weight species that are larger than the conventionally considered uremic toxins and smaller than albumen, ($> 500 < 60,000$ daltons) [6]. The line of reasoning that makes these deliberations relevant to our topic of membrane selection is as follows. If time may be considered surrogate for middle molecule clearance, then membrane selection for a more open transport structure will also enhance middle molecule removal and will translate into the options of shorter treatment time or "more adequate" (read lower mortality) treatment [6]. In considering the limitations placed on extrapolations from the NCDS, both urea and its surrogate solutes and time and its surrogate solutes must be carefully considered. Good quality kinetic modeling that encompasses not only urea but index solutes in the middle molecular weight range level is helpful in understanding these interactions (see for example, [25]).

Nutritional status as an index of adequacy: It is important to note the observation by Lowrie (Figure 19.3), that identifies a powerful inverse correlation between plasma albumen concentration and death rate in the ESRD population under treatment with conventional hemodialysis [18]. Teehan et al. as did Churchill et al. confirm this observation for patients on CAPD [26, 7]. Albumin concentration is widely believed to be one objective, if not very sensitive, measure of nutritional status. A low or falling serum albumin is consistent with negative nitrogen balance and a

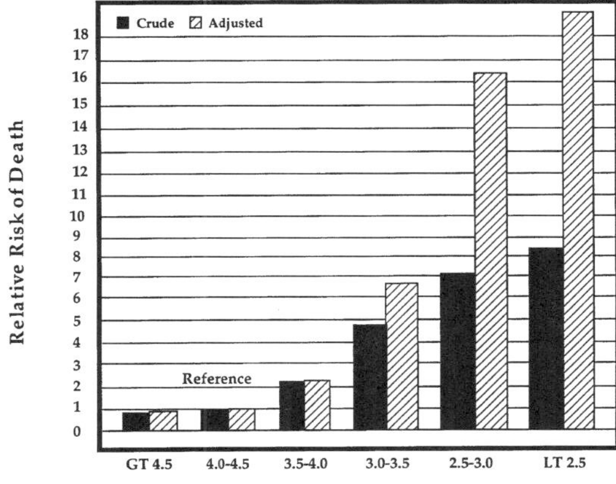

Fig. 19.3. Relative risk of death is plotted against serum albumin concentration with the reference concentration of 1 being the 4 to 4.5 g/dL. Those with serum albumin concentrations of greater than 4.5 (GT 4.5) were not significantly different from the reference standard. The powerful inverse correlation for the crude data is even more significant when the ratios are adjusted for the case mix predictors of death.

diagnosis of malnutrition. This is by no means a new observation, only a recent rigorous correlation in a large ESRD population on treatment with dialysis. The importance of sustaining a satisfactory protein intake is noted in the recommendations of the NCDS that intake of 1 gram of protein/kg of lean body wt. per day is necessary for an adequate treatment prescription.

Lindsay [27, 28] offers an hypothesis that suggests that the conventional wisdom as drawn from the NCDS is backwards with regard to the interpretation of this nutritional information i.e. that we must prescribe enough dialysis to remove the metabolites generated by the breakdown of the ingested protein. He suggests that the amount of dialysis and metabolite removal is the primary driver of protein intake through a direct modulation of the appetite. This remains an hypothesis. However, Bergstrom et al. have recently identified such a retained metabolite (not leptin) and are in the process of characterizing it [21]. This places the patient's state of nutrition at the very center of any judgment on dialysis adequacy. Studies of patients on both peritoneal dialysis and hemodialysis show that mild to severe malnutrition may be documented in some 30–40% of study subjects [18, 29, 30].

Elevated leptin levels have also been noted [31–33]. The marginal nature from the nutritional perspective of the therapy we now offer is pointed up by these distressing figures. If Lindsay et al. are right, and I believe they are, selection of a larger and/or more open membrane in the treatment prescription will enhance appetite and reduce both morbid and mortal events [21, 27, 28, 32].

TREATMENT STRATEGIES AND QUALITY ASSURANCE

The Choice of Hemodialysis Membrane

Table 19.3 lists the experimental parameters and their test ranges used in the NCDS [1]. I will specifically explore the following treatment prescriptions which employ different membranes that fall outside the test ranges noted in Table 19.1[2] and indicate how these prescriptions may affect the quality of the treatment rendered:

A. Large area and/or highly permeable membrane

B. High flux membrane

C. The peritoneal "membrane"

Large area and/or highly permeable membrane
High efficiency hemodialysis is commonly conducted using a large membrane area (1.5–2.0 m^2) and high flow rates of blood (> 400 mL/min) and dialysate (500 mL/min) to effect a more efficient removal of uremic toxins. In the U.S. this form of therapy has usually been employed in conjunction with urea kinetic modelling (UKM) and shortened treatment time (2.5–3 hours/treatment 3 times per week). In its pure form, cuprophane or its equivalent rather than more open high flux membrane is utilized. Studies by Collins et al. are fine examples of this technique [34, 35].

By expanding membrane area and flow rates beyond that employed in the NCDS, we encounter the circumstance where urea clearance would increase rather dramatically. The NCDS qualified the use of the variable volume single pool urea kinetic model which presupposes that the rate of mass transfer across the cell wall significantly exceeds that across the dialyzer membrane, i.e.

Table 19.3. Data describing therapy control for the NCDS [1]

| Long time | Long time | | Long time | | Short time | | Short time | |
| | Group I | | Group II | | Group III | | Group IV | |
	Control	Exp.	Control	Exp.	Control	Exp.	Control	Exp.
Dialysis length (min)	274 ± 10	271 ± 8	274 ± 10	268 ± 6	278 ± 13	200 ± 15	275 ± 15	190 ± 17
TAC_{urea} (mg/dL)	52.0 ± 3.9	51.1 ± 4.1	51.4 ± 4.2	87.8 ± 11.6	50.8 ± 3.7	54.7 ± 5.3	52.0 ± 3.1	93.6 ± 7.2
Midweek BUN (mg/dL)	74 ± 6	76 ± 6	75 ± 6	108 ± 14	72 ± 6	77 ± 7	75 ± 6	115 ± 9
Dialyzer urea clearance (mL/min)	158 ± 41	171 ± 41	161 ± 36	77 ± 20	162 ± 32	206 ± 30	165 ± 30	107 ± 21
PCR (g/kg)	1.04		1.04		0.96		1.08	

TAC_{urea} = time averaged concentration of urea; PCR = protein catabolic rate

Membranes: cuprophan, cellulose acetate

Area: 1.2–2.5 m^2

the cell wall does not significantly limit transport. Figure 19.4 is taken from Frost and Kerr [15] and is one of the few attempts to examine the overall area mass transfer resistance product across the cell, taken on average across all of the body cells. They recognize, of course, that the red cell membrane will have a different value than the cells dividing blood from brain. This average value is only a mathematical construct but it offers us useful insight, nonetheless. The shaded area of Figure 19.4 represents the realm of dialyzer clearance. By doubling membrane area and increasing flows it is apparent that the assumption of a single pool for urea will be violated. As previously noted, increased membrane area (less so blood flow rate) increases the clearance of middle molecules but the major impact is to increase small molecular weight solute clearance. By shortening treatment time the ratio of the mass of middle molecules that are removed per mg of urea is reduced even as the increase in membrane area increases middle molecule clearance. Short of measuring the clearances of both urea and a middle molecule such as β_2-microglobulin (11,800 daltons) or vitamin B_{12} (1,355 daltons), it is not possible to say whether the treatment rendered is adequate as defined by the NCDS or not, as removal of both large and small toxins is clinically important. Modeling these transport patterns also offers useful insight [25, 36]. Work by Collins et al. [34] in more than

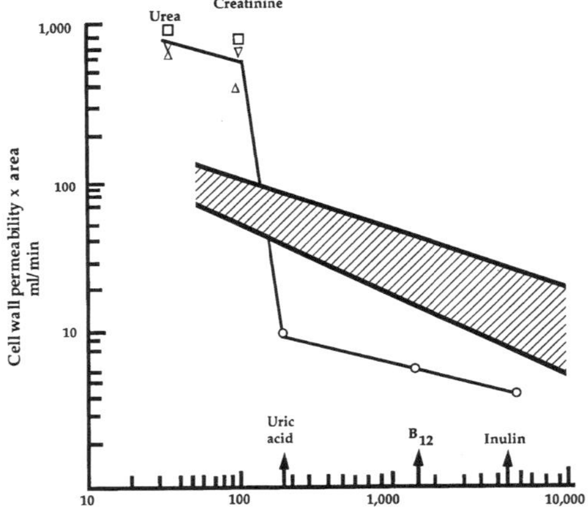

Fig. 19.4. The log of the average cell wall mass transfer coefficient (permeability times area) is plotted against the log of solute molecular weight. Data points are represented by symbols and have been taken from a variety of workers. The shaded area represents the domain of hemodialyzer clearance for 1 m^2 cuprophan membrane. Clearance across the cell wall exceeds that for the dialyzer for solutes small in molecular weight, such as urea and creatinine. Uric acid, B_{12} and inulin are measured to fall significantly below dialyzer clearance.

1,000 patients over a 4 year time frame (1986–1990) where both urea and modeled vitamin B_{12} clearances were sustained shows that survival with short (<3 hours/treatment), large surface area bicarbonate hemodialysis is statistically significantly improved in overall mortality if the Kt/V for urea is maintained 1.2,[3] a value comparable to the value of 1.0 to 1.19 for the age and risk factor adjusted control subjects. This work indicates that by using a large area dialyzer to increase urea clearance to values that sustain Kt/V comparable to the control group and concomitantly increasing middle molecule clearance, there is an improved survival rate. The possible role of the use of bicarbonate in this improved survival rate needs to be further evaluated. This work is of great importance as it shows that shortening treatment time can be safely done with high efficiency hemodialysis, i.e. proper selection of the membrane to sustain the Kt product for both urea and a middle molecule such as vitamin, B_{12} at or above NCDS standards.

High flux membrane

By this, I mean the use of membranes that have a far higher hydraulic permeability than the more commonly used cellulosic membranes, cuprophane or cellulose acetate. Use of such a membrane (e.g. polyacrylonitrile, cellulose triacetate or high flux polysulphone) requires special fluid cycling equipment to permit control of ultrafiltration. Significant ultrafiltration may occur even in the absence of net ultrafiltration rates that are high, simply by a form of "Starling's capillary flow" that produces ultrafiltrate at the arterial end of the membrane and backfiltration of fluid (dialysate mixed with ultrafiltered plasma water) at the venous end. Hemodiafiltration fits within this definition, i.e. the deliberate enhancement of ultrafiltration during a dialysis and then replacing ultrafiltrate volume that exceeds the requisite fluid loss to restore excess body water volume to normal. The convective element to transport perturbs the relationship of urea to larger solutes as it is not size discriminatory (i.e. urea's surrogate status as qualified by the NCDS for diffusive transport is perturbed). If urea kinetic modeling (single or multiple pool) is applied to this form of therapy and the Kt/V value is adjusted equal to NCDS standards for adequacy, one can assume a larger clearance of middle molecules and hence a dialysis prescription that is "more adequate" than the same Kt/V obtained using cuprophane and solely diffusive transport. The fraction of overall mass

transport that is convective in mechanism may be considered to be surrogate for treatment time. I speculate that a suitable mix of shortening treatment time, sustaining urea removal, and increasing convective transport would result in a treatment that is comparably adequate to conventional full length hemodialysis. If adequacy is comparable, the shorter treatment time by definition offers a higher quality of therapy.

At present there are only a few prospective studies that give clear qualification of this treatment strategy. See, for example, studies such as that of Channard et al. [37] using the more open complement kind polyacrylonitrile membrane (AN69) in which patients ($n = 31$) treated for 9.3 ± 0.2 hours/week are contrasted with a control group ($n = 31$) treated for 16.2 ± 0.3 hours/week with cuprophane. A significantly lower hospitalization rate and number of hospitalization days for dialysis related complications was achieved with the AN69 membrane in spite of carrying a higher pretreatment blood urea nitrogen concentration (1.16 ± 0.05 mmol/L for short treatment vs. 1.01 ± 0.03 mmol/L for conventional treatment). There are likely 2 mechanisms at work here, i.e. differences of complement activation (this will subsequently be discussed) and the augmentation of middle molecule clearances achieved with the PAN membrane. Von Albertini et al. [38] have clinically applied the bench study of Cheung et al. [39] in a small number of patients ($n = 18$) to deliberately exploit the relationship (therapeutic equivalency) of time and middle molecule removal. They have achieved an average of 2 hours in treatment 3 times per week for a year or more, using two modules of high flux membrane and flow rates that are nearly twice the common values (Figure 19.5). His patients have not shown the cardiovascular instability, considered limiting by most, for removal of excess body water (3.6 ± 1.2 L) in a 2 hour treatment time frame with hemodialysis. His rehabilitation rate for these patients was very high at $> 90\%$. This extraordinarily high flux treatment has shown the expected urea rebound that is predicted [16] when the limiting mass transfer resistance is the cell wall and not the dialysis membrane [15]. His modeling studies support a more than adequate status of clearance for not only urea but for the middle molecule index solute Inulin (5,200 daltons) as well.

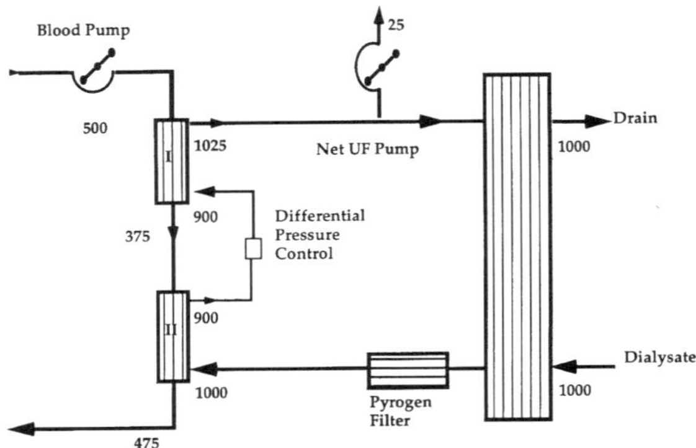

Fig. 19.5. Flow diagram and flow rates in mL/min for a hemodiafiltration circuit (von Albertini). A pair of high flux membranes is used in series with blood and dialysis fluid flowing in countercurrent manner. High flux membrane I is driven by the differential pressure controller and blood pump to ultrafilter from blood to dialysate in the amount of 125 mL/min. Sterile pyrogen free diluting fluid from the pyrogen filter and fluid cycling device is delivered to high flux membrane II and restores all but 25 mL/min of backfiltration to the blood path. Diffusive transport occurs in both membranes I and II.

At present the only safe recommendation for this form of treatment, as noted by Von Albertini, is to use a Kt/V urea of 1.2 as a minimum value. This will ensure that the mass of urea removed in spite of urea disequilibrium at high clearance rates is adequate and larger and/or more slowly diffusing solutes that are removed is comparable to, or greater than with conventional therapy [40].

An additional point of note, commented on above, may be drawn from the work of Gutierrtierez et al. [41, 42]. Their work implicates complement activation and cytokine release in the increase of catabolism noted by Borah et al. [43], and Farrell et al. [44], in response to hemodialysis. The extra catabolism that occurs on the days of dialysis with cuprophane results in a calculated urea generation rate that is approximately 20% higher than occurs on non dialysis days. As most high flux membranes are synthetic in formulation, e.g. polyacrylonitrile, polysulphone and polyamide and, as such, are complement kind, unlike cellulosic membranes that activate complement (cellulose triacetate is a notable exception being both high flux and complement kind), one may expect a lower metabolic need for treatment with these membranes.

Hemofiltration may be considered a limiting case of hemodiafiltration in which all solute transport is by convection. This technique clearly falls outside the study parameters of the NCDS and in so doing, provides some fascinating insights into the pathophysiology of uremia and has significant implications for treatment quality through membrane selection. The most substantial clinical experience with this technique may be found in the work of Quellhorst and colleagues [45]. They report on more than 100 patients maintained with post dilution hemofiltration with some having been treated for up to ten years. The majority of the study sample have been on treatment for over five years and, as such, may be satisfactorily compared with a comparable population of patients that he has followed on "routine" hemodialysis. Routine hemodialysis in this instance comprised 5 hours of hemodialysis thrice weekly, using 1.0 to 1.5 m^2 cuprophane membrane and conventional flow rates of blood (250–350 mL/min) and dialysis fluid (500 mL/min, and would likely result in an adequate Kt/V; although, neither this data nor protein intake are available in this report. The amount of hemofiltration given was calculated with the formula that one third of the total body water needed to be ultrafiltered at each treatment [45]. This would mean that a 70 kg man with 42 L of total body water would exchange 25 L of ultrafiltrate for diluting fluid, assuming a 2 L removal of excess body water. Urea clearance in post dilution hemofiltration equates to the volume of ultrafiltrate, i.e. in this example the total volume of plasma water cleared of urea would be 25 L. This, of course, provides a Kt/V for urea of only 0.6; a figure that by NCDS standards should produce major morbidity promptly. Figure 19.6 is a plot of mortality for these patients over the ten year follow up. This may be compared with similar mortality curves for his hemodialysis population and for that reported by the EDTA and French Dialysis Registries [44].

The patients in Figure 19.6 were randomly assigned to hemodialysis or hemofiltration and "poor risk" patients were excluded from the study, i.e. patients with "complications such as, diabetes mellitus, cancer, and systemic or severe cerebrovascular or cardiovascular disease" [45]. The message here is that quality assurance guidelines for treatment with hemodialysis cannot be mindlessly

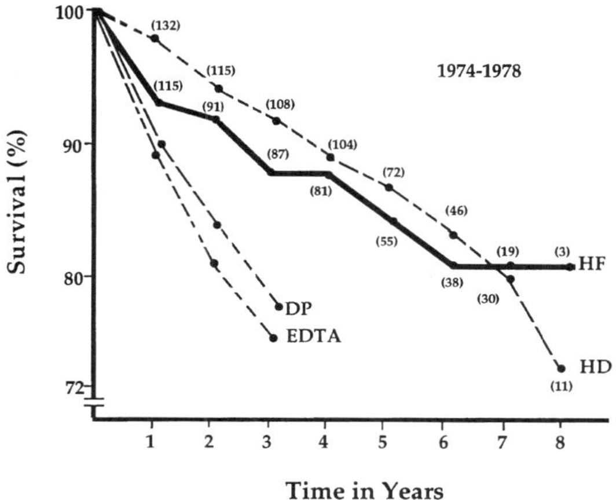

Fig. 19.6. Survival data for patients starting regular hemofiltration or hemodialysis treatment between 1974 and 1978. For comparison, data taken from both the EDTA and Diaphane registries for the same time period are shown. See text for further discussion.

applied to a therapy where the selection of a more hydraulically permeable membrane alters urea's surrogate status for uremic solute removal.

The peritoneal "membrane"

The vast majority of the literature regards the barrier to transport that divides body water and peritoneal dialysate as a semipermeable membrane. That is a pore-containing membrane that permits the ready passage of water and small solutes but restrains or blocks the passage of proteins and cell elements from entering the dialysate. Some models offer the ability to calculate mean pore radius/pore length as well as size distribution of pore radii, assuming that these pores are right circular cylinders that traverse the membrane [46]. Other writers describe serial resistances to transport each with its own physical and transport properties that sum to the earlier "unitary" description [47]. Even more recent writings offer a description of the functional properties of this barrier to transport not as a membrane at all but rather as a tissue with an "homogeneously distributed" blood vessel (this is a mathematical not a physical construct) which acts as a source for uremic solutes that find their way into the dialysate [48]. The discovery of aquaporins in the endothelium of the submesothelial capillaries of the peritoneal space lends physical reality to at least one of the three commonly construed pores in the 3-pore model [49]. While all of this work is fascinating and will permit a more incisive understanding about intimate transport mechanism, these mechanisms are not crucial to our understanding of the comparative properties on which to judge the treatment qualities offered by peritoneal dialysis. For simplicity, I shall cast what follows in terms of a simple semipermeable membrane that may be a serial or single transport resistance and/ or a homo or heteroporous structure as you would wish to conceive it.

The most glaringly inappropriate "leap of faith" in extrapolating NCDS results beyond the tested parameters occurs when the mathematics of variable volume single pool urea kinetic modeling as used in the NCDS are applied without modification to judge adequacy when the peritoneal membrane has been selected for use, i.e. chronic ambulatory peritoneal dialysis (CAPD). The NCDS used only cellulosic membrane with a range of membrane area between 1.2–2.5 m^2. An informed guess about the area of the peritoneal membrane that participates in solute and water transport (functional area) places it at less than 0.8 m^2 (i.e. 0.5–0.8 m^2) [50]. The degree of openness to diffusive solute transport between cellulosic and peritoneal membranes has been studied by several workers and the result of an early such study is shown in Figure 19.7 [51]. It is cast in terms of comparative mass transfer

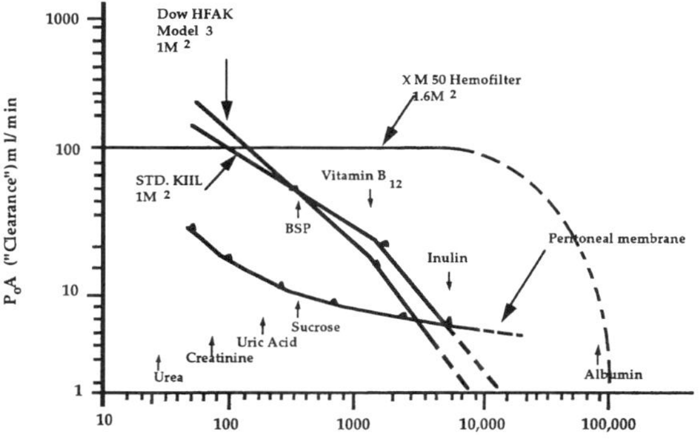

Fig. 19.7. Log plot of the permeability area product ("clearance") vs. solute molecular volume. See text for further discussion of clearance. Note the crossover point between the peritoneal membrane and the cellulosic membrane for solutes in the 5,600–6,000 dalton range.

area coefficients (P_oA) versus solute molecular weight for cellulosic dialyzers vs. the peritoneal membrane. Small solutes such as urea (< 60 d) that are swiftly diffusing are more sensitive to membrane area differences than are larger molecular weight species such as the test solute, inulin (5200 d), i.e. small solutes are more blood flow dependent than large ones when clearance is being examined. Hence, urea clearance for the peritoneal membrane falls well below that for cellulosic membrane. It is important to note that peritoneal clearance, as it is commonly measured and described, is different from the clearance term for the native kidney and that for the artificial kidney that operates by diffusion (hemodialysis) or for convective transfer (hemofiltration) or any combination of the two (hemodiafiltration) [6, 7, 52].

The common formula for peritoneal clearance is

$$\frac{D}{P} V/_t = C$$

where

C   = clearance (mL/min.)
D   = dialysate concentration (mg/dl)
P   = plasma water concentration (mg/dl)
V/t = volume (mL) of spent dialysate per exchange time in (minutes)

It has in the numerator a mass of solute (DV) that has been removed and is present in the spent dialysate over a given exchange time. (Note: Urea in the dialysate is directly measured and this is not subject to errors that occur in measuring hemodialysis clearance that result from problems of determining flow rates accurately or the presence of access recirculation.) The driving gradient for diffusion is the highest at the time when the dialysate concentration for urea is zero and progressively declines with time as equilibration between blood water and dialysate occurs (Figure 19.8). The clearance calculated with the common formula is a time averaged rate of clearance and as such will always be lower than the "instantaneous" clearance measured in a manner analogous to either the artificial or native kidney [6, 53]. The instantaneous clearance remains constant whenever measured during the course of treatment whereas peritoneal "minute to minute" clearance falls during the course of an exchange and this

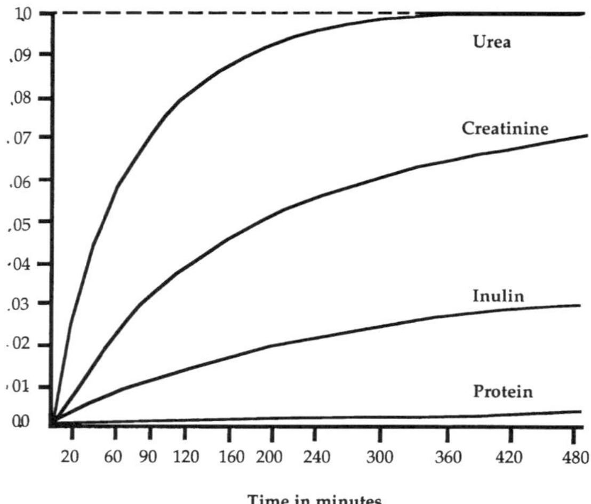

Fig. 19.8. Stylized curves for the equilibration ratio between dialysate and plasma plotted against time for a CAPD patient with average transport characteristics.

time averaged clearance falls as the exchange time is lengthened. An instructive limiting case is that for the swiftly equilibrating solute urea. With reference to Figure 19.8, for a patient with an average or high permeability peritoneal membrane, urea may well be at or near equilibrium in the last hour or two of a CAPD exchange, i.e. D/P = 1 for the final 60–120 minutes and the time averaged urea clearance drops swiftly as a result. Furthermore, no more mass is removed even through the equilibration of other solutes continues, thereby perturbing the relationship between urea clearance and the more slowly diffusing solutes for which it is surrogate.

For larger solutes the transport rate across the peritoneal membrane may be comparable to or higher than that for cellulosic membrane. It is the relationship or relative concentration that urea bares to other more toxic solutes that establishes its surrogate status. Furthermore, the NCDS employed a schedule of three times weekly treatment with each treatment ranging (by study group) from 3.0 to 4.5 hours (Table 19.1). CAPD is, of course, a continuously applied therapy. This having been said, I note for you that patients that are adequately treated on CAPD using criteria from the CANUSA Study have a measured Kt/V of 1.6–1.7 per week [8]. Dividing this by 3 to equate it to the amount of hemodialysis offered on a thrice weekly schedule identifies that CAPD at 0.5–0.6 is dramatically lower than i.e. half that required for adequate hemodialysis (1.0–1.2). (See Chapter entitled "Selection of Transport Parameters in Judging Membrane Performance" for a more detailed discussion of this discrepancy [7].)

Dr. Keshaviah emphasizes this point (i.e. the relevance of treatment application time [54]. Table 19.4 is taken from that publication and casts clearance in terms of liters per week for solutes of different molecular weight contrasting CAPD with two commonly used hemodialysis membranes. CAPD, because of its continuous nature, shows higher net weekly clearance for solutes as low in molecular weight as vitamin B_{12} when contrasted with 1.5 m^2 cuprophane (8 micron) applied for four hours, three times weekly.

Table 19.4. Weekly clearances of peritoneal and hemodialysis membranes (units = liters per week)

Solute	Mol. wt.	CAPD	Cuprophane (8 microns)	Cellulose triacetate (high flux)
Urea	60	64	119	139
Creatinine	113	57	96	126
Vitamin B_{12}	1,355	37	27	86
Inulin	5,200	17	14	51
β_2-Microglobulin	11,800	8	0	38

Cuprophane: CF 1511 (Baxter Healthcare Corporation), $Q_b/Q_d = 200/500$, 12 hours/week

Cellulose Triacetate: CT 190 (Baxter Healthcare Corporation), $Q_b/Q_d = 300/500$, 9 hours/week

At least four points of concern make it incorrect to extrapolate NCDS interpretations of urea kinetic modeling to CAPD:

- First, the impact of "saw tooth" chemistries versus steady state values has been commented on by Keshaviah et al. [54, 55]. The hypothesis that is currently being tested by these investigators states that uremic toxicity is more dependent on the predialysis peak chemistries than on trough or time average values and that CAPD with its steady state chemistries may well be exempt from some of the uremic toxicity (e.g. acidemia) that occurs intermittently in the he-

modialysis population undergoing thrice weekly treatment.

- Second, there are well understood kinetic principles that link duration of therapy with the removal of larger molecular weight solutes, i.e. time on treatment is surrogate for middle molecule removal [6, 14, 19]. With reference to Table 19.2, one notes that with the selection of the peritoneal membrane that is more open to the diffusive transport of larger solutes coupled with the continuous nature of the CAPD prescription that urea's surrogate status with regard certainly to the larger molecular weight toxins would be radically different than for hemodialysis, i.e. more middle molecules removed/gram of urea removed. I have noted previously the surprising lack of attention paid to this relationship in the published results of the NCDS. More recent analysis of data from the USRDS registry provides powerful evidence that short prescription time correlates with early mortality and likely offers one explanation of the higher death rate present in the U.S. dialysis population than that in Europe [2, 20].

- Third, as stated above, for a patient with a reasonably permeable peritoneal membrane, one may well see that the dialysate to plasma concentration ratio for urea may achieve a value of unity for the last hour or two of a six hour dwell time, i.e. no more movement of urea from blood water to dialysate. This equilibration of urea does not preclude the continued loss into the dialysate of other less swiftly diffusing toxic solutes. Again, the surrogate status that urea holds for more toxic solutes of slower diffusivity is abrogated by this event.

- Fourth, as previously noted, for non complement activating synthetic membranes, the choice of the peritoneal membrane for treatment exempts the patient from a thrice weekly activation of complement with it's release of the powerful inflammatory mediators, interleukin-1 and tumor necrosis factor which appears to result in a burst of protein catabolism with hemodialysis that is not present with CAPD [43, 44]. Recent work by the Bergstrom Group [56] points out further that the relationship for CAPD between protein catabolic rate (plotted on the axis) and Kt/V urea (on the ordinate) showed a markedly steeper slope than that for hemodialysis. This is interpreted to show that increasing dialysis dose, as measured by Kt/V urea has a "more salutory" effect on appetite in peritoneal dialysis than in hemodialysis. The recent identification of appetite-suppressing middle molecules supports this interpretation [21].

There are some common features between CAPD and hemofiltration that are instructive and may explain a clinically satisfactory outcome for both modalities at remarkably low Kt/V values:

- Both employ a complement kind membrane and hence a reduced catabolism of protein on dialysis days.

- Both have a disproportionately high clearance of middle molecules when compared with urea.

- Both techniques are conducted using only sterile pyrogen free solutions – unlike routine hemodialysis.

- Both techniques show less reduction in residual renal function over time [45, 57].

There are interesting points of difference that will require further study before fully understanding their implications:

- Hemofiltration shares with hemodialysis the common saw-toothed pattern of chemistries and fluid overload that is the "hallmark" of a three times weekly treatment schedule as contrasted with CAPD. This would argue against the peak/valley hypothesis of Keshaviah et al. [6, 55].

- Hemofiltration membranes are usually noncellulosic. The two in common use (polyacrylonitrile and polysulphone) are active adsorbers of plasma constituents, unlike the peritoneal membrane.

- Protein (5–15 gram/day) is lost in significant continuing quantities in CAPD but not hemofiltration or hemodialysis.

CLEARANCE VS. MASS REMOVED

I have a technical concern about the limitation of the clearance concept as a preferred measurement parameter for characterizing the clinical performance of a dialysis membrane [8, 52]. This concern was partially explored in relation to peritoneal dialysis in the prior section.

I again note for you that clearance for hemodialysis was designed algebraically to be constant, i.e. not change with a changing concentration of solute in the plasma water. A.V. Wolf et al. [58] by mimicking Homer Smith [59] in this trait for the equation describing clearance in hemodialysis, permitted an "apples to apples" kind of comparison for the clinician between, the then familiar native kidney performance and that of the new artificial kidney. This was useful. The disservice that results from the use of clearance, today, is that it obscures the (clinically critical) rate and/or quantity of mass removed. Take, for example, the high clearance rates for urea (500–600 mL/min) that result from high flux hemodiafiltration as practiced by von Albertini et al. [40]. While the calculated clearance is constant for the entire length of the procedure, the mass of urea removed per minute declines sharply due to the rapid fall in BUN with time. This fall is accentuated by the limited availability of intracellular urea (as previously commented upon). Said another way, the apparent distribution volume for urea is considerably less than the total body water. This, then would mean an artifactually low volume of distribution (V) for urea as computed by urea kinetic modeling.[3] As clearance (K) is not reflective of changing plasma levels, the Kt/V ratio will be artifactually high. What we really wish to track from the adequacy perspective of the NCDS, is the actual amount of urea that is removed by a given treatment. For example, a device that continuously measured the concentration of urea in the effluent stream of the dialysate could be used to provide the clinician with a minute to minute amount of urea removed. The amount (mass) of urea present pretreatment, is reasonably well determined by using a nomogram derived space of distribution for urea and the product of this volume and the pretreatment BUN unless the subject is grossly malnourished. One may then examine what fraction of urea mass is removed (FR urea) rather than

Kt/V urea. Keshaviah and Star have recently explored this approach [60], giving us the solute removal index (SRI).

$$SRI = \frac{\text{Urea mass removed}}{\text{Body content of urea pretreatment}} \times 100$$

It is easier for me to develop my clinical intuition around the fraction of solute removed than it is to have any "gestalt" about Kt/V [6, 52].

QUALITY ASSURANCE PRINCIPLES

Use of Synthetic Membrane

From the above discussion it is apparent that one may not isolate selection of the membrane from the other components of the treatment prescription when examining the quality of therapy rendered. At present we have no hard prospectively collected data from an interventional study on the comparative importance of:

A. The two physician variable components of the treatment prescription, namely, treatment time and the elements comprising artificial kidney clearance rate (i.e. membrane area, and permeability, the flow rates of blood and dialysate, and the respective components of convection and diffusion) and

B. Removal of the two broad solute domains, i.e. conventional size (<500 d) or middle molecule (>500 d and $<60,000$ d) size, which are affected differently, depending upon the choice of membrane and technique.

One may only guide patient therapy by offering, at minimum, the amount of therapy given by the best treatment group of the NCDS. This is not to say that more treatment might not be desirable. Urea kinetic modeling coupled with an understanding of the influence of treatment time on solute clearance profile is required in order to know when this minimum is achieved. Where uncertainty exists for a given prescription about middle molecule clearance it is well to kinetically model the results or better to make actual mea-

surements of a test solute such as inulin or vitamin B_{12} in order to resolve that uncertainty.

One may approach urea kinetic modeling for hemodialysis using any of a number of simplifications of the original approach that vary more in style than substance. Remember that only the single pool variable volume model employed in the NCDS has been clinically qualified as correlating with morbid and mortal outcome. Double pool models, while physiologically more attractive, have not been shown to correlate more closely with outcome. Not all patients will need to be modeled as empirical wisdom about average patients requiring an average prescription is quite strong. It is only where significant variations in patient parameters of height, weight protein catabolic rate or the treatment parameters that determine clearance, that is, A and B above, that depart from the common experience that formal modeling will be required to assure the delivery of an high quality treatment.

Use of the peritoneal membrane
With the publication of the Multicenter US Canadian Study [8], there are now clinically qualified guidelines for therapy adequacy using the peritoneal membrane involving both Kt/V urea, net weekly clearance of creatinine and nutritional parameters such as plasma albumin and global clinical assessment of nutritional status. It should be noted that the concerns about disequilibrium across cell walls (number of pools) drops away for CAPD due to the steady state chemistries. In addition, recent work by Villano and Amin have customized these criteria using data on peritoneal membrane transport characteristics as characterized by conventional testing as well as body mass and gender [61]. It is apparent that detailed individualization of therapy is important to successful outcome and that modulation upwards of the amount of therapy rendered is crucial as residual renal function declines. Large body mass in slow transport characteristics, coupled with male gender, may render a small percentage of patients unable to be adequately treated using the peritoneal membrane. This must be factored in by the physician in choosing the appropriate membrane for treatment.

NOTES

[1] Clinical assessment such as changes of lean body mass, subjective well being, complication rate and the like, coupled with serial measurement of blood urea nitrogen, creatinine, calcium phosphate, CO_2 content, plasma proteins, hemoglobin, etc. are still more commonly used to assess treatment adequacy worldwide than is urea kinetic modeling. The quality of treatment rendered using these parameters is sufficiently high to make subtle distinctions in quality impossible to detect at the clinical level simply because the number of study subjects required to show significant trends likely exceeds that available to even the director of a large clinic. I note, for your persuasion to this point, the surprise engendered in the U.S. dialysis community in 1984 by the identification of a substantially increased mortality rate in the U.S. dialysis patient population as contrasted with those of Europe and Japan when national population bases were examined [2, 3].

[2] It should be noted that since completion of the NCDS, technical advances have permitted the reduction by 50% in membrane thickness of hollow fibers made of cuprophane. This translates into a near doubling of small solute transport.

[3] The popular use of 58–60% of body weight in kg or normogram values involving height, weight, sex, to compute total body water will obviate this problem but has problems of its own. A malnourished patient will be assigned a lower body water volume and hence make his calculated Kt/V artifactually high.

REFERENCES

1. National Cooperative Dialysis Study. Kidney Int 1983; 23(13).
2. Held PJ, Brunner F, Odaka M, Garcia J, Port FK and Gaylin DS. Five year survival for end stage renal disease patients in the U.S., Europe and Japan, 1982–1987. Am J Kidney Dis 1990; 15:451–7.
3. Hull AR and Parker TF, editors Proceedings from the morbidity, mortality and prescription of dialysis symposium, Sept 15–17, 1989, Dallas. Am J Kidney Dis 1990; 15:5.
4. Gotch FA and Sargent JA. A mechanistic analysis of the National Cooperative Dialysis Study. Kidney Int 1985; 28:526–34.
5. DOQI Clinical Practice Guidelines. Am J Kidney Dis 1997; 30:3(2).
6. Henderson LW, Leypoldt JK, Lysaght MJ and Cheung AK. Death on dialysis and the time/flux trade-off. Blood Purif 1997; 15:1–14.
7. Henderson LW. Selection of transport parameters in judging membrane performance. In Henderson LW and Thuma RS, editors. Quality assurance in dialysis, vol 2. Dordrecht, Kluwer Academic Publishers, 1998; 20.
8. Churchill DN, Taylor W and Keshaviah PR. Adequacy of dialysis and nutrition in continuous peritoneal dialysis: association with clinical outcomes. J Am Soc Nephrol 1996; 7:198–207.
9. Johnson WJ, Hagge WW, Wagoner RD, Dinapoli RP and Rosevear JW. Effects of urea loading in patients with far advanced renal failure. Mayo Clinic Proc 1972; 47:21–9.
10. Gorevic PD, Casey TT, Stone WJ, DiRiaimondo CR, Presli FC and Fragione B. Beta-2 microglobulin is an amyloidogenic protein in man. J Clin Invest 1985; 76:2425–9.
11. Hörl WH, Haag-Weber M, Georgopoulos A and Block LH. Physicochemical characterization of a polypeptide present in uremic serum that inhibits the activity of polymorphonuclear cells. Proc Natl Acad Sci 1990; 87:6353–7.
12. Bergstrom J, Furst P and Zimmerman L. Uremic middle molecules exist and are biologically active. Clin Nephrol 1979; 11:229–38.
13. Henderson LW. Of time, TAC_{urea} and treatment schedules. Kidney Int 1988; 24: S105–6.
14. Leypoldt JK, Cheung AK, Carroll CE, Stannard D, Pereira B, Agadoa L et al. Removal of middle molecules enhances survival in hemodialysis (HD) patients. Am J Kid Dis (in press).
15. Frost TH and Kerr DNS. Kinetics of hemodialysis: a theoretical study of the removal of solutes in chronic renal failure compared to normal health. Kidney Int 1977; 12:41–50.
16. Miller JH, von Albertini B, Gardiner PW and Shinaberger JH. Technical aspects of high-flux hemodiafiltration for adequate short (under 2 hours) treatment. Trans Am Soc for Art Int Organs 1984; 30:377–81.
17. Laird NM, Berkey CS and Lowrie EG. Modeling success or failure of dialysis therapy: The National Cooperative Dialysis Study. Kidney Int 1983; 13:S101–6.
18. Lowrie EG and Lew NL. Death risk in hemodialysis patients: The predictive value of commonly measured variables and an evaluation of death-rate differences betwen facilities. Am J Kidney Dis 1990; 15:458–82.
19. Held PJ, Levin NW, Bovbjerg RR, Pauly MV and Diamond LH. Mortality and duration of hemodialysis treatment. JAMA 1992; 265:871–5.
20. Held PJ, Blagg CR, Liska DW, Port FK, Hakim R and Levin N. The dose of hemodialysis according to dialysis prescription in Europe and the United States. Kidney Int 1992; 42:S16–21.
21. Anderstam B, Mamoun A-H, Södersten P and Bergström J. Middle-sized molecule fractions isolated from uremic ultrafiltrate and normal urine inhibit ingestive behavior in the rat. J Am Soc Nephrol 1996; 7:2453–60.
22. Shinzato T, Nakai S, Akiba T, Yamazaki C, Sasaki R, Kitaoka T et al. Survival in long-term haemodialysis patients: results from the annual survey of the Japenese Society for Dialysis Therapy. Nephrol Dial Transplant 1997;12:885–8.
23. Maeda et al. Personal communication 1997.
24. Babb AL, Popovich RP, Christopher TG and Scribner BH. The genesis of the square meter hour hypothesis. Trans Am Soc for Artif Int Organs 1971; 17:81–91.
25. Henderson LW and Clark W. Modeling and the middle molecule. Semin Dial 1998; 11:228–30.
26. Teehan BP, Schleifer CR, Brown JM, Sigler MH and Raimondo J. Urea Kinetic analysis and clinical outcome on CAPD. A five year longitudinal study. Adv in PD 1990; 6:181–5.
27. Lindsay RM and Spanner E. A hypothesis: the protein catabolic rate is dependent upon the type and amount of

treatment in dialyzed uremic patients. Am J Kidney Dis1989; 13:382–9.

28. Lindsay RM, Spanner E, Heidenheim RP, LeFebvre JM, Hodsman A, Baird J et al. Which comes first Kt/V or PCR – chicken or egg. Kidney Int 1992; 42:S32–6.

29. Young A, Kopple J, Lindholm G, Vonesh E et al. Nutritional assessment of CAPD patients: an international study. Am J Kidney Dis 1991; 17:462–71.

30. Held PJ, Port FK, Gaylin DS, Wolfe RA, Levin NW, Blagg CR et al. Evaluation of initial predictors of mortality among 4387 new ESRD patients: the USRDS case mix study. (abstract) JASN 1991; 2:328.

31. Considine RV, Beckie M, Dunn SR, Weisberg LS, Brenda RC, Kurnik P et al. Plasma leptin is partly cleared by the kidney and is elevated in hemodialysis patients. Kidney Int 1997; 51:1980–5.

32. Coyne E, Marabet S, Dagogo-Jack S, Klein S, Santiago JV, Hmiel SP et al. Increased leptin concentration in hemodialysis (HD) patients (abstract) JASN 1996; A1908.

33. Sharma K, Michael B, Dunn S, Weisberg L, Kurnik B, Kurnik P et al. Plasma leptin is cleared by the kidney and is markedly elevated in hemodialysis patients. (abstract) JASN 1996; A3085.

34. Collins A, Liao M, Umen A, Hanson G and Keshaviah P. High efficiency bicarbonate hemodialysis has a lower risk of death in standard acetate dialysis. J Am Soc Nephrol 1991; 2:318.

35. Collins A, Liao M, Umen A, Hanson G and Keshaviah P. Diabetic hemodialysis patients treated with a high Kt/V have a lower risk of death than standard Kt/V. J Am Soc Nephrol 1991; 2:318.

36. Clark WR, Leypoldt JK, Henderson LW, Sowinski KM, Scott MK, Mueller BA et al. Effect of changes in dialytic frequency duration and flow rates on solute kinetics and effective clearances. JASN 1998; in press.

37. Channard J, Brunois JP, Melin JP, Lavaud S and Toupance O. Long term results of dialysis therapy with a highly permeable membrane. Artif Organs 1982; 6:261–6.

38. von Albertini B, Barlee V and Bosch JP. High flux hemodialfiltration: Long term results. (abstract). J Am Soc Nephrol 1991; 2:354.

39. Cheung AC, Kato Y, Leypoldt JK and Henderson LW. Hemodiafiltration using a hybrid membrane system for self-generation of diluting fluid. Trans Am Soc for Art Int Organs 1982; 28:61–5.

40. von Albertini B. High-efficiency hemodialysis: an overview. Contrib to Nephrology 1988; 61:37–45.

41. Gutierrez A, Alvestrand A, Wahren J and Bergstrom J. Effective in vivo contact between blood and dialysis membranes on protein catabolism in humans. Kidney Int 1990; 38:487–94.

42. Gutierrez A, Alvestrand A and Bergstrom J. Membrane selection and muscle protein catabolism. Kidney Int 1992; 42:S86-90.

43. Borah MF, Shoenfeld P, Gotch FA, Sargent JA, Wolfsom M and Humphreys MH. Nitrogen balance during intermittent dialysis therapy of uremia. Kidney Int 1978;14:491–500.

44. Farrell PC and Hone PW. Dialysis induced catabolism. Am J Clin Nutr 1980; 33:1417–22.

45. Quellhorst E. Long-term survival. In Henderson LW, Quellhorst EA, Baldamus CA and Lysaght MJ, editors. Hemofiltration. Berlin, Springer-Verlag, 1986; 221.

46. Rippe B and Stelin G. Simulations of peritoneal solute transport during CAPD. Application of the two-pore formalism. Kidney Int 1989; 35:1234–44.

47. Nolph KD and Twardowski Z. The peritoneal dialysis system. In Nolph KD, editor. Peritoneal dialysis, 3rd edition. Dordrecht, Kluwer Academic Publishers, 1989; 13–27.

48. Dedrick RL, Flessner MF, Collins JM and Schultz JS. Is the peritoneum a membrane? Am Soc Artif Ini Organs 1982; 5:1–8.

49. Pannekeet MM, Mulder JB, Weening JJ, Struijk DG, Zweers MM and Krediet RT. Demonstration of aquaporin-chip in peritoneal tissue of uremic and CAPD patients. Proceedings VIIth Congress ISPD, June 18–21, Stockholm. Perit Dial Bull 1995; 16:S54–57.

50. Henderson LW. The problem of peritoneal area and permeability. Kidney Int 1973; 3:409–10.

51. Babb AL, Johansen PJ, Strand MJ, Tenckhoff H and Scribner BH. Bi-directional permeability of the human peritoneum to middle molecules. Proceedings of the European Dialysis and Transplantation Association 1973; 10:247–62.

52. Henderson LW. Why do we use clearance. Blood Purif 1995; 13:283–8.

53. Henderson LW and Nolph KD. Altered permeability of the peritoneal membrane after using hypertonic peritoneal dialysis fluid. J Clin Invest 1969; 48:992–1001.

54. Keshaviah P. Urea kinetic and middle molecule approaches to assessing the adequacy of hemodialysis and CAPD. Kidney Int 1992; 43:S28–38.

55. Keshaviah PR, Nolph KD and VanStone JC. The peak concentration hypothesis: a urea kinetic approach to comparing the adequacy of continuous ambulatory peritoneal dialysis and hemodialysis. Perit Dial Bull 1989; 9:257–60.

56. Bergstrom J, Alvestrand B, Lindholm B, and Tranaeus A. Relationship between Kt/V and protein catabolic rate (PCR) is different in continuous peritoneal dialysis (CPD) and haemodialysis (HD) patients. JASN 1991; 2:358 (abstract).

57. Lysaght MJ, Vonesh E, Gotch F, Ibels L, Keen M, Lindholm B et al. The influence of dialysis treatment modality on the decline of remaining renal function. Trans Am Soc Artif Intern Organs 1991; 27:598–604.

58. Wolf AV, Remp DG, Kiley JE and Currie GD. Artificial kidney function: kinetics of hemodialysis. J Clin Invest 1951; 30:1062–70.

59. Smith HW. Principles of renal physiology. New York, Oxford University Press, 1956; 25–35.

60. Keshaviah PR and Star RA. A new approach to diaysis quantification: an adequacy index based on solute removal. Semin Dial 1994; 7:85–90.

61. Villano R and Amin N. Assigning severity indices to outcome. Quality Assurance in Dialysis, vol 2, 1998.

20. Selection of transport parameters in judging membrane performance

LEE W. HENDERSON

SYMBOLS

C = concentration. $\overline{\mathrm{C}}$ = average concentration (mg/mL); D/P = ratio of solute concentration in peritoneal dialysate/plasma; K = clearance (mL/min); Q = flow rate. $\overline{\mathrm{Q}}$ = average flow rate (mL/min); S = sieving coefficient; UV = rate of solute delivery in the urine (mg/min); V/t = flow rate of effluent peritoneal dialysate (mL/min); t = time (min)

SUBSCRIPTS

B = blood; D = dialysate; DF = diluting fluid; F = ultrafiltrate; i = inflow; o = outflow; HD = hemodialysis; PD = peritoneal dialysis; HF = post dilution hemofiltration; PW = plasma water

INTRODUCTION

The measurement of solute clearance has historical roots for the nephrologist and has contributed materially to the quantitative understanding of the performance of the native kidney in both glomerular and tubular function [1]. The logic then of designing an analogous term for use with the artificial kidney was persuasive for A.V. Wolf et al. [2]. While initially helpful the interpretation of artificial kidney clearance has become overly complex as a result of the proliferation of artificial kidney techniques with subsequent "customization" of the clearance term for the new techniques. This has led to confusion and conceptual errors in intermodality comparisons of performance and outcome when clearance based terms like Kt/V urea are used to quantitate the amount of therapy rendered [3].

What follows is a setting down of the basic definitions of clearance (emphasizing the conceptual rather than the mathematical) for the various modalities of renal replacement therapy with a critical comparison of these definitions and how they differ from each other and from that for the native kidney. It will become apparent that we are not well served by the clearance term either in quantification of transport or in clarity of understanding of transport mechanisms. New methodology for extracorporeal artificial kidney techniques makes direct quantification of solute removed from blood an easy reality in a way that has not here-to-fore been the case (see for example, Depner et al. [4]). The direct measurement of mass transport derived from direct quantification is already the common method for computing clearance by peritoneal dialysis [3]. Putting clearance on a direct quantification basis for all other renal replacement modalities while correcting the conceptual errors in intermodality comparisons does not offer the conceptual clarity that using fractional solute removal would provide. Abandoning clearance and using fractional solute removal should be our goal.

DEFINITIONS OF CLEARANCE

Hemodialysis

For single pass hemodialysis where dialysate "sees" the membrane, but once the calculation of clearance for the hemodialyzer (by design) is totally analogous to that for the native kidney:

$$\text{Native renal clearance} = \text{UV/P} \qquad (1)$$

L.W. Henderson and R.S. Thuma (eds.), Quality Assurance in Dialysis, 2nd Edition, 215–222.
© 1999 *Kluwer Academic Publishers. Printed in Great Britain*

the mass of solute appearing in the urine/minute (UV) divided by the plasma concentration (P) of solute.[1] For hemodialysis, (with reference to Figures 20.1 and 20.2) the calculation would be:

$$\text{Dialyzer solute clearance} = K_{HD}\ \frac{(C_{Do}-C_{Di})Q_D}{C_{Bi}} \quad (2)$$

That is, the mass of solute arriving in the dialysate per minute (outflow–inflow concentration X dialysate flow rate) divided by the inflowing plasma concentration of solute (C_{Bi} or P in the classical formulation for the native kidney). While these calculations are the same, the interpretation of the resulting clearance number is not. Note for starters that one of the constraints for a valid native kidney clearance measurement is that of a steady state plasma level during the urine collection period. Stability of plasma concentration renders the calculated clearance insensitive to the length of time over which urine is collected. The mass of solute removed per minute over time is also constant. This constraint is violated during hemodialysis where there is a rapid fall in plasma level for small solutes like urea, creatinine, uric acid, etc. Does this then mean that the clearance at the

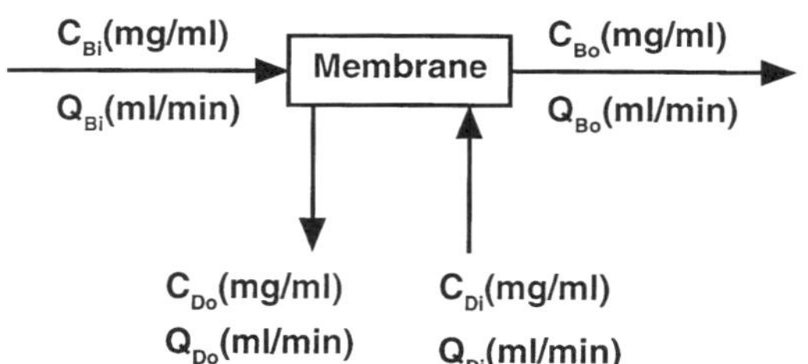

Fig. 20.1. Hemodialysis symbols.

$$K_{HD} = \frac{Q_B\ (C_{Bi}-C_{Bo})}{C_{Bi}^{*}} = \frac{Q_D(C_{Do}-C_{Di})}{C_{Bi}^{*}}$$

Unit analysis

$$K_{HD}\ (\text{ml/min}) = \frac{(\text{ml/min})\ (\text{mg/ml})}{\text{mg/ml}} = \frac{\text{mg/min}}{\text{mg/ml}} = \frac{\text{Removal rate}}{\text{Driving gradient}}$$

$$* K_{Blood} > K_{Plasma} > K_{Plasma\ water}$$

Fig. 20.2. Urea clearance for hemodialysis (K_{HD}) (ultrafiltration rate = 0).

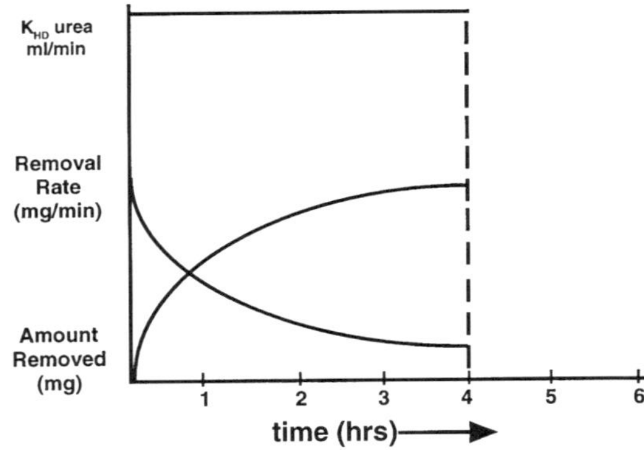

Fig. 20.3. Single pass hemodialysis ($Q_f = 0$).

beginning of a dialysis is higher than that at the end? No, it does not. The arithmetic of ratios, i.e. the concentration of solute arriving in the dialysate divided by the plasma solute concentration remains constant even as the driving concentration gradient is rapidly falling with the removal of the cleared solute in question. This characteristic of dialyzer clearance masks the falling rate of mass removed as time on treatment passes (as shown in Figure 20.3). To interpret clearance as it describes clinical result for the artificial kidney then requires the clinician to employ an empirical body of experience that gives her or him the expected reduction in body content (usually carried forward only as far as to estimate the change in plasma concentration) that may be expected for a given treatment time in a patient with the physical characteristics of the individual studied. As arti-physiologists we need to know more than Homer Smith [1] did when he measured inulin clearance. Smith simply wanted to determine the performance of the glomeruli, i.e. the glomerular filtration rate (GFR) in milliliters per minute. That is not our need. We presumably already have this performance number from the supplier of the dialyzer for several relevant solutes. What we need to know is what derives from the artificial kidney 'GFR', i.e. the amount (number of milligrams) of toxic solute removed during the course of a dialysis. The GFR is in quotes here because, of course, it is not a filtration but rather a diffusive process that we are dealing with during conventional hemodialysis.

Clearance by the native kidney for a solute that is neither secreted nor reabsorbed by the tubule, nor restrained by the glomerular basement membrane, does, in point of fact, equate to GFR. Is loss across the glomerular membrane dependent on molecular weight or size (or charge)? Certainly the clearance of creatinine (113 daltons) is the same[2] as that of inulin (5,200 daltons) and even β_2-microglobulin (11,800 daltons) is not restrained by the glomerular membrane. Were it not for proximal tubular reabsorption, this latter solute would serve as an excellent endogenous measure of GFR as well. Clearly then, transport by filtration is not size discriminatory unless the pores of the filtering membrane impinge on and restrain movement of the solute in question. A creatinine clearance for the native kidney of 100 mL/min, then, does not equate in terms of clinical implication to 100 mL/min of creatinine clearance for a cuprophane hemodialyzer where inulin may be cleared simultaneously at the rate of 10–15 mL/min and β_2-microglobulin not at all. Another point of difference stems from the convective nature of glomerular filtrate formation. For solutes that are not restrained by the glomerular basement membrane, there is no change in plasma water solute concentration from one end of the glomerular capillary to the other. This is, of course, not true for the diffusive process across the dialyzer membrane where there is an exponential decline in concentration from afferent to efferent ends. If a small swiftly diffusing solute like urea is exhausted from the blood part way down the blood path we refer to urea clearance as blood flow limited because it equates to blood flow rate through the dialyzer. As blood flow rate is increased, the clearance for urea plotted against blood flow rate reaches a plateau where further increases in flow rate do not result in an increase in clearance, i.e. membrane-limited conditions. These familiar artiphysiological concepts have no analog for solute transport in the native kidney.

There is little ambiguity as to what solute concentration should be placed in the denominator of the native kidney clearance equation as there is little or no change in plasma water concentration over the time of urine collection or from afferent to efferent end of the glomerular capillary.[3] For the 'instantaneous' nature (all samples are commonly drawn almost simultaneously) of artificial kidney clearance with the solute concentration falling (not only along the course of the blood path but during the course of treatment) there are several logical choices: 1) the arterial concentration as blood is about to enter the dialyzer or, 2) the log mean value of the inflowing and outflowing plasma concentrations or the log mean value of the pre to post treatment values. The latter two will provide information that is more closely related to the mass transport accomplished during treatment. The former which is commonly used will underestimate the transport work accomplished. The degree of underestimation will vary proportionally with the fall in solute concentration per unit length of blood path. The judgment algorithm (gestalt) used by the clinician to estimate the outcome of selecting a dialysis prescription (clearance rate and time) adjusts for this disparity as it is built on serial observations of solute concentration change as a result of treatment when this prescription is used for patients with body characteristics analogous to that of the prescriptee.

Lastly, Descombes et al. [6] describe a difference in transport properties of the uremic red cell when contrasted with the non uremic control erythrocyte. The slower transport of creatinine across the red cell membrane would make little difference in the measurement of native kidney clearance where there is little afferent-to-efferent change in plasma water concentration of creatinine and, hence, no cell membrane constraint on the availability of solute for removal. This is unlike the dialyzer circumstance where the overall limiting resistance to transport may, for a large-area thin membrane dialyzer, lie at the cell membrane both of the erythron and the somatic cell. This, again, points up the difference in native kidney clearance that requires a steady state concentration of solute in blood during the clearance interval. Said another way, at steady state, there is no need to worry about the number of compartments into which the solute is distributed within the body, unlike the very real concern about "disequilibrium" and "rebound" that accompanies treatment with hemodialysis.

Peritoneal Dialysis

The calculation of peritoneal clearance K_{PD} is quite analogous to that for the native kidney. With reference to Figures 20.4 and 20.5, the mass of solute arriving in the dialysate per minute divided by the plasma concentration equals the plasma clearance:

$$\text{Plasma clearance} = K_{PD} = \frac{D}{P} \, V/t \qquad (3)$$

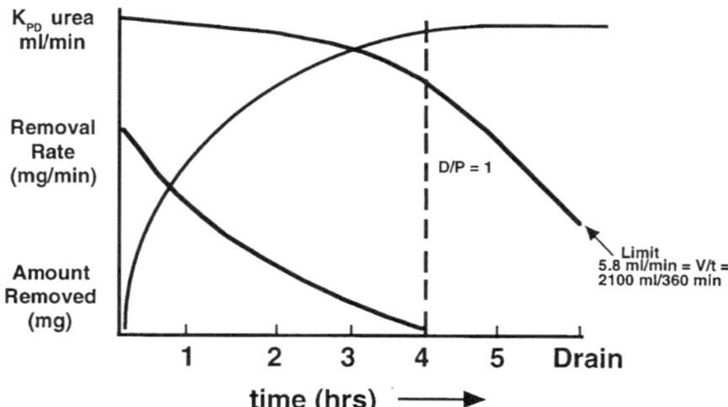

$$K_{PD} = \frac{D}{P} \, V/t = \frac{\overline{C}_{Do} \, \overline{Q}_{D}}{C_{Bi}}$$

Fig. 20.4. CAPD symbols.

$$K_{PD} = \frac{D}{P} \, V/t = \frac{\overline{C}_{Do} \, \overline{Q}_{D}}{C_{Bi}}$$

Unit analysis

$$K_{PD} \, (\text{ml/min}) = \frac{(\text{mg/ml})\,(\text{ml/min})}{\text{mg/ml}} = \frac{\text{mg/min}}{\text{mg/ml}} = \frac{\text{Removal rate}}{\text{Driving gradient}}$$

However, measurements made at time of drain (t = 360 min)

Fig. 20.5. Urea clearance for CAPD (K_{PD}) (ultrafiltration rate = 0).

Fig. 20.6. Isotonic CAPD exchange (volume = 2,100 mL, $Q_F = 0$).

The interpretation of the number is quite different however. Unlike the native kidney clearance and unlike that for hemodialysis, the peritoneal clearance is a time averaged clearance. The solute that arrives in the dialysate over the time interval of the exchange, i.e. 6 hours for continuous ambulatory peritoneal dialysis (CAPD), is computed in the above equation as an average rate of arrival in milligrams per minute; that is, the solute concentration in the spent dialysate is measured in an aliquot of the drained volume at the conclusion of the exchange. This average rate of arrival is reflective of both time elapsed and deterioration of the driving gradient for transport. Take urea for instance: (with reference to Figure 20.6) the rate of urea movement across the membrane at the instant of infusion of a CAPD exchange is the most rapid, and for a patient with a relatively normal or high membrane permeability may be expected to taper off and be in equilibrium with the urea concentration in the plasma water for the last portion of the 6 hour dwell time, i.e. no net mass transport occurring at all during this last 1–2 hours. In plotting the clearance rate per minute over time for urea, or for that matter any solute, we see a fall in rate as the solute gradient is rapidly discharging. The mass (amount) of solute removed (as with the artificial kidney) is, however, on the rise. Unlike the artificial or native kidneys the diffusion gradient falls towards equilibrium and the increasing time factor in the denominator takes its toll on this time averaged clearance which falls even though net solute (mass) removed continues to rise. This points up another difference between the blood-cleansing performance of peritoneal dialysis, hemodialysis, and the native kidney. For the native kidney the relationship of the clearance of one solute to another with widely differing size (creatinine vs. inulin) will remain constant over time as will the mass transport rate for all solutes that at constant plasma levels pass the glomerular basement membrane unstrained. For dialysis there will be a change in the spectrum of solute removed over time, such that small solute mass removed falls more sharply over time than that of larger solutes (see Figure 20.7). Take the extreme case of CAPD for example. The dialysate to plasma ratio for urea may approach unity at 4 hours, whereas, that for uric acid or β_2-microglobulin would remain less than 1 and their rate of

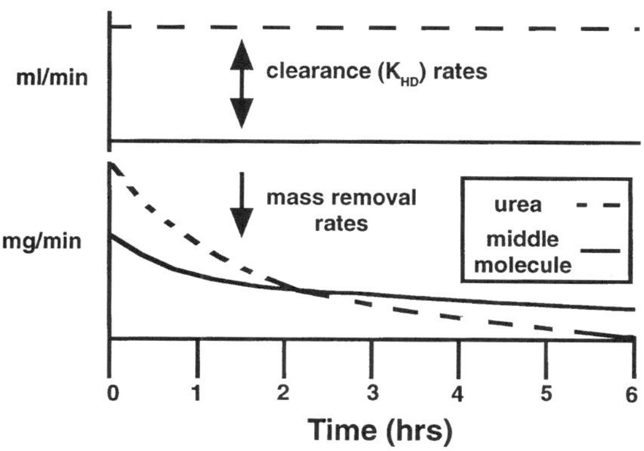

Fig. 20.7. Treatment time as surrogage for middle molecule removal.

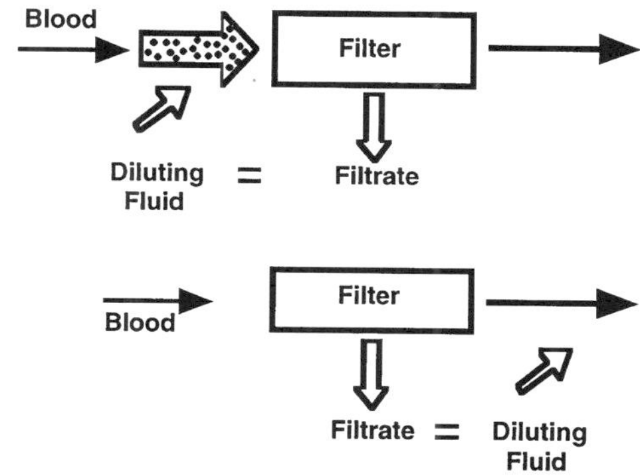

Fig. 20.8. Predilution/post dilution.

mass removed (unlike their clearance) will exceed that of urea in the remaining 2 hours of the exchange. A comparable example for hemodialysis may be seen in the work from Tassin where 8 hour dialysis, three times weekly, is the routine prescription. The clinical correlation between a clearance based parameter (Kt/V) and morbid/mortal outcome, which for 3–4 hours treatment time has shown powerful clinical correlation, drops away [7]. In the light of the above comments, this should not come as a surprise. Clearance, in masking these time-related changes in relative mass removed, set the stage for the square meter hour/ middle molecule 'discovery' which would not have been newsworthy, had mass removal been the means of the day for measuring dialysis performance.

Hemofiltration

This purely convective form of artificial kidney treatment may be conducted in pre or post dilution mode (see Figure 20.8). I will confine myself to a discussion of the post dilution mode for conceptual clarity. With reference to Figures 20.9 and 20.10, clearance defined for post dilution hemofiltration (K_{HF}) for a solute such as urea that traverses the filtration membrane unimpeded, i.e. with a sieving coefficient of one, is quite simple. It equates to the ultrafiltration rate (Q_F) [5].

K_{HF} may be considered to be an instantaneous value analogous in physical connotation to the calculation for K_{HD} (note the identity of Figures

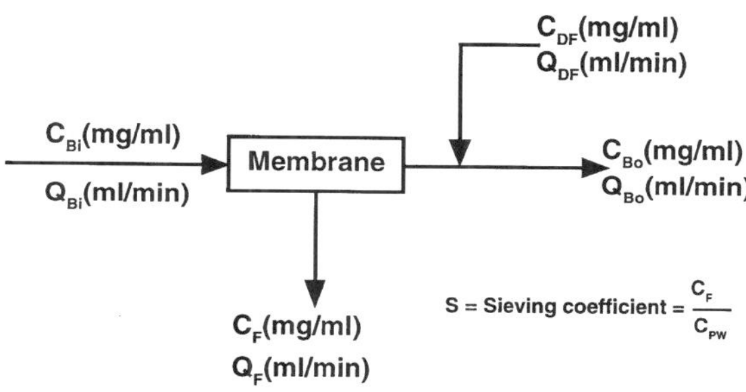

Fig. 20.9. Post dilution hemofiltration symbols.

$$K_{HF} = \frac{C_F\,Q_F}{C_{PW}} = SQ_F$$

For urea the sieving coefficient $\left(\dfrac{C_F}{C_{PW}}\right) = 1$ as $C_F = C_{PW}$

$$\therefore\ K_{HF} = Q_F$$

Unit analysis

$$K_{HF}\,(\text{ml/min}) = \frac{(\text{mg/ml})\,(\text{ml/min})}{\text{mg/ml}} = \frac{\text{mg/min}}{\text{mg/ml}} \neq \frac{\text{Removal rate}}{\text{Driving gradient}}$$

= meaningless, except as a clearance analogous to native kidney clearance (K_k)

Fig. 20.10. Urea clearance for hemofiltration (K_{HF}) (post dilution, net ultrafiltration = 0).

20.3 and 20.11 for urea) but different in its implications for outcome due to the difference in solute clearance profile that attends hemofiltration. Improved survival value has recently been shown to attend the enhanced removal of solutes

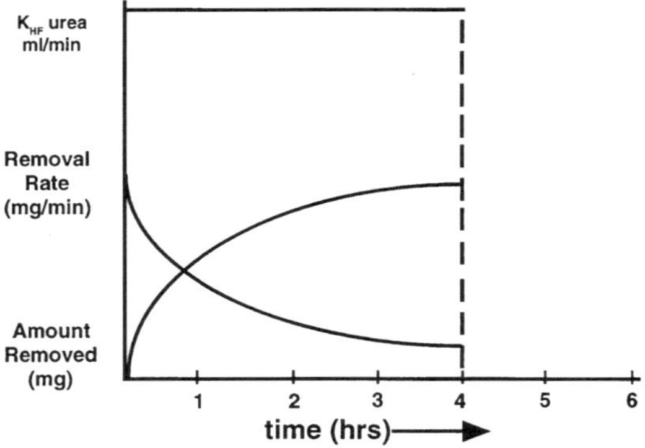

Fig. 20.11. Post dilution hemodialysis (S = 1, Q_F = constant, Q_F = 0).

larger in molecular weight than conventional uremic solutes such as urea, creatinine, phosphate etc., i.e. middle molecule removal contributes to longevity in the ESRD population [3, 8].

IMPLICATIONS

Clearance as it is commonly measured for each renal replacement modality bears a different quantitative relationship to the mass of urea removed for each of these modalities. As such:

$$K_{HD} \neq /K_{PD} \neq /K_{HF} \tag{4}$$

for urea. Furthermore, the surrogate status that urea holds for other uremic toxins must be uniquely defined for each modality as it will differ. As such the implications for the amount of therapy rendered as an index of treatment adequacy will be modality specific.

$K_{HD}t/V$ urea was developed by Gotch and Sargent in their paper describing a mechanistic analysis of the national cooperative dialysis study [9]. It has been widely used both by these investigators and others to describe quantitatively the amount of therapy rendered. There appears to be considerable misunderstanding about what $K_{HD}t/V$ urea represents. It is a fractional volume cleared and not a fractional solute clearance as many suppose. The latter by definition ranges from 0 to 1 and cannot exceed unity and still make physical sense. $K_{HD}t/V$ urea can and does exceed unity as a

fractional volume cleared simply because the virtual (as contrasted with an actual and identifiable specific volume) volume of blood that is cleared may be considered to circulate by the dialysis membrane more than once and hence may be cleared more than once. The dimensionless ratio $K_{HD}T/V$ for urea in conjunction with the protein catabolic rate has been widely used to provide a quantitative description of the amount of therapy rendered in comparing the outcome of for example hemodialysis and chronic ambulatory peritoneal dialysis (CAPD) (see, for example, Keshaviah et al. [10], Gotch and Keen [11] and Depner [12]). As has been examined in detail elsewhere [3], there is an underlying assumption in this intermodality comparison; namely, that K_{HD} and K_{PD} have the same physical meaning with regard to the mass of urea removed by each modality. As can be judged at a glance from the shape of the curves in Figures 20.3 and 20.6 this is a conceptual error. As noted above for urea,

$$K_{HD} \neq K_{PD} \neq K_{HF}. \tag{5}$$

hence:

$$K_{HD}T/V \neq K_{PD}T/V \neq K_{HF}T/V \tag{6}$$

See Figure 20.12 for clinical confirmation that using Kt/V urea as an adequacy criterion is modality specific.

This having been said, what can we make of the considerable time and effort put into providing the clinical correlation between $K_{HD}t/V$ urea and morbid and mortal outcome? Within a given modality and within the study parameters that

Using 2 year mortality as the normalizing parameter

Modality	Frequency	Weekly KT/V_{urea}	2yr mortality
HD[1]	t.i.w.	3.6	72%
CAPD[2]	continuous	1.7	78%
HF[3]	t.i.w.	1.5	95%

1. Held et al. KI 42 (suppl 38): S16-S21:92
2. Churchill et al. JASN 7:198-207:96
3. Quelhorst et al. ASAIO J 4:185-191:83

Fig. 20.12. Interpretation of Kt/V is modality specific.

have provided the clinical correlation with morbid and/or mortal outcome, the use of $K_{HD}t/V$ urea makes a satisfactory tool for use in prescribing adequate therapy. Out side those parameters or across modalities where solute clearance profiles differ it is not satisfactory.

Measurement of solute in the effluent dialysate over time, for any mode of treatment in order to quantify it's net removal, permits the clinical observer to calculate the fraction of that solute that has been removed from the patient for that therapy. As noted above the only mode of therapy for which direct quantification is currently standard practice is peritoneal dialysis. Our present habit is then to back calculate a time averaged PD clearance. A preferred practice that would facilitate accurate intermodality comparison would be to calculate the fractional removal of that solute as it would have direct conceptual clarity in terms of what the therapy had accomplished. e.g. 50% of the urea was removed. A happy arithmetic circumstance causes the term $K_{PD}\,t/V$ to equate to the fractional reduction in urea as calculated from direct quantification [13]. What is required, in addition, to arrive at a fractional reduction from the amount of solute removed during therapy with hemodialysis or hemofiltration is knowledge of the starting amount of solute within the body. For long procedures like CAPD the generation rate for the solute being studied will enhance the accuracy of this figure. In the simplest case of a 4 hours artificial kidney treatment in which the urea removed is measured, we may make some reasonable assumptions that the amount of urea generated will be small and relatively constant and the starting amount will be distributed throughout the total body water. With measurement of the pre-dialysis urea concentration in the plasma water it will permit us (with the use of common formulas, (e.g. Watson's formula [14] or some of the newer measuring techniques) to calculate the patient's total body water. A very reasonable estimate of the starting amount of urea may be then obtained as a simple product. With this as the denominator and the amount removed during therapy in the numerator we may express the impact of therapy in terms of a fractional reduction. Keshaviah and Star [15] have explored this approach in detail. It should be apparent that many of the limitation of clearance are avoided by use of the solute removal

index. Specifically, for hemodialysis recirculation of the blood and/or differences in regional perfusion are both accounted for in the direct quantification of urea removed as are the concerns about slow transcellular transport and disequilibrium. In addition urea removed by convection with ultrafiltered plasma water is taken into account unlike the circumstance with the common clearance measurement. Lastly, with the direct quantification of the amount of two common metabolites, urea and creatinine, we may derive significant insight into the nutritional status of the patient [16].

Technology is already available that measures urea on line in the effluent dialysate [12] it will soon be available to measure creatinine and as other relevant solutes are identified I would expect these to come on line as well. Direct quantification should be our 'gold standard' for assessing the clinical performance of our renal replacement therapy, not clearance or clearance-derived parameters.

NOTES

[1] I shall write about plasma clearance as that is commonly measured clinically. Note, however, that whole blood clearance > plasma clearance > plasma water clearance due to the displaced volume of cell matrix and plasma protein or that of plasma protein and one may readily be converted to the other if hematocrit and plasma protein concentration are known [5].

[2] I am, for the sake of simplicity, ignoring the small amount of creatinine that arrives in the urine by tubular secretion.

[3] Plasma concentration, of course, falls as protein does not pass through the membrane and occupies an increasingly greater volume in the sample you take for analysis.

REFERENCES

1. Smith H. Measurement of the rate of glomerular filtration. In Principles of renal physiology. New York, Oxford University Press, 1956.
2. Wolf AN, Remp DG, Kiley JE and Currie JD. Artificial kidney function: kinetics of hemodialysis. J Clin Invest 1951; 39:1062–70.
3. Henderson LW, Leypoldt JK, Lysaght MJ and Cheung AK. Death on dialysis and the time/flux trade-off. J Blood Purif 1997; 15:1–14.
4. Depner TA, Keshaviah PR, Ebben JP, Emerson PF, Collins AJ, Jindal KK et al. Multicenter clinical validation of an on-line monitor of dialysis adequacy J Am Soc Nephrol 1996; 7:464–71.

5. Henderson LW. Biophysics of ultrafiltration and hemofiltration. In Maher JF, editor. Replacement in renal function by dialysis, 4th edn. Dordrecht, Kluwer, 1996; 114–45.

6. Descombes F, Perriard F and Fellay G. Diffusion kinetics of urea, creatinine, and uric acid in blood during hemodialysis: clinical implication. Clin Nephrol 1993; 40:286–95.

7. Charra B, Calemard E, Ruffet M, Chazot C, Terrat JC, Vanel T et al. Survival as an index of adequacy of dialysis. Kidney Int 1992; 41:1286–91.

8. Leypoldt JK, Cheung AK, Carroll CE, Stannard D, Pereira B, Agadoa L et al. Removal of middle molecules enhances survival in hemodialysis patients (abstract). J Am Soc Nephrol 1996; 7:1454.

9. Gotch F and Sargent JA. A mechanistic analysis of the National Cooperative Dialysis Study. Kidney Int 1985; 28:526.

10. Keshaviah PR, Nolph KD and Van Stone JC. The peak concentration hypothesis: a urea kinetic approach to comparing the adequacy of continuous ambulatory peritoneal dialysis (CAPD) and hemodialysis. Perit Dial Int 1989; 9:257–60.

11. Gotch FA and Keen ML. Kinetic modeling in peritoneal dialysis. In Nissenson AR, Fine AR and Gentile DE, editors. Clinical dialysis, 3rd edn. Norwalk, Appleton & Lange, 1995; 343–75.

12. Depner TA. Quantifying hemodialysis and peritoneal dialysis: examination of the peak concentration hypothesis. Semin Dial 1994; 7:315–17.

13. Keshaviah P. The solute removal index: a unified basis for comparing disparate therapies. Perit Dial Int 1995; 15:101–4.

14. Watson PE, Watson ID and Batt RD. Total body water volumes for adult males and females estimated from simple anthropometric measurements. Am J Clin Nutr 1980; 33:27–39.

15. Keshaviah PR and Star RA. A new approach to dialysis quantification: An adequacy index based on solute removal. Semin Dial 1994; 7:85–90.

16. Keshaviah PR, Nolph KD, Moore HL, Prowant B, Emerson PF, Meyer M et al. Lean body mass estimation by creatinine kinetics J Am Soc Nephrol 1994: 4:1475–85.

21. Quality in peritoneal dialysis: achieving improving outcomes

BARBARA F. PROWANT, KARL D. NOLPH, LEONOR PONFERRADA, RAMESH KHANNA
AND ZBYLUT J. TWARDOWSKI

The goal of this chapter is to discuss the characteristics of systems (structure) and activities (process) within a peritoneal dialysis (PD) program which contribute to optimal outcomes (quality) for peritoneal dialysis patients.

PROGRAM PHILOSOPHIES

PD Provides Effective Therapy

One value imperative for achieving quality in a PD program is the conviction that chronic peritoneal dialysis is an acceptable treatment for end-stage renal disease (ESRD). With appropriate adjustments for age and population risk factors, Cox proportional hazards model comparisons of hemodialysis and continuous ambulatory peritoneal dialysis patient survivals show no consistent survival advantage of either dialysis therapy [1–3]. A very recent analysis of Canadian Registry Data [2] shows survival advantages for CAPD over intermittent HD for the first three years. This is true for different age groups as well as diabetics and non-diabetics. Recent analyses of trends in United States Renal Data System data show improving survival trends for both HD and CAPD and no consistent survival advantages of one over the other [4]. Most comparisons have not adjusted for dialysis adequacy and compliance with therapy which can also influence survivals and need to be considered in future comparisons.

Philosophy of Self Care

A parallel value is that PD can be successfully managed as a home or self-care therapy. Although not all patients are totally responsible for self-care, most PD patients dialyze at home either independently or with the assistance of a partner. It is imperative that the administrative staff and all team members believe that patients and their families can learn to dialyze safely and effectively at home, and that self-care, home dialysis may offer advantages to the patient in terms of independence, scheduling, control, and quality of life.

Program Integration

Another value embraced by successful peritoneal dialysis programs is that it is essential for the peritoneal dialysis program to be integrated with acute and chronic hemodialysis units [5] and a renal transplantation program. There are many advantages of a truly integrated program. Decisions concerning optimal therapy can be made without the bias of how it will affect the income to the program and/or physician. The patient can transfer back and forth between therapies when necessary with relative comfort and ease. This philosophy of integration can be carried a step further to include liaisons with long-term care facilities. Short term placement in a residential care facility may be required following surgery or an acute illness. Permanent placement may be indicated for patients who are no longer able to do self-care or lose a dialysis partner.

Patient Involvement in Choosing a Chronic Dialysis Therapy

Another value inherent to successful peritoneal dialysis programs is that the patient and family should be encouraged to participate in the choice

L.W. Henderson and R.S. Thuma (eds.), Quality Assurance in Dialysis, 2nd Edition, 223–243.
© 1999 *Kluwer Academic Publishers. Printed in Great Britain*

of a therapy which best meets their needs and fits their lifestyles [6–10]. Ninety-three percent of the 32 centers of excellence for modality selection practices identified by Baxter Healthcare allowed the patient to make the final choice of chronic dialysis modality after receiving professional assessment, education and recommendations. These centers had an impressive technique survival of 85% at three years [11]. Data from predialysis programs indicate that significantly more patients who received predialysis education choose a self-care home dialysis therapy compared to patients who presented with uremic symptoms and in need of immediate dialysis [9, 12–14]. A number of models for dialysis modality selection have been developed [9, 13–17]. Key features of successful predialysis education programs are listed in Table 21.1. Ideally, education is initiated when the creatinine clearance approaches 25 mL/minute, 3–6 months prior to the need for dialysis therapy.

Table 21.1. Key components of successful predialysis patient education programs

- Education is initiated 3–6 months prior to the need for chronic dialysis

- The patient is assessed by the renal team

- There is an unbiased presentation of all treatment options

- Medical advantages and/or contraindications for a therapy are discussed

- There is a combination of classes and one-on-one sessions

- Families and significant others are included in the education process

- Predialysis patients meet individuals on various ESRD therapies

- The patient is included in the decision-making process

A review of 63 patients who selected peritoneal dialysis [12] indicated that the predominant reason (25%) was to maintain independence, activities and flexibility in scheduling. Motivation to perform one's own dialysis and maintain some control was the reason 15% chose peritoneal dialysis and an additional 12% of the patients cited the ability to continue working. Although the majority of patients chose PD for positive reasons, 14%

selected peritoneal dialysis because of long distances to a hemodialysis unit and an additional 9% because they felt travel to center hemodialysis or the demands of home hemodialysis would impose an unacceptable burden on their families [12].

Administrative Support

A PD program cannot succeed and expand without strong and unified administrative support. For a PD program to thrive both the administrator and medical director must believe that peritoneal dialysis is a legitimate dialysis therapy for the majority of patients as is hemodialysis; and that PD can be a revenue producing program. Only when there is such a philosophy will the PD program be able to obtain adequate space, personnel, equipment, budget and support.

Allowing designated nursing staff to work solely in the home dialysis program is one indicator of administrative support. Of the 18 centers of excellence for patient education and training practices identified by Baxter Healthcare, 92% assigned nurses to the peritoneal dialysis outpatient program only with no responsibilities for center hemodialysis or intermittent peritoneal dialysis [18].

Another example of strong administrative support is flexibility to choose the most appropriate PD modality and to have the option of more than one peritoneal dialysis system, so that each patient has a dialysis prescription and system which will meet his or her unique needs. For example a handicapped or visually impaired patient may require an assist device, a patient with high membrane permeability may need nightly cycler dialysis, and a large patient with average membrane permeability on CAPD may need an overnight exchange device.

Lack of strong administrative support makes it difficult, if not impossible, to provide high quality care. Three examples of the lack of administrative support follow: the first is a peritoneal dialysis program that chooses not to provide nursing back-up evenings, nights and weekends in order to avoid paying nurses for call time and/or overtime. Consequently, patients visit the emergency room or are admitted for problems which could have been prevented or easily managed at home had there been prompt reporting and early intervention. A second example is a unit that limits the use of adequacy testing to 6 monthly intervals because the laboratory tests cannot be separately billed. Additional adequacy testing cannot be done when clinically indicated or after prescription changes because of cost. The third example is a peritoneal dialysis program with more than 30 patients which operates out of two small treatment rooms, one of which is the only nurse's office. If clinic visits are scheduled during a training day the nurse has no place to speak confidentially to a patient who calls for assistance. Furthermore, patient records kept in the nurse's office are not adequately secured.

Philosophy of Excellence

Finally, for a peritoneal dialysis program to achieve a consistent quality of care the administrative, professional and support staff must share a commitment to quality. They must believe that their program can and does provide a high quality of care and caring. They must be committed to continuous quality improvement. They must be willing to go above and beyond the realm of routine activities, to try innovative approaches, and occasionally step outside the bounds of the job description. The philosophy of excellence includes a willingness to individualize dialysis prescriptions and to provide an optimal dose of dialysis, and adequate support services. The highest possible level of health and rehabilitation is truly the goal for each patient. The patient is the staff's central focus and the difficult or complex patient is seen as a challenge, rather than a problem.

PROGRAM STRUCTURE

The Peritoneal Dialysis Team

Peritoneal dialysis as a subspecialty has emphasized the importance of interdisciplinary collaboration and a team approach to patient care [19–23]. The peritoneal dialysis team becomes a continuous quality circle responsible for the quality of care provided to their patients. Typically the team responsible for the care of peritoneal dialysis

patients is composed of a physician, nurse, dietitian and social worker. Additional team members might include the surgeon responsible for peritoneal catheter placement, an exercise specialist, a rehabilitation expert or a psychologist or psychiatrist. Finally, the patient, the focus of services provided by the team, may actively participate in the team's decision making process [24]. Some institutions recommend that self-care or home dialysis patients participate in team care conferences to develop the long-term care plan. In other units the team's recommendations and/or care plan are later reviewed with the patient.

The major physician responsibilities are to prescribe appropriate therapy for ESRD and other medical problems, and to diagnose and treat complications of ESRD and dialysis therapy. The physician can also facilitate the effectiveness of the team by clarifying and/or validating the roles of the other team members, to patients, other physicians or other departments and institutions.

Table 21.2 lists the areas in which we believe a physician must be knowledgeable and competent to effectively manage peritoneal dialysis patients. In order to prescribe appropriate therapy, physicians caring for peritoneal dialysis patients must understand peritoneal dialysis kinetics and how to assess peritoneal membrane transport characteristics. Furthermore, the physician should be able to assess the adequacy of dialysis based on: a) quantifying dialysis; b) combined renal and dialysis urea

Table 21.2. Areas of physician knowledge and competence required for a successful peritoneal dialysis practice

General competence in hemodialysis
Peritoneal dialysis
– Catheter insertion protocols
– Evaluation of individual peritoneal membrane characteristics
– PD modalities
– PD systems
– PD prescription
– Evaluation of PD adequacy
– Nutritional requirements of PD patients
– Diagnosis and treatment of catheter-related infections
– Recognition, prevention and treatment of complications
– Management of diabetes mellitus
  – Regulation of blood sugar with intraperitoneal insulin

and/or creatinine clearances; c) interpretation of laboratory values; d) nutritional status, and e) patient well-being.

Roles of the nurse are to provide the education, guidance, support, supervision and assistance patients require to perform PD at home, to adhere to the treatment regimen and to experience the highest possible quality of life.

Because most nurses do not come to peritoneal dialysis programs with experience in nephrology or peritoneal dialysis an extensive orientation and education program is required in order to achieve a high level of nursing care. One such program lasts for 6 weeks during which the nurse learns theoretical information about peritoneal dialysis as well as learning to perform peritoneal dialysis procedures. A competency-based learning system which allows the learner to demonstrate the requisite knowledge and/or skills in each specific area can be used efficiently and effectively for initial orientation. The new nurse observes home dialysis education, clinic visits, home visits and outpatient nursing management. The nurse begins working with patients with a preceptor so there is a readily available resource and support. As the nurse learns or reviews ESRD, peritoneal dialysis content and principles of adult education he or she begins teaching patients in familiar topics such as monitoring blood pressure, then moves on to other topics. The number of primary patients is gradually increased, and patients requiring more complex care are added as the nurse gains experience. Nurses wait three months before taking call, and then another nurse is available for consultation.

The social worker's role is to assess the patient's (and family's) financial and psycho-social status and to provide psycho-social support, counseling and referrals as needed. Social workers are also involved in exercise and rehabilitation programs.

The dietitian's role is to assess the patient's nutritional status and make recommendations regarding the diet regimen. The dietitian teaches the patient and significant others about the therapeutic diet, assists them in meal planning, and helps them incorporate the dietary regimen into their lifestyle. To achieve a high quality of care for peritoneal dialysis patients the renal dietitian needs to have an understanding of dialysis kinetics, and how adequacy is related to nutrition, nutritional requirements of the chronic peritoneal

dialysis patient [25–28], and monitoring of nutritional indices. The dietitian also needs to understand basic principles of adult education and have adequate time to teach patients and families and to evaluate their adherence to the diet plan. The Council on Renal Nutrition provides guidelines for staff to patient ratios based upon the extent of services provided [29].

Team Interactions

Assembling an interdisciplinary group to care for patients does not necessarily ensure that they will function as a team. It is essential that the patient and family be viewed as a whole and that there is a system which will prevent fragmentation of care by promoting communication and collaboration [30, 31]. Collaboration is a joint effort involving the mutual determination of goals, pooling of resources by participants to solve problems that are larger than one person or organization could solve alone.

Team interactions take place in a variety of settings; however, some structured meetings are essential. Regularly scheduled team meetings provide opportunities to review the patient's current status, to discuss problems, to develop the team's long term plan of care, and for collaborative decision making. Hospital rounds by an interdisciplinary team also facilitate collaboration and contribute to coordinated, continuous care.

Mutual respect, similar goals, effective communication, and techniques to manage conflict among team members are essential for the team to function effectively. Physical proximity can also enhance team function. Team members with adjoining desks or offices (or even offices in the same building or facility) are likely to have much more informal interaction with each other than with physically distant team members [30].

Primary Nursing

Primary nursing is a system that assigns the nursing care of each individual patient and family to one nurse. The primary nurse is responsible and accountable for providing individual, comprehensive, and continuous nursing care for a group of patients. The primary nurse may also coordinate health care services provided by other disciplines.

A number of studies have shown that primary nursing enhances job satisfaction and professional development [32–35]. Primary nursing provides high levels of attainment on job enrichment criteria such as autonomy, direct feedback, identification with the whole product and task variability [35, 36]. In many instances primary care is also more cost effective [36, 37].

Primary care seems to be the most appropriate nursing modality for outpatient peritoneal dialysis [20, 38–40] and is the nursing modality most widely utilized in peritoneal dialysis programs in North America. Ninety-four percent of the centers of excellence for patient education and training practices utilized primary nursing during home training and 81% continued to utilize primary nursing for outpatient followup [18].

Professional Enhancement and Job Enrichment

Assigning additional projects and responsibilities to staff members who are clinically competent and efficient provides diversity, and an avenue for personal growth and professional development. Table 21.3 lists a number of such activities. Most of these tasks and activities are inherent components of a home dialysis program, so these projects do not actually add additional work.

Continuing education for all team members is essential for professional enhancement as well as optimal care. Team meetings, clinics and rounds provide opportunities for informal teaching. Working with a partner or mentor is an effective way for professionals new to peritoneal dialysis to acquire knowledge and learn to make clinical assessments, diagnoses, and management decisions. Unit inservices and professional education meetings provide more structured learning as does formal education. Professional meetings also offer opportunities to meet colleagues and do informal networking.

Peritoneal dialysis staff are frequently asked to teach others about this therapy. Such invitations provide opportunities to develop skills in planning and providing professional education and in public speaking. Opportunities to do technical or professional writing are also available to peritoneal dialysis staff members. Beginning writers may start with simple in-house projects such as policies and procedures or patient education materials.

Table 21.3. Staff projects to enhance professional growth and development

- Write or revise policies and procedures
- Evaluate new products and peritoneal dialysis systems
- Develop patient education modules
- Develop patient education materials
- Participate in quality improvement activities
- Develop clinical expertise in related specialties, e.g. gerontology, diabetes
- Serve as a liaison to long term care facility(s)
- Serve as a liaison to associated hospital(s)
- Collect and analyze infection data
- Participate in or direct research projects
- Serve on institutional committees

Encouraging membership and active participation in professional organizations can provide yet another avenue for professional enhancement, and continuing education.

PD Program Requirements

First of all, peritoneal dialysis programs have physical space requirements. Eighteen centers of excellence for patient education and training practices identified by Baxter Healthcare had significantly higher technique survival and patient survival rates than their counterparts. All of these units had space devoted solely to the home peritoneal dialysis program [18]. Eighty-two percent of these centers had a PD training room, a separate PD clinic area, and a PD nurses' office. All of the units also had separate storage and utility areas for peritoneal dialysis [18].

Another of the most basic requirements is a set of standards of clinical practice. A standard is the yardstick of the quality of a service and Mason states that nursing standards "define unequivocally what quality care is and provide specific criteria that can be used to determine whether quality care has been provided" [41]. A standard describes what should be done and how the patient will benefit from the care. The American Nephrology Nurses' Association has published standards of clinical practice for nephrology nursing [42]. Appropriate standards can be selected and adapted for use in a particular dialysis unit.

A policy and procedure manual that guides safe practice is also essential [43]. Policies for all nursing procedures, machine and equipment maintenance, emergencies, and managing problems will help ensure consistent, safe care. A unit's standards and policies and procedures are also used by inspectors and surveyors to evaluate the program. Although clinical policies and procedures are developed primarily by the nursing staff we recommend consultation with administration regarding legal issues, with the medical director regarding nursing protocols to manage complications, and with patients regarding the self-care procedures. An annual review and update of policies and procedures is appropriate. Examples of the types of policies and procedures required for a peritoneal dialysis program are listed in Table 21.4.

Medical protocols and procedures also contribute to quality. For teaching institutions a manual for housestaff and renal fellows is essential for consistent care. Examples of content are listed in Table 21.5.

Patient Education

Nurses in home PD programs should be familiar with principles of learning, and principles of adult and patient education. There are a number of excellent texts available, as well as information specific to the ESRD patient.

Each PD program needs to develop a generic curriculum for PD patient education that can be modified for each individual patient and adapted for patients with special needs. Teaching materials such as an instructor's manual, printed information for patients or a patient education manual, patient procedures, audio-visual aids (posters, slides, videos), practice supplies, a PD model or "dummy tummy" for practicing exchanges, patient record forms, need to be developed. Use of these materials will be individualized based on the characteristics of the teacher and learner.

The initial PD nursing assessment typically includes an educational assessment. Table 21.6 lists items from an educational assessment. The patient education process typically proceeds from

Table 21.4. Examples of peritoneal dialysis unit policies and procedures

General Procedures
    Handwashing
    Measuring blood pressure
    Quantitative urine collection

Peritoneal dialysis procedures
    Exit-site care procedures
    Exchange procedure (for each system used)
    Cycler procedures
        Machine set up for closed drain
        Machine set up for open drain
        Connection procedure
        Cycler operation
        Disconnection procedure
        Dialysate sampling procedure
    Administration of intraperitoneal medication
    Catheter adapter change procedure
    Peritoneal equilibration test

Protocols for managing problems and complications
    Obstruction of flow
    Fibrin in dialysate
    Contamination of the system
    Crack or hole in catheter
    Hypervolemia
    Peritonitis

Emergency procedures
    Cardio-pulmonary arrest
    Fire
    Hurricane or tornado

Table 21.5. Selected content from manual for renal fellows (or housestaff)

Chronic catheter insertion
    Catheter selection
    Pre-surgical assessment
    Marking catheter exit site
    Preoperative orders
    Catheter break-in

Peritoneal equilibration test (indications, orders, interpretation of results)

Prescriptions for chronic dialysis (CAPD, CCPD nightly intermittent cycler dialysis)

Measurement and evaluation of dialysis adequacy

Infection treatment protocols (diagnosis, treatment, followup)
    Exit-site infection
    Peritonitis
    Tunnel infection

Table 21.6. Components of initial nursing assessment related to education

- Educational background
- Work experience
- Previous involvement in self-care activities
- General level of health
- Physical disabilities which could affect learning
- Factors that interfere with health care or following the medical regimen
- Level of cognitive function
- Psychiatric/emotional status
- Level of activity and independence
- Dialysis partner or backup support
- Current knowledge of PD
- Concerns regarding ESRD and/or dialysis
- Expectations of PD education program
- Current stressors and symptoms of stress
- Motivation to learn and perform PD
- Best way to learn
- Best time to learn
- Assessment of reading skills
- Assessment of memory

Table 21.7. Topics required for initial PD training at 18 facilities [18]

Asepsis*
Handwashing
Exchange procedure*
Exit site care*
Recommended diet, meal planning
Fluid balance
Record keeping
Procedure for system contamination
Causes of peritonitis
Peritonitis prevention
Peritonitis symptoms*
Reporting peritonitis to unit
Peritonitis treatment
Catheter complications
Supply inventory
Vital signs
Laboratory values
Patient responsibilities
Communications and call system

*Minimum knowledge required for all patients

assessment of the patient's ability and readiness to learn to developing an individualized plan for the patient's education. The plan includes developing behavioral objectives, outlining content, identifying specific teaching and learning activities, and planning for evaluation. The process continues through the actual implementation and evaluation phases. Teaching can be done in classes, with 2 or 3 patients or individually. Most PD programs use a 1:1 nurse patient ratio for at least part of the initial patient education.

Table 21.7 lists topics covered by over 90% of 18 facilities evaluated for the best demonstrated practices in patient education [18]. Lecture and discussion were the primary modes of patient teaching among the best demonstrated practice centers. Demonstration, return demonstration, and simulated problem solving were also used by all of these facilities.

The patient education process may be documented a number of ways. An account of the assessment, goals and progress is recorded in the progress notes or nurse's notes. In addition, annotations are often made on the patient objectives or an education checklist to document a patient's mastery of the subject, that a topic has been omitted, or that the routine approach or procedure has been modified. At the completion of training there is a comprehensive evaluation of the patient's (and/or partner's) knowledge and skills. A variety of testing methods are used: verbal and written testing, return demonstration of procedures, and/or simulated problem solving. Training time ranges from 5–10 days.

The process of patient education is ongoing, so review, reassessment of learning needs and/or teaching should take place at almost every patient contact. Ongoing patient education may take place in several formats: review or update sessions for large groups of patients; smaller groups for patients with similar interests or diagnoses; and individual teaching related to specific clinical problems.

Follow-Up Care

PD patients require frequent monitoring, assessment, guidance, and support as they begin to dialyze independently at home [20]. This is most efficient and cost effective if the frequency and type of followup is tailored to the patient's specific needs. Many programs contact newly discharged patients two or three times during the first week and then gradually increase the intervals between telephone calls. The first clinic visit is usually scheduled a week or two post discharge and, thereafter, the frequency is adjusted depending upon how well the patient is coping and the number and type of problems. Clinic visits for nursing assessment and further teaching are sometimes scheduled independently of medical clinic visits.

Most peritoneal dialysis programs require patients to be seen in the clinic every 4 to 8 weeks. Activities during a routine clinic visit might include a review of home records (or otherwise documenting the home dialysis regimen), measurement of vital signs (including supine and upright blood pressures), assessment of fluid balance, physical examination, evaluation of the catheter exit site, selected blood chemistries and hematology, review of medications, evaluation of activity level and rehabilitation status.

A more comprehensive assessment which may include more extensive bloodwork, X-rays, an electrocardiogram is usually done biannually. The National Kidney Foundation Dialysis Outcomes Quality Initiative (DOQI) Clinical Practice Guideline for Peritoneal Dialysis Adequacy [44] recommend that adequacy testing be done at least twice in the first six months and every four months thereafter (See Table 21.8).

Table 21.8. Dialysis outcomes quality initiative recommendations for measuring dialysis adequacy [44]

- Within 1 month of initiating dialysis
- Two or three times within the first 6 months of dialysis
- Every four months after the 6th month
- After a change in dialysis prescription
- As clinically indicated

Home visits are a valuable adjunct to center followup. Assessing the patient and family in the home provides valuable insights about family interactions, the degree of self care, supply inventory and storage, general management of health, emotional adjustment and dietary practices [45]. Home visits to both patients with perceived problems and those doing well resulted in recommendations for change [45]. Repeated home visits have been used to count supplies and document compliance [46].

Liaison with Hospitals

Outpatient peritoneal dialysis programs must work closely with affiliated hospitals, in order to assure that hospitalized patients receive continuous, coordinated care [47, 48]. Ideally, all PD patients would be admitted to a renal ward where the entire nursing staff understands ESRD and could perform PD procedures. Few programs enjoy such a luxury, or in fact, have a chronic dialysis population large enough to support a renal ward. Other options are a hospital PD or dialysis staff; contractual arrangements allowing the outpatient PD nurses to provide PD and exit-site care for hospitalized patients; or a few medical-surgical nurses trained to do PD procedures. It is also imperative that hospitals have supplies and PD systems compatible with those the patients use at home and that PD procedures are consistent with the procedures used and taught in the outpatient unit.

Medical-surgical nurses caring for PD patients in the hospital need to understand basic principles of peritoneal dialysis and the routine medication regimens. Some dialysis units have formal programs where ESRD is included in staff orientation and continuing education programs are regularly scheduled. In large hospitals a renal clinical nurse specialist can provide consultation and education on an ongoing basis.

When catheters are inserted at the hospital (either on an inpatient or outpatient basis) the nursing staff must be familiar with the preoperative care, the operative procedure and postoperative catheter care and communicate with the outpatient peritoneal dialysis staff at discharge [47].

Communication between the nurses responsible for outpatient and inpatient dialysis is essential

[20]. The current dialysis regimen, current medications, fluid status, PD related infections and other complications must be provided to the staff taking over the patient's care. The use of a standard form for hospital admission and discharge can facilitate effective communication of such details.

Liaison with Extended Term Care Facilities

As the age and comorbidities of dialysis patients increase, some chronic dialysis patients require continuous, skilled nursing care and reside in long-term care facilities [49–51]. Peritoneal dialysis programs have successfully taught the staff at nursing homes to perform PD procedures and manage fluid balance and other aspects of care [51]. The education outline is similar to that used for patient and family education. The patient receiving chronic PD in a long term care facility still requires followup by the PD staff, and continuing education and support are also provided to the facility staff.

Back-Up Support or On-Call Program

Patients performing dialysis and managing their ESRD at home require 24-hour, professional staff support to guide and assist them in identifying and managing problems or complications. Support is also essential for newly trained patients just beginning to dialyze independently at home. Both a nurse and physician must be on call 24 hours/day. Because most questions or problems are related to dialysis procedures and/or are within the realm of nursing practice, in most programs the nurse is the initial contact. For medical problems the nurse consults with or refers to the physician on call.

KEY CLINICAL ELEMENTS

Catheter Type and Insertion

A well-functioning, permanent access is a critical component of quality care in peritoneal dialysis. Increasing data are available to support traditional clinical recommendations for catheter insertion and care. Principles of good surgical technique and healing can be combined with replicated research results to develop research-based protocols for catheter selection, insertion and care.

Two large, national registries have reported data to support the use of double-cuff catheters for chronic PD therapy, because they are associated with fewer peritonitis episodes [52], a lower incidence of exit site complications [53], and longer survival times [53] compared to single cuff catheters. These findings have been confirmed in a prospective multi-center analysis in pediatric patients [54].

There are also data to confirm that a downward direction of the catheter tunnel and exit site are associated with fewer severe exit and tunnel infections [55, 56], a lower relative risk of the first peritonitis episode [52] and a lower rate of peritonitis in pediatric patients [54].

Single center studies evaluating the effect of prophylactic antibiotics at catheter insertion have had conflicting findings. Although the 1992 United States Renal Data System (USRDS) report [52] showed no benefit of prophylactic antibiotics in delaying the onset of the *first* peritonitis episode; Network 9 data reported by Golper et al. [56] found that patients who received prophylactic antibiotics had a lower relative risk of peritonitis and of peritonitis with concomitant exit site and tunnel infection. This may be explained by findings of Twardowski and Prowant [57] in an observational study of exit-site healing in 43 catheters post insertion, that exit sites which were not colonized for 5 weeks post catheter insertion had significantly lower peritonitis rates and fewer recurrent episodes. Furthermore, catheters with exit-sites colonized after 5 weeks were not as likely to be removed for either tunnel infections or refractory peritonitis. Thus, prophylactic antibiotic therapy may not always have an impact on time to first peritonitis, which may be due to contamination of the PD system but, by reducing the risk of colonization at the cuffs or in the tunnel between cuffs during healing, may reduce the risk of later, complicated peritonitis due to contamination from tunnel infection.

Table 21.9 summarizes elements of catheter insertion believed to be associated with improved outcomes. Delaying the use of peritoneal dialysis or using small volumes in the supine position to lower intraabdominal pressure will reduce the risks of leaks postimplantation [58].

Table 21.9. Recommended techniques for peritoneal catheter insertion [58]

- Limit catheter placement to experienced surgeon or ne-phrologist
- Assess abdomen and determine exit site preoperatively (avoid belt line, scars, fat folds)
- Use a lateral or paramedian approach
- Soak catheter in sterile solution to saturate cuffs and expel air
- Exit site should face downward
- Excellent hemostasis to avoid hematoma
- Avoid sutures at the exit site
- Infuse and drain solution prior to closing to assess function
- Absorbent, sterile, dressings
- Immobilize catheter

Catheter Care

The impact of exit site care procedures on the incidence of exit site infection has been evaluated post catheter insertion [59–61] and an expert panel has made recommendations for post operative exit care [58]. Common elements of these post operative exit site care procedures are listed in Table 21.10.

The chronic exit site care procedures which have been recommended [58] and studied [62–65] are more varied. Common elements include cleansing with an antibacterial soap or a medical disinfectant, rinsing and drying the exit site and securing the catheter. The ideal cleansing agent is not known and recommended frequency varies from daily to several times weekly.

Preventing Infections

Staphylococcus aureus carriers have been shown to be at increased risk for peritonitis and exit-site infection [66–71] and catheter loss [72]. Treatment of *Staphylococcus aureus* nasal carriers by use of systemic rifampin [73], other systemic antibiotics [70], and application of mupirocin ointment to the nares [74, 75] or to the exit site [76] have consistently shown significant reductions in the inci-

Table 21.10. Recommendations for post operative exit site care

- Restrict dressing changes to trained staff, patient or partner
- Aseptic technique (masks and sterile gloves)
- Sterile dressings
- Keep strong oxidants out of the wound
- Rinse with sterile water or normal saline
- Do not submerge the exit until healed
- Immobilize the catheter

dence of *Staphylococcus aureus* exit site infections and peritonitis with an overall decrease in the incidence of infections.

There are a number of other approaches to peritonitis prevention. Matching the peritoneal dialysis system to the patient's physical and mental abilities will reduce the risk of contamination to the system. Reevaluation of the patient's abilities and procedure technique after peritonitis has occurred enables the nurse to identify a problem with technique or determine if the current system is no longer appropriate for the patient. Even if no technique problems are identified, changing to a y-set [77, 78] may reduce the incidence of peritonitis.

Effectively teaching the patient how to identify a break in technique or contamination of the system and the appropriate responses will reduce the incidence of peritonitis. The use of prophylactic antibiotics for known contamination of the system is recommended [80]. Baxter Healthcare's best demonstrated practices program found that ten of 15 centers with a 1986 peritonitis rate of 1 episode every 18.7 months routinely used prophylactic antibiotics for a break in technique [80]. Thirteen of the fifteen centers routinely prescribed prophylactic antibiotics for a known contamination of the system. Ten of the same 15 centers also prescribed prophylactic antibiotic therapy for invasive dental procedures to prevent hematogenous contamination of the peritoneal cavity [80].

Recently there has been increased emphasis on preventing peritoneal catheter exit-site infection by avoiding trauma and massive contamination [81, 82].

Prescribing Adequate Dialysis

A number of studies have shown that quantitatively more dialysis is associated with less morbidity and lower mortality rates [83–88]. Although it is more difficult to achieve adequate dialysis after loss of residual renal function and in large patients [88–97], an expert committee concluded that adequate PD therapy can be achieved in almost all individuals if the patient's size (BSA), residual renal function, and peritoneal membrane transport characteristics are considered when developing the dialysis prescription [96].

In order to determine the most efficient dialysis modality and the optimal dialysis schedule for an individual patient the physician needs information regarding the patient's peritoneal membrane characteristics. Several tests can be used to characterize the peritoneal membrane. These include determination of mass transfer area coefficient [98–105], the peritoneal equilibration test (PET) [106, 107] and the peritoneal function test [108]. The most widely used, the abridged peritoneal equilibration test [107, 109–111], measures the dialysate to plasma ratio of creatinine at 0, 2, and 4 hours dwell time, dialysate glucose/dialysate glucose at 0 dwell time at 2 and 4 hours, and ultrafiltration volume. These values can be compared to or plotted on published curves to determine if solute transport is average, high or low [107–112]. A standardized pediatric adaptation of the PET which uses an exchange volume of 1000 mL/m^2 has been developed for use in children [113].

It is recommended that studies to characterize the peritoneal membrane be done shortly after initiating chronic peritoneal dialysis therapy [114–116]. The assessment does not need to be routinely repeated, but reassessment is necessary when there are clinical problems or indications that there may be a change in membrane transport characteristics (Table 21.11). Such indicators include an increase or decrease in ultrafiltration, an unexplained change in serum chemistries, a severe peritonitis episode, or an unexplained increase or decrease in adequacy of dialysis..

Knowledge of individual peritoneal membrane characteristics can be used to predict clinical dialysis clearances and fluid removal, and thus guide the choice of treatment modality [112, 114–116]. Table 21.12 outlines the most appropriate or

Table 21.11. Clinical use of PET results

- Classification of peritoneal membrane transport
- Choice of peritoneal dialysis regimen
- Estimate dialysis dose
- Estimate D/P ratio at time *t*
- Monitor peritoneal membrane function
- Diagnose acute injury to the peritoneal membrane
- Evaluate cause of inadequate ultrafiltration
- Evaluate cause of inadequate solute clearances
- Diagnose early ultrafiltration failure
- Assess influence of systemic disease on membrane

Table 21.12. Dialysis characteristics and optimal modalities based on peritoneal equilibration test results [109,110, 112, 114]

Solute transport	Fluid removal	Clearances	Preferred prescription(s)
High	Poor	Good	NIPD, tidal NIPD, DAPD
High average	Adequate	Adequate	Any regimen
Low average	High	Borderline	Standard or high dose continuous
Low	Excellent	Inadequate	CAPD with evenly distributed dwells, hemodialysis

preferred dialysis modalities based on solute transport characteristics. Computerized kinetic modeling programs can further evaluate the effect of exchange volume, distribution of exchanges (day and night) and dwell times on clearances according to patient's size and membrane characteristics [94, 95, 117] Table 21.13 lists common PD prescription mistakes [96].

Obviously, if physicians are to prescribe the most appropriate therapy based on peritoneal membrane transport rates, there must be administrative and nursing support for a wide variety of PD modalities (CAPD, CAPD with an additional overnight exchange, CCPD, CCPD with an additional daytime exchange, intermittent cycler dialysis (for patient's with high transport characteristic), and for the use of more dialysis solution. Unit

Table 21.13. Common peritoneal dialysis prescription error. Adapted from Burkart et al. [95]

CAPD
    Mismatch of dwell time and transport type
    Infused volume is not maximized
    Inappropriately short daytime dwell(s)
    Inadequate glucose concentration for overnight dwell

Cycler therapy
    Failure to set a higher target dose for intermittent therapy
    Use of nightly, intermittent dialysis without daytime dwells
    Failure to consider a second, daytime dwell in CCPD
    Inappropriately long drain times
    Too many overnight cycles in patients with average or low permeability
    Inadequate glucose concentration for long, daytime dwell

Table 21.14. Dialysis outcomes quality initiative recommendations for weekly dialysis dose [116]

	Weekly Kt/V urea[a]	Weekly Cr clearance[b]
CAPD (Continuous ambulatory peritoneal dialysis)	2.0	60 L
CCPD (Continuous cycling peritoneal dialysis)	2.1	63 L
NIPD (Nightly intermittent peritoneal dialysis)	2.2	66 L

[a]Normalized to total body water

[b]Normalized to 1.73 m^2 of body surface area

support also includes appropriate policies and procedures, availability of machine installation and maintenance, nurses skilled in operating cyclers, an educational curriculum and teaching materials, and billing and accounting systems.

Evaluating Dialysis Adequacy

The National Kidney Foundation Dialysis Outcomes Quality Initiative (DOQI) Clinical Practice Guideline for Peritoneal Dialysis Adequacy recommends that both weekly Kt/V urea and weekly creatinine clearance be routinely used to measure dialysis adequacy [116]. Twenty-four hour dialysate collections are recommended because abbreviated collections and other sampling techniques may be inaccurate [118, 119]. DOQI recommendations for the timing of adequacy measurements are listed in Table 21.8, and the recommended doses of PD therapy are shown in Table 21.14 [116]. Clinical assessment of adequacy is summarized in Table 21.15. Data from The Health Care Financing Administration's End Stage Renal Disease Core Indicators Project show that, although the proportion of patients who meet DOQI guidelines for adequate dialysis is gradually increasing, for the collection period of November 1996–April 1997 only 36% of a randomly selected national sample met the DOQI guidelines for adequate dialysis (Table 21.16) [120, 121].

Table 21.15. Clinical assessment of adequacy of dialysis. Adapted from Twardowski [115]

Clinical criteria
    Patient "feels well and looks good"
    Blood pressure controlled
    Good fluid balance
    Stable lean body mass
    Stable nerve conduction velocities

Absence of uremic symptoms
    Anorexia
    Dysgeusia
    Nausea
    Vomiting
    Asthenia
    Insomnia

Laboratory criteria
    Electrolytes within normal range
    Serum creatinine   < 20 (muscular persons)
                     < 15 (non muscular persons)

It is critical that residual renal function is monitored closely during the early months of dialysis therapy, that loss of residual renal function is anticipated, and that the decline in residual renal function is balanced by an increase in the dialysis prescription.

Table 21.16. Adequacy of dialysis – health care financing administration ESRD core indicators. Data from randomized samples of adult (> 18 yrs) peritoneal dialysis patients [120, 121]

| | 1995 | | 1996 | | 1997 | |
	Value	%Meeting DOQI (guidelines)	Value	%Meeting DOQI (guidelines)	Value	%Meeting DOQI (guidelines)
Mean weekly Kt/V[a]						
CAPD	1.91	(23)	2.00	(27)	2.12	(36)
Cycler			2.12	(28)	2.24	(36)
Mean weekly creatinine clearance (L)						
CAPD	61.48	(21)	64.35	(30)	65.84	(34)
Cycler	63.37	(26)	67.45	(33)		

[a]V determined by Watson's formulae

[b]Corrected to body surface area (BSA) of 1.73 m^2; BSA calculated using the formulae of Dubois and Dubois

Increasing Dialysis

Dialysis prescriptions can be quantitatively enhanced by increasing the daily dialysate drainage volume and/or maximizing dwell times [95, 96, 109]. Increasing the dialysate volume can be accomplished by the use of 2.5 or 3.0 L fill volumes or an increase in the number of exchanges. A daytime dwell may be added for overnight cycler patients, or an additional nighttime exchange using an automated exchange device may be added for CAPD patients [122]. Blake et al. believe that with the exception of patients with high transport rates, all cycler patients will require daytime exchange(s) in the absence of residual renal function [96]. Whereas increasing the number of exchanges will improve adequacy in patients with high peritoneal transport rates, patients with low peritoneal transport may benefit most from increased exchange volume and a more even distribution of dwell times [94–96].

Maintaining Adequate Nutrition

Malnutrition in PD patients is associated with increased morbidity [85, 88, 123–128] mortality [85, 88, 123, 125–131] and increased risk of transfer from PD therapy [125, 126]. Many patients are already malnourished and have some wasting when they begin PD [132, 133]. Although appetite and nutritional status may improve after initiating dialysis therapy, many markers of nutri-

tion remain abnormal [132, 134, 135]. Cross-sectional studies of CAPD patients have shown the prevalence of protein-energy malnutrition to ranges from 18–56% [134–137].

Routine, period assessment of nutritional status is recommended for patients with chronic renal failure and those on chronic dialysis therapy. The nutritional assessment is typically done at the same time dialysis adequacy is assessed. Diet history, subjective global assessment, assessment of weight and body composition, and measurement of serum proteins and cholesterol, are recommended and commonly performed [26, 138, 139]. Urea kinetic modeling with calculation of PNA and PCR has also been recommended, and may be helpful, but should not substitute for clinical assessment [140].

The etiology of malnutrition in PD patients is multifactorial and is related to the kidney failure, other systemic diseases, and the dialysis therapy [26–28, 134, 138, 139, 141–150]. Although the nutritional requirements for peritoneal dialysis patients have been defined [25, 134, 142, 149], there is no evidence that the nutritional status of chronic peritoneal dialysis patients has improved over time. The Health Care Financing Administration (HCFA) Core Indicators data from a random, national sample of peritoneal dialysis patients does not show a consistent improvement in serum albumin for CAPD patient (Table 21.17) [120]. Lowrie suggests that this is because we do not have the same type of nutrition-related knowl-

Table 21.17. Health care financing administration ESRD core indicators. Data from randomized samples of adult (> 18 yrs) peritoneal dialysis patients [120]

	1995 %Meeting DOQI guidelines	1996 %Meeting DOQI guidelines	1997 %Meeting DOQI guidelines
Mean %Hct			
CAPD	32.48 (30)	33.14 (34)	33.89 (40)
Cycler	33.06	33.17 (37)	33.67 (40)
Serum albumin gm/dL (BCG[a])			
CAPD	3.46	3.53	3.49
Cycler	3.39	3.51	3.52
Serum albumin gm/dlL(BCP[b])			
CAPD	3.18	3.16	3.29
Cycler	2.94	3.28	3.32
%Patients with hypertension[c]			
CAPD	34	34	34
Cycler	11	31	32

[a]Bromcresol green method
[b]Bromcresol purple method
[c]Hypertension defined as either systolic BP > 150 mm HG or diastolic BP > 90 mm Hg

edge or model that provides guidelines to improve albumin that we have for improving dialysis adequacy [151]. Another factor may be inadequate clinical dietary support. A recent analysis of 19 centers in Network 16 found that from 1983 to 1992 that the older, sicker patients required on average an additional 18 minutes per month of the renal dietitian's time [152]. There are, however, a number of recommendations for improving malnutrition in PD patients [141, 142, 149, 150, 153–157]. These are summarized in Table 21.18. Anecdotal reports of quality improvement activities describe improvements in serum albumin related to exercise [158] and innovative patient education combined with nutritional supplementation [159].

QUALITY IMPROVEMENT ACTIVITIES

Benchmarking Outcomes

The HCFA Core Indicators Project has collected data from a random, national sample of U.S. PD patients annually for three years [121, 160–163]. The resulting data for dialysis prescription, ade-

Table 21.18. Treatment of protein energy malnutrition [141, 142, 149, 150, 153–157]

- Increase protein and energy intake

    - Intensive dietary counseling
    - Oral supplements
    - Enteral supplements
    - Temporary administration of oral amino acids or their keto analogs (for hypercatabolism)
    - Parenteral supplementation during peritonitis or other serious, acute illness

- Identify and avoid specific inhibitors to hunger or stimulators of satiety.

- Correct acidosis

- Correct anemia

- Increase the dialysis dose

- Treat depression

- Use biocompatible PD solutions

- Use amino acid dialysis solutions

- Anabolic steroids

- Growth hormone and insulin-like growth factor-1

quacy, hematocrit, albumin and blood pressure values may be used by dialysis providers to benchmark their performance, to establish target ranges and to identify opportunities for improving their care delivery process to improve outcomes. Examples of the HCFA Core indicators data are shown in Tables 21.16 and 21.17.

The United States Renal Data System Annual Reports contain data from HCFA for ESRD patients in the U.S. Information in the 1997 report [164] includes the distribution of patients to dialysis modalities and transplantation, patient characteristics and comorbidities, PD modalities, PD prescriptions, PD patient compliance, survival, cause of death, and frequency of hospitalizations. Unit specific data have also been sent to each HCFA dialysis facility. This allows comparison of program data to the national data.

Continuous Quality Improvement

Evaluation of the incidence of peritonitis and characteristics of peritonitis episodes is a useful indicator of quality within a peritoneal dialysis program. A simple ratio of the number of peritonitis episodes over the patient months of exposure may be used to calculate the peritonitis rate, or life table analysis may be used to determine the probability of the first (or subsequent) peritonitis episodes [165–167]. A comparison of infection rates for each peritoneal dialysis modality and each type of peritoneal dialysis system may also be of value. Identifying the presumed etiology of each infection may help in identifying trends and developing strategies to reduce the incidence of peritonitis. CQI projects have resulted in improved peritonitis rates through improved patient education, prophylactic antibiotic therapy for contamination of the system, changes in exit site care procedures, and changing individual patient to other systems either alone or in combination with other strategies [168–175].

The incidence of exit site infection and distribution of causative organisms are also useful indicators. Trends in infection rates in a single program can be compared over time if the definition of exit site infection is consistent. The rates of and reasons for catheter removal should also be monitored. These data may then be used to identify the most frequent causes of exit site infection and

serve to focus CQI activities. Recent reports document that CQI projects have effectively decreased the incidence of exit site infections through changes in exit site care procedures and patient education activities [175–177].

Patient survival and technique survival (the proportion of patients remaining on peritoneal dialysis therapy), determined by actuarial techniques, should also be monitored as general indicators of program quality. High mortality rates may indicate a poor quality of care. Reasons for excessive transfer to hemodialysis therapy may also direct attention to problems with quality.

A number of CQI projects have reported improvement in indices of dialysis adequacy through staff and patient education, improving patient compliance with adequacy collections, more frequent monitoring of adequacy, and prescription changes [178–186].

CQI activities must also include routine evaluation of the patients' quality of life and satisfaction with the care they receive. Patient' perceptions of quality may be quite different from those of the staff providing care.

There are many facets to establishing and maintaining a peritoneal dialysis program. A comprehensive and integrated approach to building in quality increases the chances for and degree of success. The strong support and participation of administrators and physicians is essential. Communication of CQI data and results to the entire staff will enhance the likelihood that they will understand the rationale for change and support the process.

REFERENCES

1. Maiorca R, Cancarini GC, Zubani R et al. CAPD Viability: a long-term comparison with hemodialysis. Perit Dial Int 1996; 16:276–87.
2. Fenton SS, Schaubel DE, Desmeules M et al. Hemodialysis versus peritoneal dialysis: a comparison of adjusted mortality rates. Am J Kidney Dis 1997; 30:334–42.
3. Bloembergen WE, Port FK, Mauger EA, Wolfe RA. A comparison of mortality between patients treated with hemodialysis and peritoneal dialysis. J Am Soc Nephrol 1995; 6:177–83.
4. Vonesh E. Further comparisons of mortality between hemodialysis and PD. Presentation at the 18th Annual PD Conference, Nashville, TN, February 25, 1998.

5. Boen ST. Integration of continuous ambulatory peritoneal dialysis into endstage renal failure programmes: present and future. In Atkins RC, Thomson NM and Farrell PC, editors. Peritoneal dialysis. Edinburgh, Churchill Livingstone, 1981; 424–9.

6. Coover D and Conlon S. ESRD treatment modalities: The patient does have the right to choose. Nephrol Nurse 1982; 4:13–16,18.

7. Orr ML. Pre-dialysis patient education. J Nephrol Nursing 1985; 2:22–4.

8. Nitz J and Shayman D. A model for patient education. ANNA J 1986; 13:253–5.

9. Starzomski RC. Patient and staff involvement in decisions for ESRD treatment. ANNA J 1986; 13:325–8.

10. Tiedke J, Bielski C, Kinas J and Marquardt B. Dialysis treatment: are patients aware of their options? Nephrol News Issues 1992; 6(11):52–3, 58.

11. Baxter Healthcare Corporation. The Best Demonstrated Practices Program: Modality Selection Practices. Deerfield, IL: Author, 1988.

12. Campbell AR. Choosing an appropriate chronic dialysis therapy: a study of decisions by nephrology staff and patients (abstract). Perit Dial Int 1991; 11:40.

13. Grumke J and King K. Missouri Kidney Program's patient-education program: a 10-year review. Dial Transplant 1994; 23:691–9, 712.

14. Stephenson K and Villano R. Results of a predialysis patient education program. Dial Transplant 1993; 22:566-7, 570.

15. Campbell A. Strategies for improving dialysis decision making. Perit Dial Int 1991; 11:173–8.

16. Hayslip DM and Suttle CD. Pre-ESRD patient education: a review of the literature. Adv Renal Replace Ther 1995; 1:217–26.

17. Kochavi S. Implementing a pre-dialysis education program for patients and families. Dial Transplant 1990; 19:526–7,531.

18. Baxter Healthcare Corporation. The best demonstrated practices program: patient education and training practices. Deerfield, IL: Author, 1987.

19. Nolph KD, Sorkin MI, Prowant B and Webb J. National conference of continuous ambulatory peritoneal dialysis. Perit Dial Bull 1981; 1:65–66.

20. Uttley L and Prowant B. Organization of the peritoneal dialysis program – the nurses' role. In Gokal R and Nolph KD, editors. The textbook of peritoneal dialysis. Dordrecht: Kluwer Academic Publishers, 1994; 335–56.

21. Harvey E, Secker D, Braj B, Picone G and Balfe JW. The team approach to the management of children on chronic peritoneal dialysis. Adv Renal Replace Ther 1996; 3:3–13.

22. Chinn C. Collaborative practice of renal nutrition in endstage renal disease patient care. Adv Renal Replace Ther 1997; 4:397–9.

23. Kelly MP. Introduction: Diagnostic Reasoning: maximizing the strength of an interdisciplinary approach. Adv Renal Replace Ther 1997; 4:95–6.

24. Burnell MS. The hemodialysis patient: object of diagnosis or part of the treatment team? Adv Renal Replace Ther 1997; 4:145–51.

25. Kopple JD, and Blumenkrantz MJ. Nutritional requirements for patients undergoing continuous ambulatory peritoneal dialysis. Kidney Int 1983; 24:S295–302.

26. Lindholm B and Bergström J. Nutritional requirements of peritoneal dialysis patients. In Gokal R and Nolph KD, editors. The textbook of peritoneal dialysis. Dordrecht, Kluwer Academic Publishers, 1994; 443–72.

27. Blumenkrantz MJ. Nutrition. In Daugirdas JT and Ing TS, editors. Handbook of dialysis, 2nd edn. Boston, Little, Brown and Company, 1994; 374–400.

28. Wolfson M and Shuler C. Nutrition in patients with chronic renal failure and patients on dialysis. In Nissenson AR, Fine RN and Gentile DE, editors. Clinical dialysis, 3rd ed. Norwalk, CT, Appleton & Lange, 1995; 518–34.

29. Council on Renal Nutrition NKF, Inc. Guidelines for estimating renal dietitian staffing levels. New York, National Kidney Foundation, 1993.

30. Ducanis AJ and Golin AK. The interdisciplinary health care team. Germantown, MD, Aspen, 1979.

31. Lecca PJ and McNeil JS, editors. Interdisciplinary team practice: issues and trends. New York, Praeger, 1985.

32. Marram G, Barrett MW and Bevis EMO. Primary nursing, a model for individualized care. St. Louis, CV Mosby, 1979.

33. Giovanetti P. Evaluation of primary nursing in the nursing literature. Annu Rev Nurs Res 1986; 4:127–51.

34. Reed SE. A comparison of nurse-related behavior, philosophy of care and job satisfaction in team and primary nursing. J Adv Nurs 1988; 13:383–95.

35. Gardner KG. The effects of primary versus team nursing on quality of patient care and impact on nursing staff and costs: a five year study. Rochester NY, Rochester General Hospital, 1989.

36. Thomas LH and Bond S. Outcomes of nursing care: the case of primary nursing. Int J Nurs Stud 1991; 28:291–314.

37. Marram G, Flynn K. Abaravich W and Carey S. Cost-effectiveness of primary and team nursing. Wakefield, MA, Contemporary Publishing, 1976.

38. Perras ST, Mattern ML and Zappacosta AR. The integration of primary nursing into a chronic care program. Nephrol Nurse 1982; 4:23–4.

39. Zappacosta AR and Perras ST. CAPD. Philadelphia, J.B. Lippincott, 1984; 24–65.

40. Perras S, Mattern M, Hugues C, Coyer J and Zappacosta A. Primary nursing is the key to success in an outpatient CAPD teaching program. Nephrol Nurse 1983; 5:8–11.

41. Mason EJ. How to write meaningful nursing standards, 3rd ed. New York, John Wiley & Sons, 1994.

42. Burrows-Hudson S, editor. Standards of clinical practice for nephrology nursing. Pitman, NJ, American Nephrology Nurses' Association, 1993.

43. Hekelman FP. A framework for organizing a CAPD training program. J Nephrol Nurs 1985; 2:56–60.

44. NKF-DOQI clinical practice guidelines for peritoneal dialysis adequacy. Am J Kidney Dis 1997; 30(Suppl. 2): S67–136.

45. Ponferrada L, Prowant B, Schmidt LM, Burrows L, Satalowich RJ and Bartelt C. Home visit effectiveness for peritoneal dialysis patients. ANNA J 1993; 20:333–6.

46. Bernardini J, Piraino B. Compliance in CAPD and CCPD patients as measured by supply inventories during home visits. Am J Kidney Dis 1998; 31:101–7.

47. Thaler MK and Sasak C. Cooperative nursing care for patients using peritoneal dialysis. ANNA J 1988; 15:237–40

48. Lewandowski L. Developing collaborative partnerships between inpatient nephrology and outpatient dialysis units. Adv Renal Replace Ther 1995; 2:371–2.

49. Anderson JE, Sturgeon D, Lindsay J and Schiller A. Use of continuous ambulatory peritoneal dialysis in a nursing home: patient characteristics, technique success, and survival predictors. Am J Kidney Dis 1990; 16:137–41.

50. Anderson JE, Kraus J and Sturgeon D. Incidence, prevalence, and outcomes of end-stage renal disease patients placed in nursing homes. Am J Kidney Dis 1993; 21:619–27.

51. Jorden L. Establishing a peritoneal dialysis program in a nursing home. Adv Renal Replace Ther 1996; 3:266–8.

52. U.S. Renal Data System. USRDS 1992 annual data report, The National Institutes of Health, National Institute of Diabetes and Digestive and Kidney Diseases, Bethesda, MD, August 1992.

53. Lindblad AS, Hamilton RW, Nolph KD and Novak JW. A retrospective analysis of catheter configuration and cuff type: a National CAPD Registry report. Perit Dial Int 1988; 8:129–33.

54. Warady BA, Sullivan EK and Alexander SR. Lessons from the peritoneal dialysis patient database: a report of the North American pediatric renal transplant cooperative study. Kidney Int 1996; 49(Suppl. 53):S68–71.

55. Twardowski ZJ and Khanna R. Peritoneal dialysis access and exit site care. In Gokal R and Nolph KD, editors. The textbook of peritoneal dialysis. Dordrecht, Kluwer Academic Publishers, 1994; 271–314.

56. Golper TA, Brier ME, Bunke M et al. for the Academic Subcommittee of the Steering Committee of the Network 9 Peritonitis and Catheter Survival Studies. Risk factors for peritonitis in long-term peritoneal dialysis: the Network 9 peritonitis and catheter survival studies. Am J Kidney Dis 1996; 28:428–36.

57. Twardowski ZJ and Prowant BF. Exit-site healing post catheter implantation. Perit Dial Int 1996; 16(Suppl. 3): S51–70

58. Gokal R, Alexander S, Ash S et al. Peritoneal catheters and exit site practices toward optimum peritoneal access: 1998 update. Perit Dial Int 1998; 18:11–33.

59. Copley JB, Smith BJ, Koger DM, Rodgers DJ and Fowler M. Prevention of postoperative peritoneal dialysis catheter-related infections. Perit Dial Int 1998; 8:195–7.

60. Schmidt L, Prowant B, Schaefer R et al. An evaluation of nursing intervention for prevention of post operative peritoneal catheter exit site infections (abstract). ANNA J 1986; 13:98.

61. Jenson SR, Pomeroy M, Davidson M, Cox M and McMurray SD. Evaluation of dressing protocols that reduce peritoneal dialysis catheter exit site infections. ANNA J 1989; 16:425–31.

62. Starzomski R. Three techniques for peritoneal catheter exit site dressings. ANNA J 1984; 11:9–16.

63. Prowant BF, Schmidt LM, Twardowski ZJ et al. Peritoneal dialysis catheter exit site care. ANNA J 1988; 15:219–23.

64. Luzar MA, Brown C, Balf D et al. CAPD exit site care and exit-site infection in continuous ambulatory peritoneal dialysis (CAPD): results of a randomized multicenter trial. Perit Dial Int 1990; 10:25–9.

65. Fuchs J, Gallagher ME, Jackson-Bey D, Krawtz D and Schreiber MJ. A prospective randomized study of peritoneal catheter exit-site care. Dial Transplant 1990; 19:81–4.

66. Sewell CM, Clarridge J, Lacke C, Weinman EJ and Young EJ. Staphylococcal nasal carriage and subsequent infection in peritoneal dialysis patients. JAMA 1982; 248:1493–5.

67. Sesso R, Draibe S, Castelo A et al. Staphylococcus aureus skin carriage and development of peritonitis in patients on continuous ambulatory peritoneal dialysis. Clin Nephrol 1989; 31:264–8.

68. Davies SJ, Ogg CS, Cameron JS, Poston S and Noble WC. Staphylococcus aureus nasal carriage, exit-site infection and catheter loss in patients treated with continuous ambulatory peritoneal dialysis (CAPD). Perit Dial Int 1989; 9:61–4.

69. Luzar MA, Coles GA, Faller B et al. Staphylococcus aureus nasal carriage and infection in patients on continuous ambulatory peritoneal dialysis. New Engl J Med 1990; 322:505–9.

70. Swartz R, Messana J, Starmann B, Weber M and Reynolds J. Preventing Staphyloccus aureus infection during chronic peritoneal dialysis. J Am Soc Nephrol 1991; 2:1085–91.

71. Piraino B, Perlmutter JA, Holley JL and Bernardini J. Staphylococcus aureus peritonitis is associated with *Staphylococcus aureus* nasal carriage in peritoneal dialysis patients. Perit Dial Int 1993; 13(Suppl. 2):S332–4.

72. Zimmerman SW, O'Brien M, Wiedenhoeft FA and Johnson CA. Staphlococcus aureus peritoneal catheter-related infections: a cause of catheter loss and peritonitis. Perit Dial Int 1988; 8:191–4.

73. Zimmerman SW, Ahrens E, Johnson CA et al. Randomized controlled trial of prophylactic rifampin for peritoneal dialysis-related infections. Am J Kidney Dis 1991; 18:225–31.

74. Pérez-Fontán M, García-Falcón T, Rosales M et al. Treatment of Staphyloccus aureus nasal carriers in continuous ambulatory peritoneal dialysis with mupirocin: long-term results. Am J Kidney Dis 1993; 22:708–12.

75. Mupirocin Study Group. Nasal mupirocin prevents Staphylococcus aureus exit-site infection during peritoneal dialysis. J Am Soc Nephrol 1996; 2403–8.

76. Bernardini J, Piraino B, Holley J, Johnston JR and Lutes R. A randomized trial of Staphylococcus aureus prophylaxis in peritoneal dialysis patients: mupirocin calcium ointment 2% applied to the exit site versus cyclic oral rifampin. Am J Kidney Dis 1996; 27:695–700.

77. Maiorca R, Cantaluppi A, Cancarini GC et al. Prospective controlled trial of a Y-connector and disinfectant to prevent peritonitis in continuous ambulatory peritoneal dialysis. Lancet 1983; ii:642–4.

78. Canadian CAPD Clinical Trials Group. Peritonitis in continuous ambulatory peritoneal dialysis (CAPD): a multi-centre randomized clinical trial comparing the Y connector disinfectant system to standard systems. Perit Dial Int 1989; 9:159–63.

79. Keane WF, Alexander SR, Bailie GR et al. Peritoneal dialysis-related peritonitis treatment recommendations: 1996 update. Perit Dial Int 1996; 16:557–73.

80. Baxter Healthcare Corporation. The best demonstrated practices program peritonitis management and antibiotic therapy practices. Deerfield, IL; 1987.

81. Prowant BF and Twardowski ZJ. Recommendations for exit care. Perit Dial Int 1996; 16(Suppl. 3):S94–9.

82. Prowant BF. Nursing interventions related to peritoneal catheter exit-site infections. Adv Renal Replace Ther 1996; 3:228–31.

83. Teehan BP, Schleifer CR and Brown J. Adequacy of continuous ambulatory peritoneal dialysis: morbidity and mortality in chronic peritoneal dialysis. Am J Kidney Dis 1994; 24:990–1001.

84. Brandes JC, Piering WF, Beres JA, Blumenthal SS and Fritsche C. Clinical outcome of continuous peritoneal dialysis predicted by urea and creatinine kinetics. J Am Soc Nephrol 1992; 2:1430–5.

85. Maiorca R, Brunori G, Zubani R et al. Predictive value of dialysis adequacy and nutritionalindices for morbidity and mortality in CAPD and HD patients: a longitudinal study. Nephrol Dial Transplant 1995; 10:2295–305.

86. Lameire NH, Vanholder R, Veyt D, Lambert MC and Ringoir S. A longitudinal, five year survey of urea kinetic parameters in CAPD patients. Kidney Int 1992; 42:426–32.

87. Genestier S, Hedelin G, Schaffer P and Faller B. Prognostic factors in CAPD patients: a retrospective study of a 10-year period. Nephrol Dial Transplant 1995; 10:1905–11.

88. CANADA-USA (CANUSA) Peritoneal Dialysis Study Group. Adequacy of dialysis and nutrition in continuous peritoneal dialysis: association with clinical outcomes. J Am Soc Nephrol 1996; 7:198–207.

89. Nolph KD, Jensen RA, Khanna R and Twardowski ZJ. Weight limitations for weekly urea clearances using various exchange volumes in continuous ambulatory peritoneal dialysis. Perit Dial Int 1994; 14:261–4.

90. Twardowski ZJ and Nolph KD. Is peritoneal dialysis feasible once a large muscular patient becomes anuric? Perit Dial Int 1996; 16:20–3.

91. Jindal KK, Hirsch DJ. Long-term peritoneal dialysis in the absence of residual renal function. Perit Dial Int 1996; 16:78–89.

92. Tzamaloukas AH, Murata GH, Malhotra D, Fox L, Goldman RS and Avasthi PS. The minimal dose of dialysis required for a target KT/V in continuous peritoneal dialysis. Clin Nephrol 1995; 44:316–21.

93. Harty J, Boulton H, Venning M and Gokal R. Impact of increasing dialysis volume on adequacy targets: a prospective study. J Am Soc Nephrol 1997; 8:1304–10.

94. Keshaviah P. Establishing kinetic guidelines for peritoneal dialysis modality selection. Perit Dial Int 1997; 17(Suppl. 3):S53–7.

95. Burkart JM, Schreiber M, Korbet SM et al. Solute clearance approach to adequacy of peritoneal dialysis. Perit Dial Int 1996; 16:457–70.

96. Blake P, Burkart JM, Churchill DN et al. Recommended clinical practices for maximizing peritoneal dialysis clearances. Perit Dial Int 1996; 16:448–56.

97. Afthentopoulos IE, Oreopoulos DG. Is CAPD an effective treatment for ESRD patients with a weight over 80 kg? Clin Nephrol 1997; 47:389–93.

98. Henderson LW and Nolph KD. Altered permeability of the peritoneal membrane after using hypertonic peritoneal dialysis fluid. J Clin Invest 1969; 48:992–1001.

99. Garred LJ, Canaud B, Farrell PC. A simple kinetic model for assessing peritoneal mass transfer in chronic ambulatory peritoneal dialysis. ASAIO J 1983; 6:131–7.

100. Randerson DH and Farrell PC. Mass transfer properties of the human peritoneum. ASAIO J, 1980; 3:140–6.

101. Pyle WK. Mass transfer in peritoneal dialysis [dissertation]. Austin, Texas: University of Texas, 1981.

102. Pyle WK, Moncrief JW and Popovich RP. Peritoneal transport evaluation in CAPD. In Moncrief JW and Popovich RP, editors. CAPD Update: Continuous ambulatory peritoneal dialysis. New York, Masson Publishing, 1981; 35–52.

103. Popovich RP, Moncrief JW and Pyle WK. Transport kinetics. In Nolph KD, editor. Peritoneal dialysis, 3rd edn. Dordrecht, Kluwer Academic 1989; 96–116.

104. Rippe B and Stelin G. Simulations of peritoneal solute transport during CAPD. Application of a two-pore formalism. Kidney Int 1989; 35:1234–44.

105. Rippe B and Krediet RT. Peritoneal physiology-transport of solutes. In Gokal R and Nolph KD, editors. The textbook of peritoneal dialysis. Dordrecht, Kluwer Academic Publishers, 1994; 69–113.

106. Verger C, Larpent L and Dumontet M. Prognostic value of peritoneal equilibration curves in CAPD patients. In Maher JF and Winchester JF, editors. Frontiers in peritoneal dialysis. New York, Field, Rich and Associates, 1986; 88–93.

107. Twardowski ZJ, Nolph KD, Khanna R et al. Peritoneal equilibration test. Perit Dial Bull 1987; 7:138–47.

108. Gotch FA and Keen ML. Kinetic modeling in peritoneal dialysis. In Nissenson AR, Fine RN and Gentile DE, editors. Clinical dialysis, 3rd ed. Norwalk, CT, Appleton & Lange, 1995; 343–75.

109. Twardowski ZJ. Clinical value of standardized equilibration tests in CAPD patients. Blood Purif 1989; 7:95–108.

110. Twardowski ZJ. New approaches to intermittent peritoneal dialysis therapies. In Nolph KD, editor. Peritoneal dialysis, 3rd edn. Dordrecht, Kluwer Academic Publishers, 1989; 133–51.

111. Schmidt LM, Prowant BF. How to do a peritoneal equilibration test. ANNA J 18:368–70.

112. Diaz-Buxo JA. Peritoneal permeability in selecting peritoneal dialysis modalities. Perspectives in peritoneal dialysis 1988; 5:6–10.

113. Warady BA, Alexander SR, Hossli S et al. Peritoneal membrane transport function in children receiving long-term dialysis. J Am Soc Nephrol 1996; 7:2385–91.

114. Twardowski ZJ, Khanna R and Nolph KD. Peritoneal dialysis modifications to avoid CAPD drop-out. Adv Cont Ambul Perit Dial 1987; 3:171–8.
115. Twardowski ZJ. PET – A simpler approach for determining prescriptions for adequate dialysis therapy. Adv Perit Dial 1990; 6:186–91.
116. NKF-DOQI Clinical practice guidelines for peritoneal dialysis adequacy. Am J Kidney Dis 30 1997; (No.3 Suppl. 2): S67–136.
117. Vonesh EF, Burkart J, McMurray SD and Williams PF. Peritoneal dialysis kinetic modeling: validation in a multi-center clinical study. Perit Dial Int 1996; 16:471–81.
118. Burkart JM, Jordan JR and Rocco MV. Assessment of dialysis dose by measured clearance versus extrapolated data. Perit Dial Int 1993; 13:184–88.
119. Ponferrada L, Moore H, Van Stone J and Prowant B. Is there an alternative dialysate sampling method for Kt/V determination in CAPD patients (abstract). ANNA J 20:281.
120. Adequacy measures for adult peritoneal dialysis patients: supplemental Report No. 2, 1997. End stage renal disease (ESRD) core indicators project. Baltimore: Department of Health and Human Services Health Care Financing Administration Office of Clinical Standards and Quality, In press.
121. Health Care Financing Administration. 1997 annual report, end stage renal disease core indicators project. Baltimore: Department of Health and Human Services, Health Care Financing Administration, Office of Clinical Standards and Quality, December 1997.
122. Diaz-Buxo JA. Enhancement of peritoneal dialysis: the PD plus concept. Am J Kidney Dis 1996; 92–8.
123. Teehan BP, Schleifer CR, Brown JM, Sigler MH and Raimondo J. Urea kinetic analysis and clinical outcome on CAPD. A five year longitudinal study. Adv Perit Dial 1990; 6:181–5.
124. Spiegel DM, Anderson M, Campbell U et al. Serum albumin: a marker for morbidity in peritoneal dialysis patients. Am J Kidney Dis 1993; 21:26–30.
125. Blake PG, Flowerdew G, Blake RM and Oreopoulos DG. Serum albumin in patients on continuous ambulatory peritoneal dialysis – predictors and correlations with outcomes. J Am Soc Nephrol 1993; 3:1501–7.
126. Pollock CA, Allen BJ, Warden RA et al. Total-body nitrogen by neutron activation in maintenance dialysis. Am J Kidney Dis 1990; 16:38–45.
127. Sreedhara R, Avram MM, Blanco M, Batish R, Avram MM and Mittman N. Prealbumin is the best nutritional predictor of survival in hemodialysis and peritoneal dialysis. Am J Kidney Dis 1996; 28:937–42.
128. Chertow GM and Lazarus JM. Malnutrition as a risk factor for morbidity and mortality in maintenance dialysis patients. In Kopple JD and Massry SG, editors. Nutritional management of renal disease. Baltimore, Williams & Wilkins 1997; 257–76.
129. Gamba G, Mejia JL, Saldivar S, Pena JC and Correa-Rotter R. Death risk in CAPD patients. Nephron 1993; 65:23–7.
130. Spiegel DM and Breyer JA. Serum albumin: a predictor of long-term outcome in peritoneal dialysis patients. Am J Kidney Dis 1994; 23:283–5.
131. Avram MM, Goldwasser P, Erroa M and Fein PA. Predictors of survival in continuous ambulatory peritoneal dialysis patients: the importance of prealbumin and other nutritional and metabolic markers. Am J Kidney Dis 1994; 23:91–8.
132. Lindholm B and Bergström J. Nutritional management of patients undergoing peritoneal dialysis. In Nolph, KD, editor. Peritoneal dialysis, 3rd edn. Dordrecht, Kluwer Academic Publishers, 1989; 230–60.
133. Marckmann P. Nutritional status of patients on hemodialysis and peritoneal dialysis. Clin Nephrol 1988; 29:75–8.
134. Lindholm B and Bergström J. Nutritional aspects on peritoneal dialysis. Kidney Int 1992; 42:S165–71.
135. Schilling H, Wu G, Pettit J et al. Nutritional status of patients on long-term CAPD. Perit Dial Int 1985; 5:12–18.
136. Fenton SSA, Johnston N, Delmore T et al. Nutritional assessment of continuous ambulatory peritoneal dialysis patients. Trans Am Soc Artif Intern Organs 1987; 33:650–3.
137. Young GA, Kopple JD, Lindholm B et al. Nutritional assessment of continuous ambulatory peritoneal dialysis patients: an international study. Am J Kidney Dis 1991; 17:462–71.
138. Wolfson M. Causes, manifestations, and assessment of malnutrition in chronic renal failure. In Kopple JD and Massry SG, editors. Nutritional management of renal disease. Baltimore, Williams & Wilkins, 1997: 245–56.
139. Dombros NV, Digenis GE and Oreopoulos DG. Nutritional markers as predictors of survival in patients on CAPD. Perit Dial Int 1995; 15(No.5 Suppl.):S10–19.
140. Bargman JM. The rationale and ultimate limitations of urea kinetic modelling in the estimation of nutritional status. Per Dial Int 1996; 16:347–51.
141. Ikizler TA, Wingard RL and Hakim RM. Malnutrition in peritoneal dialysis patients: etiologic factors and treatment options. Perit Dial Int 1995; 15(No.5 Suppl.):S63–6.
142. Heimbürger O, Lindholm B and Bergström J. Nutritional effects and nutritional management of chronic peritoneal dialysis. In Kopple JD and Massry SG, editors. Nutritional management of renal disease. Baltimore, Williams & Wilkins, 1997; 619–68.
143. Nolph KD, Moore HL, Prowant B et al. Cross sectional assessment of weekly urea and creatinine clearances and indices of nutrition in continuous ambulatory peritoneal dialysis patients. Perit Dial Int 1993; 13:178–83.
144. Kagan A, Bar-Khayim Y, Schafe Z et al. Heterogeneity in peritoneal transport during continuous ambulatory peritoneal dialysis and its impact on ultrafiltration, loss of macromolecules and plasma level or proteins, lipids and lipoproteins. Nephron 1993; 63:32–42.
145. Struijk DG, Krediet RT, Koomen GCM et al. Functional characteristics of the peritoneal membrane in long term continuous ambulatory peritoneal dialysis. Nephron 1991; 59:213–20.
146. BurkartJM. Effect of peritoneal dialysis prescription and peritoneal membrane transport characteristics on nutritional status. Perit Dial Int 1995; (No.5 Suppl.):S20–35.

147. Malhotra D, Tzamaloukas AH, Murata GH, Fox L, Goldman RS and Avasthi PS. Serum albumin in continuous peritoneal dialysis: Its predictors and relationship to urea clearance. Kidney Int 1996; 50:243–9.

148. Churchill DN, Thorpe KE, Nolph KD, Keshaviah PR, Oreopoulos DG and Pagé D for the Canada-USA (CANUSA) peritoneal dialysis study group. Increased peritoneal membrane transport is associated with decreased patient and technique survival for continuous ambulatory peritoneal dialysis patients.

149. Schmicker R. Nutritional treatment of hemodialysis and peritoneal dialysis patients. Artificial Organs 1995; 19:837–41.

150. Schreiber MJ Jr. Nutrition and dialysis adequacy. Per Dial Int 1995; 15(No.5 Suppl.):S39–49.

151. Lowrie EG. Chronic dialysis treatment: clinical outcome and related processes of care. Am J Kidney Dis 1994; 255–66.

152. Daines MM, Wilkens K and Cheney C. Comparison of 1983 and 1992 renal dietitian staffing levels with patient morbidity and mortality. J Renal Nutrition 1996; 6:94–102.

153. Kopple JD. Uses and limitations of growth factors in renal failure. Perit Dial Int 1996; S63–6.

154. Soliman G and Oreopoulos DG. Anabolic steroids and malnutrition in chronic renal failure. Perit Dial Int 1994; 362–5.

155. Dombros NV, Digenis GE, Soliman G and Oreopoulos DG. Anabolic steroids in the treatment of malnourished CAPD patients: a retrospective study. Perit Dial Int 1994; 14:344–7.

156. Walls J. Metabolic acidosis and uremia. Perit Dial Int 1995; (No.5 Suppl.):S36–8.

157. Graham KA, Reaich D, Channon SM et al. Correction of acidosis in CAPD decreases whole body protein degradation. Kidney Int 1996; 49:1396–400.

158. McGriff C, Goodman D, Ting Ko W et al. CQI process decreases malnutrition in peritoneal dialysis patient population (abstract). Perit Dial Int 1996; 16(Suppl. 1):S85.

159. Sasak C. Patient participation in a CQI process to improve serum albumin. Presentation at the 18th Annual PD Conference, Nashville, TN, February 25,1998.

160. Health Care Financing Administration. Highlights from the 1995 ESRD core indicators project for peritoneal dialysis patients. Baltimore, Department of Health and Human Services, Health Care Financing Administration, Office of Clinical Standards and Quality, May 1996.

161. Health Care Financing Administration. Highlights from the 1996 ESRD core indicators project for peritoneal dialysis patients. Baltimore, Department of Health and Human Services, Health Care Financing Administration, Office of Clinical Standards and Quality, January 1997.

162. Health Care Financing Administration. Highlights from the 1997 ESRD core indicators project for peritoneal dialysis patients. Baltimore, Department of Health and Human Services, Health Care Financing Administration, Office of Clinical Standards and Quality, October 1997.

163. Rocco MV, Flanigan MJ, Beaver S et al. Report form the 1995 core indicators for peritoneal dialysis study group. Am J Kidney Dis 1997; 20:165–73.

164. The U.S. Renal Data System. USRDS 1997 annual data report. Bethesda, MD, National Institutes of Health, National Institute of Diabetes and Digestive and Kidney Diseases, April 1997.

165. D'Apice AJF and Atkins RC. Analysis of peritoneal dialysis data. In Atkins RC, Thomson NM and Farrell PC, editors. Peritoneal dialysis, Edinburgh, Churchill Livingstone, 1981:440–4.

166. Corey P. An approach to the statistical analysis of peritonitis data from patients on CAPD. Perit Dial Bull 1981; 1:S29–32.

167. Pierratos A, Amair P, Corey P, Vas SI, Khanna R and Oreopoulos DG. Statistical analysis of the incidence of peritonitis on continuous ambulatory peritoneal dialysis. Perit Dial Bull 1982; 2:32–6.

168. Gray JS and Nickles JR. Improving infection control in a PD unit. Nephrol News Iss 1995; 9:14–18.

169. Benson B and Lutz N. CQI process helps identify patient training as a requirement for improving peritonitis management (abstract). Perit Dial Int 1997; 17(Suppl. 1):S42.

170. Pagnotta-Lee R, Hershfeld S, Fitzsimmmons D and Manners D. Implementing changes in a PD program to improve peritonitis rates (abstract). Perit Dial Int 1998;18(Suppl. 1):S33.

171. Hall G., Lee S, Davachi F et al. Continuous quality improvement (CQI) process helps to improve peritonitis rates (abstract). Perit Dial Int 1998; 18(Suppl. 1):S58.

172. Holland LP. Implementation of a quality improvement (QI) audit to improve episodes of peritonitis (EOP) (abstract). Perit Dial Int 1998; 18(Suppl. 1):S58.

173. Street JK, Krupka DL, Broda L et al. Utilizing the CQI process to decrease episodes of peritonitis (abstract). Perit Dial Int 1998; 18(Suppl. 1):S59.

174. Chemleski B, Enrico R, Montes P et al. Continuous quality improvement (CQI) demonstration project: peritonitis rate in the home dialysis unit (abstract). Perit Dial Int 1996; 16(Suppl. 2):S84.

175. Thompson MC and Speaks DD. Exit site infections reduced through CQI exit site care study (abstract). Perit Dial Int 1997; 17(Suppl. 1):S46.

176. Boorgu NR and Liles V. CQI initiated focusing on exit-site infection (abstract). Perit Dial Int 1998; 18(Suppl. 1):S59.

177. Martin P, McGauvran J and Reimer L. CQI impacts exit-site infection (abstract). Perit Dial Int 1998; 18(Suppl. 1): S59

178. Wageman J, Martin M, Mathews M et al. CQI impacts peritoneal dialysis adequacy (abstract). Perit Dial Int 1997; 17(Suppl. 1):S77.

179. Zilber M, Bander S and Marion R. Applying the CQI process to improve adequacy outcomes (abstract). Perit Dial Int 1997; 17(Suppl. 1):S78.

180. Alvarado N, Mendez N, Roberts BW and Dukes C. CQI process helps improve dialysis adequacy in adult and pediatric peritoneal dialysis population (abstract). Perit Dial Int 1997; 17(Suppl. 1):S12.

181. Quinonez IM, Bencomo ME, Candelaria G, Hage D and Olsen K. CQI process helps define relationship between PD adequacy and dialysis-related hospitalizations and dropout rate (abstract). Perit Dial Int 1997; 17(Suppl. 1):S21.

182. Richmond DJS, Poseno M, Shea S, Schultz K, Kutchey C and Smith P. What can we do to improve Kt/V's? (abstract). Perit Dial Int 1997; 17(Suppl. 1):S22.
183. Viker D, Gill P, Faley G Hartvikson S, Morrissey M. Improving adequacy markers utilizing the CQI process (abstract). Perit Dial Int 1997; 17(Suppl. 1):S25.
184. Hebah N. The challenge to improve adequacy markers in noncompliant PD patients (abstract). Perit Dial Int 1998; 18(Suppl. 1):S17.
185. Brothers SE, Saylor ZE, Heacock PM et al. Continuous quality improvement of peritoneal dialysis: improving adequacy through patient and staff education (abstract). Perit Dial Int 1998; 18(Suppl. 1):S57.
186. Faley G, and Viker DM. Restructuring patient training to improve patient outcomes (abstract). Perit Dial Int 1998; 18(Suppl. 1):S60.

22. The critical role of prescription management in a peritoneal dialysis program

ROSALIE VILLANO, TERESA DUNHAM AND SALIM MUJAIS

INTRODUCTION

Prescription management for patients on renal replacement therapy requires consideration of a wide range of interrelated conditions including dialysis therapy, medications for co-morbid conditions and nutrition. Optimal outcomes cannot be achieved by focusing on solute clearances alone because outcomes are dependent on a constellation of factors related to control of the patient's disease. Hence, the adequacy of dialysis involves attention to controling co-morbid conditions as well as correction of the consequences of renal failure. Table 22.1 contains a partial list of the components of adequacy in renal replacement therapy. While dialysis addresses many of these components, additional measures are necessary to attain optimal outcomes. Blood pressure control, improved anemia, and better calcium-phosphate metabolism are achievable through adequate dialysis prescription, but additional antihypertensive therapy, erythropoietin administration and increased vitamin D intake are essential for optimal care. Thus, while the present chapter focuses on the elements of dialysis prescription management, the recommendations discussed herein must always be taken in the context of overall patient management.

PRESCRIPTION AND OUTCOMES

The correlation between peritoneal dialysis prescription and patient outcome is not as certain as common sense would imply. While it can be readily accepted that volume control by dialysis is crucial to optimal outcome, the dose of solute removal required for such outcomes remains a subject of debate. Except for transplantation, renal replacement therapies can hardly approach the functions delivered by the native kidney. Historically, we have attempted to provide a level of renal function replacement that may mimic a level of endogenous renal function compatible with survival. Because of technical limitations, this goal has until recently been modest. With improvements in our understanding of dialysis delivery and advances in dialysis technology, higher levels of replacement can be achieved along with improved outcomes.

While the relationship between clearance levels and patient outcomes may continue to be debated (and the best indicators of clearance even more), sound clinical practice would dictate that patients be offered the best care within the constraints of available technology, knowledge and cost. Several authoritative recommendations have been presented towards this goal, and it is generally agreed that we should strive to attain a clear set of goals. These goals were first formulated by the Ad Hoc Committee on Peritoneal Dialysis Adequacy, a

Table 22.1. Components of dialysis adequacy

- Cardiovascular risk reduction
- Control of co-morbid conditions
- Solute removal
- Volume control
- Nutrition
- Anemia correction
- Bone disease prevention

L.W. Henderson and R.S. Thuma (eds.), Quality Assurance in Dialysis, 2nd Edition, 245–256.
© 1999 *Kluwer Academic Publishers. Printed in Great Britain*

group convened to recommend clinical practices that would improve PD as a long term renal replacement therapy. The Ad Hoc Committee concluded that rather than focus on a single numerical target, "the recommended clinical practice is to provide the most dialysis that can be delivered to the individual patient, within the constraints of social and clinical circumstances, quality of life, life-style and cost" [1]. The National Kidney Foundation Dialysis Outcome Quality Initiative (NKF-DOQI™) attempted to develop clearance targets for PD as part of their effort to define optimal clinical practices. The NKF-DOQI™ guidelines for PD Adequacy are shown in Table 22.2 [2].

Table 22.2. Weekly total solute clearance targets recommended by the NKF-DOQI™ clinical practice guidelines for PD adequacy

	CAPD	CCPD	NIPD
Kt/V_{urea}	≥ 2.0/wk	≥ 2.1/wk	≥ 2.2/wk
$C_{cr}/1.73\ m^2$	≥ 60 L/wk	≥ 63 L/wk	≥ 66 L/wk

It has become apparent that many patients do not achieve these clearance targets with the outdated standard PD prescription of four 2 L exchanges (4×2 L). The new targets have focused attention on individualized prescriptions as an essential component for the long term success of PD.

THE IMPORTANCE OF PRESCRIPTION MANAGEMENT

Peritoneal dialysis (PD) was introduced as a simple way to dialyze patients at home in the late 1970s. At that time, the basic four exchange by 2 L regime (4×2L) was used as a "one size fits all" prescription philosophy. With the advent of knowledge comes change, and the need to individually prescribe PD according to specific patient characteristics has become clear with the recognition of the significant effect clearance, achieved by altering prescription, has on patient outcome. In finding that higher total clearances (renal and peritoneal) are associated with superior patient survival and lower hospitalization, attention focused on the need to achieve higher clearances through individually tailored prescription management issue. This recognition has resulted in a significant change in the way PD is prescribed. Today, product improvements including automated exchange systems and alternate osmotic agent solutions, give physicians and patients more flexibility in prescription choices.

THE PRESCRIPTION MANAGEMENT PROCESS

Prescription management, including consideration of clinical, nutritional and clearance parameters, must be an ongoing and integral part of everyday patient management [3]. Thus, a process that integrates prescription management into the daily unit routine will focus attention on good prescription management practices which are essential to the long term success of every PD program.

The prescription management process involves three basic steps (Figure 22.1) [4]:

1. assessing the patient,

2. individualizing the prescription based on the patient's BSA, amount of residual renal function (RRF) and peritoneal membrane type, and

3. monitoring the patient regularly, adjusting the prescription as necessary.

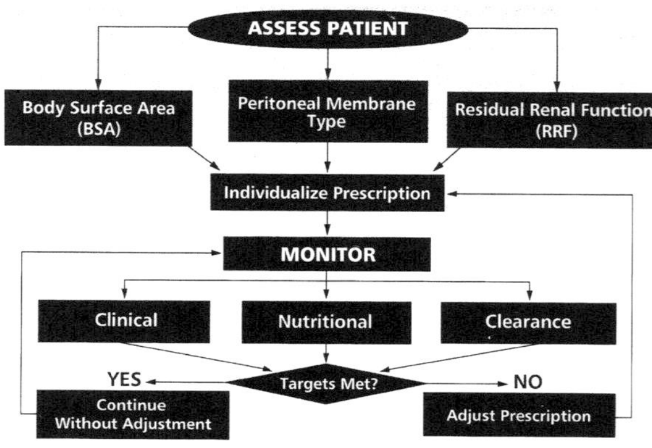

Fig. 22.1. The prescription management process.

Step One: Assessing the Patient for Appropriate Prescription

Patient factors affecting prescription
The peritoneal dialysis prescription is affected by patient factors which cannot be altered such as body size, amount of residual renal function, peritoneal membrane characteristics and co-morbid conditions. While these factors cannot be changed, they do need to be considered when establishing the prescription. While lifestyle is not a "fixed" factor per se, lifestyle considerations are a critical factor in patient compliance and thus therapy success.

Determining the prescription involves assessing the patient's body size, level of RRF and peritoneal membrane type, as well as performing a clinical and nutritional assessment of the patient's condition. At subsequent visits, patient assessment includes clinical, nutritional and clearance components.

Body size
Body size has a fundamental effect on the amount of dialysis required. Larger patients require more dialysis than smaller patients in order to achieve equivalent clinical benefits. Body surface area (BSA) as a determinant of patient size, can be easily determined from the patient's height and weight using the formula developed by DuBois [5]. Historically, 1.73 m^2 has been used as the average body size when discussing prescriptions; however, in a study of 806 adult U.S. patients, 75% were larger than this with 1.85 m^2 the median BSA [1]. This finding supports the importance of individualized rather than standard "one size fits all" prescriptions.

Residual renal function
The CANUSA Study [6] found that renal clearance made a significant contribution to total solute clearance and highlighted the need for dialysis practitioners to adjust prescriptions as RRF declines. Even small amounts of RRF make it easier to obtain clearance targets and are thus very important. For example, each one mL/min of creatinine clearance adds approximately 10 L/week of clearance for a 70 kg person and 1 mL/min of urea clearance adds 0.25 to the total weekly Kt/V urea for a person of this same size [3]. While the equivalence of renal and peritoneal clearance has not been formally proven, it is generally accepted that an increase in peritoneal clearance will compensate for a decline in residual renal clearance. RRF must be monitored regularly so that the prescription can be adjusted as needed. Thus, every measure to protect residual renal function should be considered. The inadvertent use of non-steroidal drugs, unnecessary prolonged gentamicin administration, avoidable contrast dye studies and volume contraction should be assiduously avoided.

Peritoneal membrane transport characteristics
The rate at which a patient's peritoneal membrane transports solutes has a significant impact on clearance and hence prescription. Membrane transport characteristics vary between individuals and must be assessed in each patient. The Peritoneal Equilibration Test (PET) [7] is used to classify the patient's peritoneal membrane into one of four types, each with unique transport characteristics (Figure 22.2). The PET should be performed after the first month of therapy. Of the four membrane types, high transport membranes are the most efficient and transport solutes the quickest. However, patients with high transport membranes may have difficulty achieving ultrafiltration because of

Patients (%)	Membrane type	4 hour D/P creatinine	Characteristics
10	High	0.81–1.03	– Very efficient membrane – Transports solutes quickly – Increased glucose absorption – May have difficulty achieving ultrafiltration – At risk for low serum albumin
53	High average	0.65–0.81	– Efficient membrane – Transports solutes well – Ultrafilters well
31	Low average	0.50–0.64	– Less efficient membrane – Transports solutes somewhat slowly – Ultrafilters well
6	Low	0.34–0.49	– Inefficient membrane – Transports solutes slowly – Difficult to obtain clearances when RRF equals zero – Ultrafilters very well

Fig. 22.2. Peritoneal membrane characteristics.

the rapid dissipation of the osmotic gradient (glucose). At the other extreme, low transport membranes are inefficient and transport solutes slowly. These low transport membranes, however, are efficient at ultrafiltration because they maintain the osmotic gradient for a longer period due to the low absorption of glucose. In between the two extremes are the high average and low average membranes. The vast majority of patients (84%) have high average or low average membranes [4]. If the initial prescription assumes an average transport, a large percentage of patients will achieve the target clearance even before their transport type is known.

Therapy factors affecting prescription

Fill volume

Higher fill volume achieves three important effects: 1) it assures recruitment of the whole peritoneal surface; 2) it prevents rapid buildup of removed solutes thereby allowing further removal of toxins; 3) it attenuates the dissipation of the glucose gradient, thus more glucose is present which promotes ultrafiltration. A limitation of increases in fill volume is a slight increase in intra-abdominal pressure. Increasing fill volume from 2 to 3 L increases intra-abdominal pressure by 2.12 cm H_2O, a value too small to have significant physiologic impact [8].

The main barriers to increasing fill volume are residual dogmas that when tested are clearly conjectural. Clinical studies have shown that when tested under blinded conditions, patients are unable to accurately predict fill volume [9]. Further, while there has been a major increase in

Table 22.3. Strategies for increasing fill volume

- Increase fill volume at times of least activity (e.g. night)
- Use lower percent dextrose with larger fill volumes to decrease total drained volumes
- Change fill volumes in 200 cc increments to help the patient acclimate
- Positively reinforce success
- Educate patients regarding benefits of using larger fill volumes

the use of larger fill volume solutions in recent years, there has been no increase in reported associated complications. There are several approaches to increase fill volume (Table 22.3).

Dwell time

Diffusive transport is time dependent, particularly for larger solutes, but even for urea. Failure to appreciate the importance of appropriate dwell time is a common error in APD prescriptions. Figure 22.3 illustrates the impact of prolonging dwell time on the number of exchanges required to reach a target Kt/V of 2.1 in a 70 kg male [10].

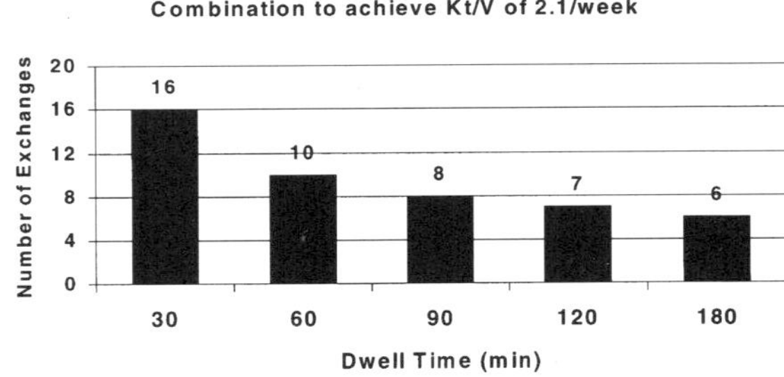

Fig. 22.3. Dwell time and clearance targets.

Solution type

Modern peritoneal dialysis solutions employ a variety of osmotic agents. In their current formulation all of these solutions have on average similar diffusive properties. They do differ in ultrafiltration profile and as such can influence convective transport as well as attainment of proper fluid balance management that is an important component of prescription management. Figure 22.4 illustrates the impact of various concentrations of glucose on ultrafiltration [11]. A higher ultrafiltration rate is translated into increased clearance. Figure 22.5 illustrates the ultrafiltration profile and achieved solute clearance in CCPD patients using icodextrin instead of a standard glucose solution during the daytime dwell [12]. The newer high molecular weight osmotic agent icodextrin allows maintenance of sustained osmotic gradient for a longer time period due to its action by colloid osmosis and its very slow reabsorption (by the lymphatic system) are ideal for long dwell periods with both CAPD and APD. Newer solutions, such

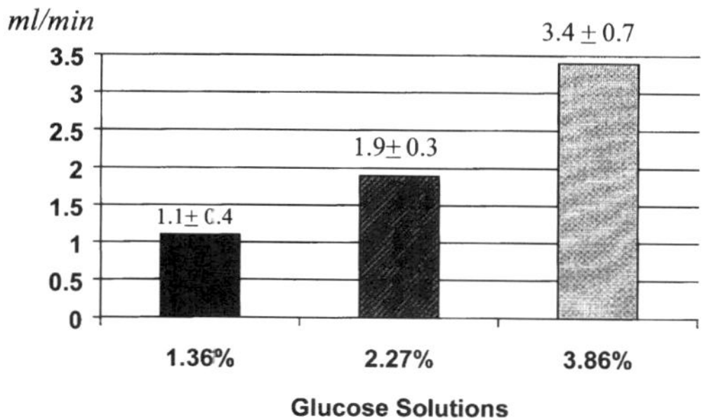

Fig. 22.4. Effects of different solutions on ultrafiltration.

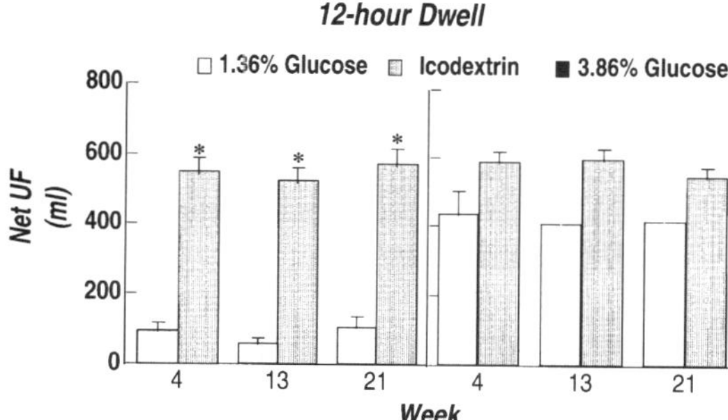

Fig. 22.5. Net overnight ultrafiltration with glucose icodextrin exchanges.

as amino acid solutions, hold promise for patients with more demanding nutritional needs. Use of these solutions should be evaluated in the context of patient needs.

Step Two: Individualizing the Prescription

The initial prescription should be based on the patient's body size and level of residual renal function and an average membrane type should be assumed. BSA can be easily determined from standard tables and RRF residual renal function can be easily determined using a 24 hour urine collection. Peritoneal membrane transport type using the PET should be assessed at the first month's clinic visit.

Prescriptions can be individualized using algorithms that consider patient size, membrane type and amount of residual renal function or computer

models such as PD Adequest can be used. Computer models make it possible to predict the amount of clearance that would be achieved with various prescription options. PD Adequest has been repeatedly validated on large patient databases for both CAPD and APD, and its use is highly recommended [13].

In an attempt to determine if clearance targets could be achieved with prescriptions that would not place an unreasonable burden on patients, data from 806 randomly selected adult PD patients from 39 U.S. centers was used to identify 12 "typical" patients for modeling. The 12 patients were based on 4 PET classifications (high, high average, low average and low) and three patient BSA categories. The modeling results revealed that by individualizing prescriptions, target adequate clearance could be achieved in almost all patients, including patients with no RRF and patients with large body size, contrary to frequently cited dogma

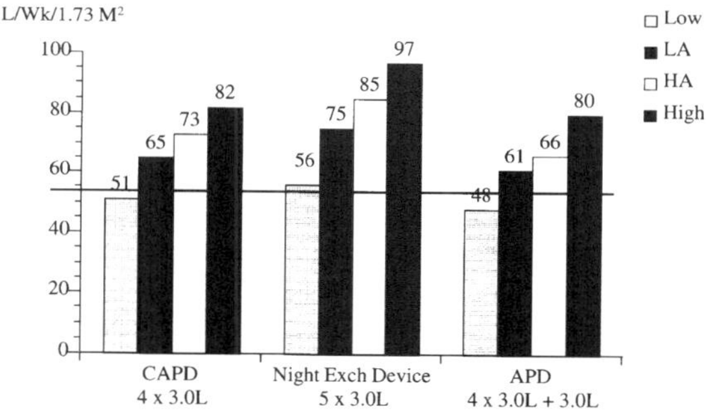

Fig. 22.6. Creatinine clearance: BSA 1.71–2.0 m^2; no RRF

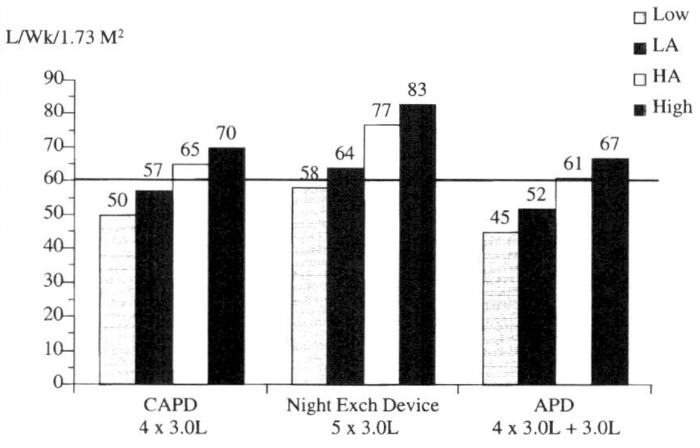

Fig. 22.7. Creatinine clearance: BSA >2.0 m^2; no RRF

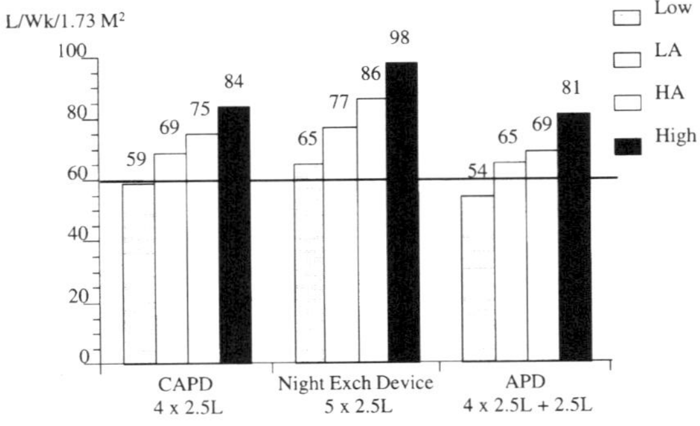

Fig. 22.8. Creatinine clearance: BSA > 2.0 m^2; 14 L RRF

[1]. For the majority of patients, several prescriptions allowed the patient to meet acceptable clearance, lifestyle and cost criteria. Figures 22.6 and 22.7 present the results of modeling of average and large sized patients with no RRF, demonstrating that clearance targets can be met by individualizing the prescription. Figure 22.8 presents the results of modeling of a large size patient with 14 L/week residual renal creatinine clearance and illustrates the enormous impact residual renal function has on a patient's prescription options.

Step Three: Monitoring the Patient and Prescription Adjustment

Monitoring the clinical status, nutritional status and level of clearance achieved are essential components of good prescription management practices.

Clinical assessment
Routine clinical assessment of the PD patient should include review and management of the following:

- co-morbid disease

- anemia

- weight and fluid balance

- patients' ultrafiltration response to dextrose

- routine labs

- presence/absence of: nausea/vomiting, insomnia, muscle weakness, anorexia, excess fatigue

- Ca/PO$_4$ balance

- blood pressure control

- exit site and catheter function

- current medications

Nutritional assessment
Nutritional status plays a key role in patient well-being and can be assessed by monitoring serum albumin level, dietary protein intake and performance of the subjective global assessment (SGA). SGA and serum albumin have been statistically correlated with outcomes. Serum albumin measurements are affected by dietary protein intake, rate of albumin synthesis and catabolism, albumin losses in the dialysate and urine, intravascular volume, and laboratory methodology.

Nutritional assessment of the patient involves reviewing the diet history as well as an evaluation of food intake and the need for dietary intervention. There are two methods to assess nutrient intake: diet history and measurement of normalized protein appearance (nPNA). In the stable patient, nPNA reflects the dietary protein intake. Studies have shown positive nitrogen balance when nPNA is greater than or equal to 0.9–1.1 gram per kilogram per day [14–16].

The Subjective Global Assessment is a simple and reliable tool to rate the nutritional status of the patient subjectively based on the patient's medical and physical history. SGA ratings have been shown to be a reliable nutritional assessment tool for dialysis patients [17, 18], with a higher SGA score correlated with a lower risk of death [6].

Clearance assessment
Clearance assessment involves determining if the patient is achieving clearance targets that will insure good patient outcomes. A 24 hour dialysate and urine collection should be performed and weekly clearance indices calculated. For those patients with renal function, their residual function is added to the calculated dialysate clearance to determine their total clearance.

Selecting a Measure of Clearance Assessment: Kt/V and/or CrCl?

Clearance targets for urea and creatinine may not be achieved simultaneously in an individual patient. This is due to differences inherent to measurements of urea and creatinine. Measures of residual creatinine clearance overestimate the glomerular filtration rate (GFR) because of tubular secretion of creatinine. Conversely, urea clearance underestimates GFR because of tubular reabsorption of urea. Also, because transport of creatinine across the peritoneal membrane is slower than for urea, it is more difficult to achieve peritoneal creatinine clearance than peritoneal urea clearance. The shorter dwell times used in automated peritoneal dialysis (APD) accentuate this difference.

In the CANUSA study, creatinine clearance, normalized to BSA, was a stronger predictor of outcomes than was Kt/V [6]. No data definitively supports the use of one measure of clearance over another at this time. Kt/V as an accurate assessment of clearance is affected by the difficulty in measuring body water (V). V can be calculated using anthropomorphic formulae; however, these result in gender-specific targets for equal sized males and females. On the other hand, reliance on creatinine clearance for measurement of required clearance may lead to delays in initiation of dialysis.

At the current recommendations of starting dialysis when endogenous creatinine clearance is 10–15 mL/min, weekly clearance is clearly above the target to be achieved by dialysis. To reconcile the target to be achieved with endogenous clearance, renal Kt/V needs to be used at these higher levels of residual renal function. Each of the two measures has serious limitations, and the search for better ways of measuring delivered solute clearance needs to continue. Whatever measure is used to assess therapy effectiveness, it is essential that the measure of clearance target is used in conjunction with an ongoing assessment of the patient's clinical state.

A guide for monitoring the care of PD patients beginning with when the patient is first seen in the dialysis center is shown in Figure 22.9 [4]. This guide contains recommendations for assessing the

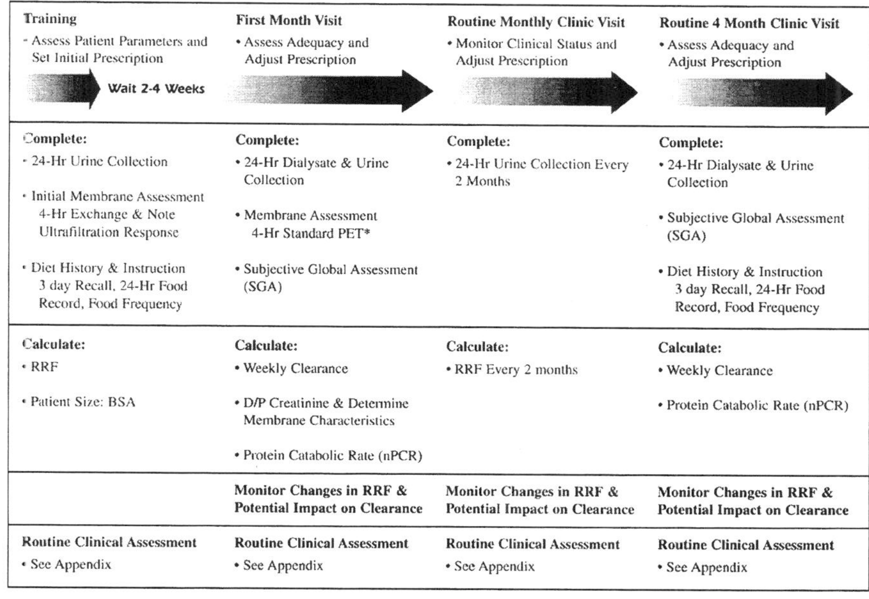

Training	First Month Visit	Routine Monthly Clinic Visit	Routine 4 Month Clinic Visit
- Assess Patient Parameters and Set Initial Prescription **Wait 2-4 Weeks**	• Assess Adequacy and Adjust Prescription	• Monitor Clinical Status and Adjust Prescription	• Assess Adequacy and Adjust Prescription
Complete: - 24-Hr Urine Collection • Initial Membrane Assessment 4-Hr Exchange & Note Ultrafiltration Response • Diet History & Instruction 3 day Recall, 24-Hr Food Record, Food Frequency	**Complete:** • 24-Hr Dialysate & Urine Collection • Membrane Assessment 4-Hr Standard PET* • Subjective Global Assessment (SGA)	**Complete:** • 24-Hr Urine Collection Every 2 Months	**Complete:** • 24-Hr Dialysate & Urine Collection • Subjective Global Assessment (SGA) • Diet History & Instruction 3 day Recall, 24-Hr Food Record, Food Frequency
Calculate: • RRF • Patient Size: BSA	**Calculate:** • Weekly Clearance • D/P Creatinine & Determine Membrane Characteristics • Protein Catabolic Rate (nPCR)	**Calculate:** • RRF Every 2 months	**Calculate:** • Weekly Clearance • Protein Catabolic Rate (nPCR)
	Monitor Changes in RRF & Potential Impact on Clearance	**Monitor Changes in RRF & Potential Impact on Clearance**	**Monitor Changes in RRF & Potential Impact on Clearance**
Routine Clinical Assessment • See Appendix	**Routine Clinical Assessment** • See Appendix	**Routine Clinical Assessment** • See Appendix	**Routine Clinical Assessment** • See Appendix

*A baseline PET should be completed at the First Month Clinic Visit[5]. If later findings suggest changes in peritoneal transport a repeat PET will be necessary. These later findings include unexpected changes in 24-Hr D/P, 24-Hr volume, or dialysis clearance.

Fig. 22.9. Time line for PD prescription management

three components of prescription management: clinical, nutritional and clearance. Monitoring of these three components is also helpful in evaluating patient compliance. It is important to remember that all monitoring guidelines are exactly that– guidelines– and they should never be relied on to replace good clinical judgment. Depending on patient requirements, more frequent monitoring and prescription adjustment may be necessary.

Adjusting the Prescription to Meet Targets

At the routine monthly visit, a prescription adjustment may be necessary depending on the patient's clinical symptoms, nutritional status and clearance indices (Figure 22.10). If the patient is adhering to the prescription, but not meeting targets, the prescription should be adjusted.

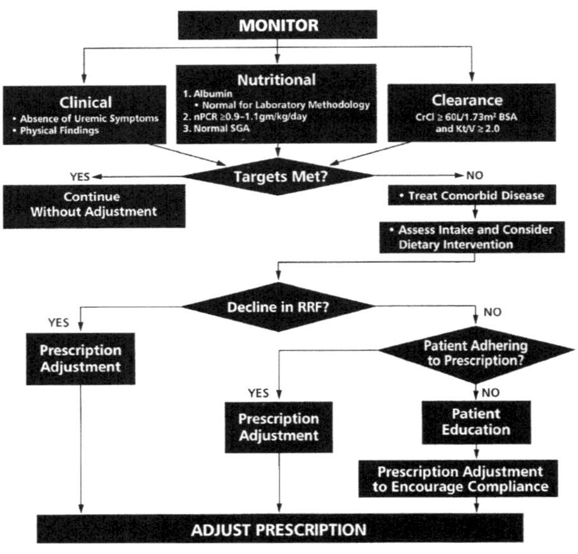

Fig. 22.10. Process for patient monitoring and prescription adjustment at the routine monthly visit.

Increasing fill volume is the most efficient way to increase clearance in CAPD patients. This approach increases delivered clearance significantly and has the advantage of not altering the therapy routine making adherence to the prescription more likely. Increasing the number of daily exchanges can also increase clearance, but this strategy is less efficient. For example, in a patient with a BSA of 1.86 m^2, with no RRF, increasing

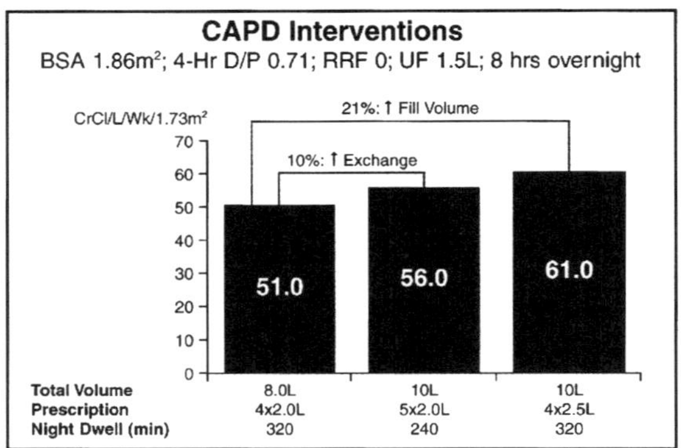

Fig. 22.11. CAPD interventions. Using larger fill volumes is a more efficient strategy for increasing weekly clearance than is adding an exchange.

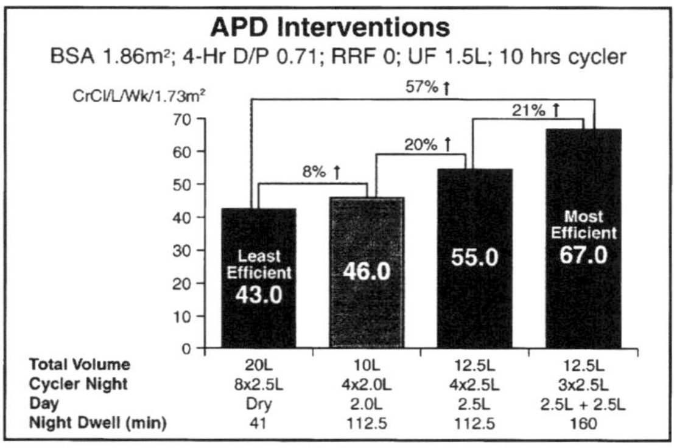

Fig. 22.12. By efficiently using the entire 24 hour day, more clearance can be achieved using 12.5 L of solution than by using 20 L.

fill volume from 2.0 L to 2.5 L increases clearance 21%. However, increasing the number of daily exchanges from 4 to 5 daily increases clearance by only 10% (Figure 22.11) [4]. CAPD patients can also increase clearance by use of a simple automated device that performs an exchange while the patient is sleeping.

For patients on APD, use of larger fill volumes and use of the peritoneal membrane during the entire 24 hour day can maximize clearance. Figure 22.12 illustrates inefficient and efficient prescriptions.[4] Efficient use of the entire 24 hours requires use of a daytime dwell (a "wet" day) and in some cases, a daytime exchange. "Dry" days result in lost dialysis time, and it is rare for a patient to achieve adequate clearance with a dry day.

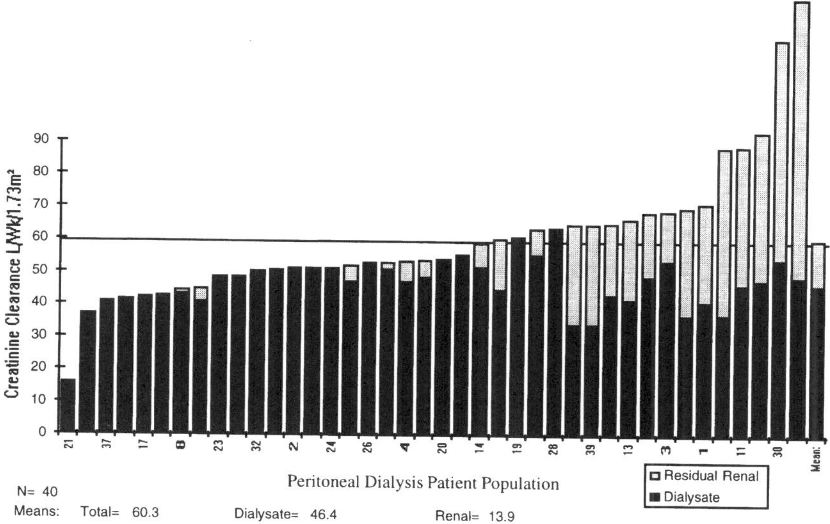

Fig. 22.13. Baseline weekly creatinine clearance in one center.

There are reports of maintaining patients with ultrafiltration failure on PD using solution containing icodextrin as the osmotic agent [19], thus its use for these patients is recommended in areas where available. Solutions containing this glucose polymer can also be used to reduce glucose load. Other new solutions should be considered a part of the dialysis prescription, and need to be included in the process when prescription changes are required. These solutions should be evaluated in the context of prescription adjustment as patient condition dictates.

EVALUATING THE PRESCRIPTION MANAGEMENT PROCESS WITH CQI

The Continuous Quality Improvement (CQI) process linked to a quality assurance program should can be used to implement, follow-up and enhance a unit's prescription management practices. The CQI process encourages assessment of current clinical practices for individual patients, as well as for the entire PD program. This process includes initial data collection of a sample of patients to establish a baseline against which future unit and patient data can be benchmarked against.

Indicators measured in the baseline analysis include creatinine clearance per 1.73 m^2 BSA and Kt/V values reported for dialysate, renal function and total clearance. Baseline weekly creatinine clearance in one center is illustrated in Figure 22.13. Graphic analyses of such parameters as BSA, weight, serum albumin and peritoneal membrane type are also useful for profiling a patient population. By repeating the data collection at a later data, the effectiveness of unit efforts to educate staff and patients on ways to improve prescription management can be evaluated.

Many professionals have used the CQI process to improve their prescription management practices as measured by an increase in the percent of their patients with a delivered Kt/V of ≥ 2.0 or a CrCl ≥ 60 L/week. In an analysis of 320 centers participating in the T.A.R.G.E.T. program (Treatement Adequacy Review for Gaining Enhanced Therapy Outcomes), a CQI process Baxter Health Care Corporation initiated to improve PD therapy outcomes, 80% of participating centers noted improvement in the percent of patients reaching desired clearance targets at the first comparison milestone (Figure 22.14) [20].

Among patients at centers participating in the T.A.R.G.E.T. process, the percent of patients

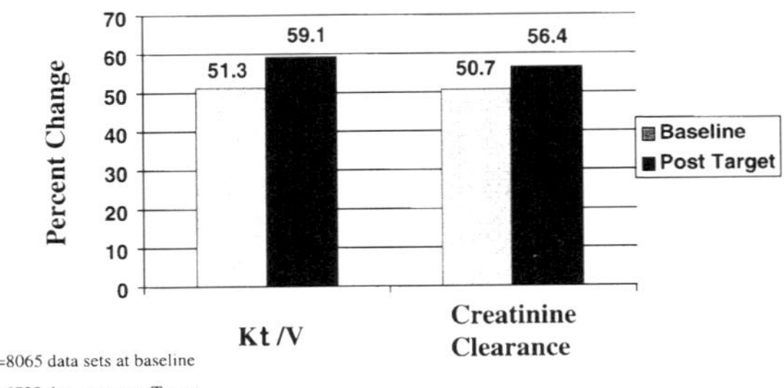

n=8065 data sets at baseline

6729 data sets post Target

Fig. 22.14. Percentage of patients achieving targets.

Table 22.4. Experience of one center using T.A.R.G.E.T.

	Pre- T.A.R.G.E.T.	Post- T.A.R.G.E.T.
% Patients with Kt/V ≥ 2.0	26%	89%
% Patients with CrCl ≥ 60	21%	61%
Mean Kt/V	1.8	2.5
Mean CrCl	52.1	74

Table 22.5. The NKF-DOQI^{TM} guidelines for dialysis initiation [2]. The NKF-DOQI^{TM} guidelines recommend initiation of dialysis when:

- Kt/V $_{urea}$ < 2.0 /week, which approximates:

  - A residual renal urea clearance <7mL/min/1.73 m^2
  - Residual renal creatinine clearance between 9–14 mL/min/1.73 m^2
  - GFR (U+Cr/2) <10.5 mL/min/1.73 m^2

  or

- nPNA <0.8 g/kg/day

achieving Kt/V's of ≥ 2.0 and CrCl of ≥ 60 L/1.73 m^2 increased on average from baseline by 15.3% and 11.3% respectively in 243 units. Individual centers may see significant improvements, such as shown in the example below (Table 22.4).

When to Initiate Dialysis

The NKF-DOQI^{TM} guidelines for PD adequacy recommend initiation of dialysis earlier than what has been the usual U.S. practice (Table 22.5). The recommendation to initiate dialysis while the patient is still healthy is based on recognition that a pre-ESRD patient's level of renal function and level of protein intake are independent predictors of clinical outcome. Patients who begin dialysis in a well nourished state have better outcomes than patients who begin dialysis in a malnourished state. The PD Adequacy committee of DOQI^{TM} concluded that it is paradoxical for dialysis practitioners to focus on clearance targets after initiation of dialysis, yet accept much lower levels of clearance during the pre-dialysis period. Although patient burn-out and infections are risks associated with earlier initiation of dialysis, the risks of late initiation of dialysis are well known and unacceptable. Incorporating healthy initiation of dialysis into the prescription management process is expected to play an increasingly significant role in improving patient outcomes.

There are two approaches to "healthy start" or timely initiation of dialysis: incremental and full therapy, each with unique advantages and disadvantages (Table 22.6). The incremental approach involves starting patients with a dose of dialysis that will bring their total weekly Kt/V to at least 2.0. This may mean that the patient receives two

Table 22.6. Therapeutic choices for healthy start

Incremental therapy		Full therapy	
Pros	Cons	Pros	Cons
– Individualized, target linked	– Frequent measurements/ prescription adjustments	– Infrequent measurements/ prescription adjustments	– Generalized, non-specific
– Gradual adaptation with less burnout		– "Bonus" clearance	– Early adaptation with more burnout
– Less costly			– More costly

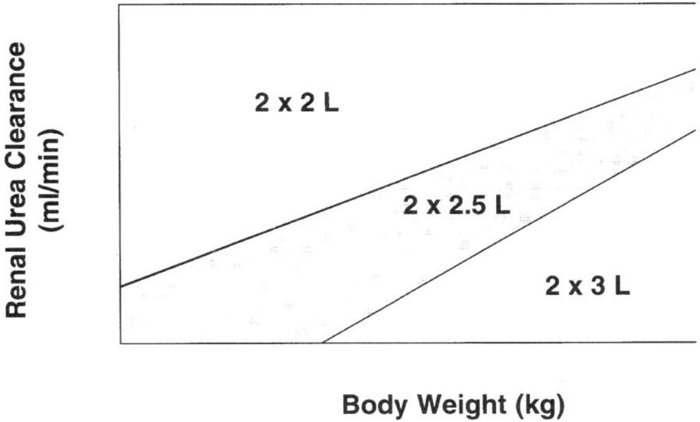

Fig. 22.15. Prescription guidelines for incremental initial PD prescription.

exchanges per day at the start of dialysis, with additional exchanges added as residual renal function declines. The alternative to incremental dosing is to initiate dialysis with a full prescription. This has the advantage of providing the patient with additional clearance and requires less prescription initial adjustment later. Guidelines for incremental initial therapy, such as the one illustrated in Figure 22.15 have been modeled and are undergoing clinical testing.

CONCLUSIONS

With our current level of understanding of peritoneal dialysis as a renal replacement therapy, it is clear that to ensure adequacy of dialysis, and thus successful patient outcomes, prescription management must be an ongoing and integral part of everyday patient management. Good prescription management practices include a comprehensive assessment of the patient, individualized prescriptions, and ongoing monitoring of the patient. It is then possible to adjust the patient's prescriptions as needed to make sure the patient meets clearance targets, is well nourished, and free of the clinical symptoms of uremia. With careful attention to prescription management, almost all patients, even large anephric patients without residual renal function, can achieve clearance targets.

A process that insures attention to good prescription management practices begins prior to dialysis initiation. This recognition demands a review and re-evaluation of current patient initia-

tion practices. Both levels of prescription management, initial and long term, are essential to the long term success of every PD program. Evaluation of prescription management begins with the individual patient, but must be amalgamated to the group level to evaluate the prescription management practices of the unit as a whole. Application of the CQI process to prescription management has been effective in improving the quality of PD patient care. As advances in PD prescription continue to be made, a prescription management process ensures that patients will receive the best therapy available.

REFERENCES

1. Blake P, Burkart JM, Churchill DN, Daugirdas J, Depner T, Hamburger RJ et al. Recommended clinical practices for maximizing peritoneal dialysis clearances. Perit Dial Int 1996; 16:448–56.
2. NKF-DOQI™ clinical practice guidelines for peritoneal dialysis adequacy. Am J Kidney Dis 1997; 30:S67–136.
3. Burkhart JM, Schreiber M, Korbet SM, Churchill DN, Hamburger RJ, Moran J et al. Solute clearance approach to adequacy of peritoneal dialysis. Perit Dial Int 1996; 16:457–70.
4. Peritoneal dialysis prescription management decision tree. Baxter Healthcare Corporation, 1997.
5. DuBois D and DuBois EF. A formula to estimate the approximate surface area if height and weight be known. Arch Intern Med 1961; 17:863–71.
6. Churchill DN, Taylor DW and Keshaviah PK. Adequacy of dialysis and nutrition in continuous peritoneal dialysis: association with clinical outcomes. Canada-USA (CANU-SA) peritoneal dialysis study group. J Am Soc Nephrol 1996; 7:198–207.
7. Twardowski ZJ, Nolph KD, Khanna R et al. Peritoneal equilibration test. Perit Dial Bull 1987; 7:138–47.
8. Durand P, Chanliau J, Gamberoni J, Hestin D and Kessler M. Measurement of hydrostatic intraperitoneal pressure: a necessary routine test in peritoneal dialysis. Perit Dial Int 1996; 16:S84–7.
9. Piraino B, Bernardini J, Sarkar S, Johnston J and Fried L. 3L exchange volumes are tolerated by most PD patients. Perit Dial Int 1998; 18:S22.
10. Wang T, Heimbürger O, Waniewski J, Bergström J and Lindholm B. Time dependence of solute removal during a single exchange. Adv Perit Dial 1997; 13:23–8.
11. Wang T, Waniewski J, Heimbürger O, Werynski A and Lindholm B. A quantitative analysis of sodium transport and removal during peritoneal dialysis. Kidney Int 1997; 52:1609–16.
12. Mistry CD, Gokal R, Peers E and the MIDAS study group. A randomized multicenter clinical trial comparing isosmo-

lar icodextrin with hyperosmolar glucose solutions in CAPD. Kidney Int 1994; 46:496–503.

13. Vonesh E, Burkart J, McMurray S and Williams P. Peritoneal dialysis kinetic modeling: validation in a multicenter clinical study. Perit Dial Int 1996; 16:471–81.

14. Jones MR. Etiology of severe malnutrition: results of an international cross-sectional study in continuous ambulatory peritoneal dialysis patients. Am J Kidney Dis 1994; 23:412–20.

15. Kopple JD and Blumenkrantz MJ. Nutritional requirements for patients undergoing continuous ambulatory peritoneal dialysis. Kidney Int 1983; 24:S295–302.

16. Bergström J et al. Protein and energy intake, nitrogen losses in patients treated with continuous ambulatory peritoneal dialysis. Kidney Int 1993; 44:1048–57.

17. Enia G, Sicuso C, Alati G and Zoccali C. Subjective global assessment of nutrition in dialysis patients. Nephrol Dial Transp 1993; 8:1094–8.

18. Oreopoulos DG, Anderson GH, Bergström J et al. Nutritional assessment of continuous ambulatory peritoneal dialysis patients: an international study. Am J Kidney Dis 1991; 17:462–71.

19. Wilkie ME. Icodextrin 7.5% dialysate solution in patients with ultrafiltration failure: extension of CAPD technique survival. Perit Dial Int 1997; 17:84–6.

20. Tebeau J, Moran J, Vonesh E and Harter M. Improvements in delivered dose utilizing a prescription management process. Perit Dial Int 1998; 18:S23.

23. Criteria for biocompatibility testing of peritoneal dialysis solutions

C.J. HOLMES

INTRODUCTION

The characterization of the biocompatibility of materials employed for medical diagnostic and therapeutic purposes is now well established as a fundamental requirement for such materials, as evidenced by the comprehensive and general guide published in the International Standard ISO-10993 [1]. In hemodialysis, the term "biocompatibility" has grown over the last decade to encompass a multitude of biological events defined either by clinical, physiological or biochemical indices that are attributable to extracorporeal blood-circuit interactions. Events such as activation of the complement, coagulation and kinin pathways, cytokine induction, neutrophil and platelet activation have all been suggested as important mediators of, not only some of the acute symptoms sometimes observed during dialysis, but also of chronic morbidities such as susceptibility to infection, osteodystrophy, amyloidosis and catabolism.

During peritoneal dialysis, the interface between the patient and the dialysis system is not a blood to membrane one but peritoneum to dialysis solution in nature. Although it is now over ten years since the *in vitro* detrimental effects of dialysis solution on phagocyte function were first described [2], in more recent years there has been an increasing number of reports on a wider variety of aspects of dialysis solution biocompatibilty. The impetus for this research is the belief by some that bioincompatible aspects of conventional PD solution formulations may be causally associated with complications of the therapy. Examples of the latter are pain upon infusion in the acute setting and loss of ultrafiltration in the long term patient. Concomitant with the increase in the number of scientific publications in this field has been the

variety of test systems and methods with which PD solution biocompatibilty has been evaluated [3]. The aim of this chapter is to discuss the various approaches available for PD solution biocompatibility testing, with an emphasis on the advantages and disadvantages of each approach. In addition, a pragmatic, hierarchical testing scheme is provided for those attempting to embark on such an exercise.

DEFINITIONS OF BIOCOMPATIBILITY

Currently, there is limited consensus as to what "biocompatibility" of peritoneal dialysis solutions refers. In 1994, the Consensus Conference on Biocompatibility defined this term as "the ability of a material, device or system to perform without a clinically significant host response in a specific application" [4]. This is an uncontroversial definition, but it is suggested that an improved version may include the term a "clinically significant *undesirable* host response," assuming all host responses are not undesirable. This definition mandates human clinical evaluation and thus, for practical purposes during the research and development phases of new PD solutions or when more immediate insight into biocompatibility characteristics is desirable, alternative definitions have been proposed. In 1993, Holmes defined PD solution biocompatibility as the biological effect that the solution exerts on the normal functioning of the tissues and cells of the peritoneum during both uninfected and infected states [3]. This definition best lends itself to acute *in vitro* testing methods. This definition was later complemented by Di Paolo who prefers "the capacity to leave the anatomical and physiological characteristics of

L.W. Henderson and R.S. Thuma (eds.), Quality Assurance in Dialysis, 2nd Edition, 257–265.
© 1999 *Kluwer Academic Publishers. Printed in Great Britain*

the peritoneum unchanged in time" [5]. Obviously this definition is tailored more to the use of animal models and clinical trials for biocompatibility evaluations, emphasizing the need to consider the effect of chronic exposure in such studies.

CURRENT APPROACHES TO BIOCOMPATIBILITY TESTING

Biocompatibilty testing approaches can be categorized into the following: *In vitro* cell culture systems; *in vivo* animal models; human *ex vivo* studies and human clinical trials. Figure 23.1 describes a hierarchical representation of these approaches in terms of clinical relevance. It is important to note that, wherever possible, one should strive to move up this hierarchical triangle. It is also suggested that as one does so, information obtained from studies higher in the hierarchy should always supersede that obtained from other studies lower in the hierarchy, where conflicts occur. A more detailed description of methods employed now follows.

In Vitro Methods

Most studies to date have employed techniques commonly used by immunologists and cell biologists to measure a variety of parameters such as cell viability, proliferation and function. Leukocytes and mesothelial cells have been the cell types subject to most research, although some studies on fibroblasts have appeared in the literature. Some debate exists on the appropriateness of using established cell lines versus primary cells. Cell lines, such as mouse fibroblast L929 or BALB 3TS clone 131, offer easy and reproducible systems for screening cytotoxicity and can be a good first line of evaluation. Primary cells result in much more variability in the data, but provide invaluable insight into the effects of solutions on cells derived from clinically relevant tissues.

Parameters selected for the *in vitro* evaluation of biocompatibility can be categorized as measures of cell viability, cell function and cell morphology. Cell viability methods are standard methods using intracellular ATP, LDH release, MTT dye assay and trypan blue exclusion. Standardized cell pro-

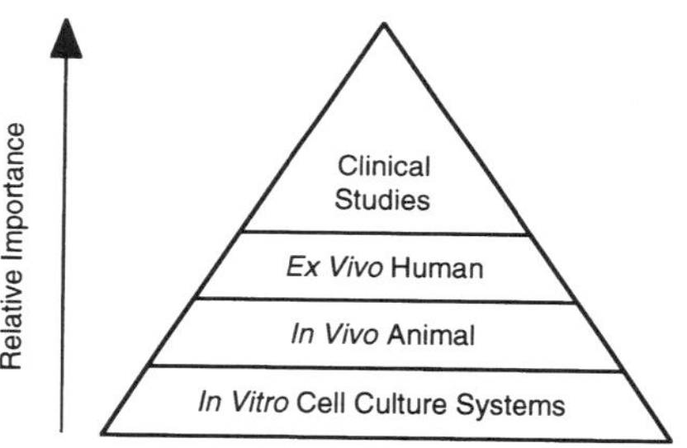

1°	Human clinical studies	Randomized, controlled in design
2°	Human *ex vivo* studies	Should be the default in absence of clinical studies.
		Should be performed whenever deemed safe to do so.
		Analogous to acute human clinical studies of biocompatibility in hemodialysis, *e.g.*, complement activation, PMN function.
3°	Animal models	More meaningful than *in vitro* studies and should be default where human exposure not possible.
4°	*In vitro* studies	Useful studies to initially evaluate biocompatibility profile of solutions prior to animal and human subjects exposure.

Fig. 23.1. A proposed hierarchical representation of biocompatibility testing for PD solutions.

Parameters Assessed in Biocompatibility Testing	
PMN	Viability (LDH, trypan blue exclusion, ATP), respiratory burst (superoxide generation, chemiluminescence), $[pH]i$, $[Ca^{2+}]i$, LTB_4, phagocytosis, chemotaxis, actin polymerization, integrin expression, respiration (O_2 uptake), bactericidal activity
MNC/PMØ	Viability, respiratory burst, $[Ca^{2+}]i$, LTB_4, phagocytosis, chemotaxis, integrin expression, respiration, bactericidal activity, cytokine synthesis
Peritoneal mesothelial cell & fibroblast	Viability, cytokine synthesis, proliferation, prostaglandin synthesis, collagen synthesis, hyaluronic acid

Fig. 23.2. Typical parameters selected for biocompatibility testing.
PMN = polymorphonuclear cells; MNC/PMØ = mononuclear cells/peritoneal macrophages; LDH = lactate dehydrogenase; LTB_4 = leukotriene B_4.

Gene Products of Cultured Mesothelial Cells	
Function	*Gene Product*
Host Defense	IL-1α, IL-1ß, IL-6, IL-8, MCP-1, RANTES, TNF-R1, ICAM-1, ICAM2, VCAM-1
Coagulation and Fibrinolysis	TF, PAI-1, PAI-2, tPA, uPA
ECM Synthesized Degradation	MMP9, TIMP-1, collagen, interstitial collagenase, 92kd gelatinase, TGF-ß, hyaluronic acid
Lubrication	Phospholipids, *e.g.,* phosphatidylcholine

Fig. 23.3. Gene products of mesothelial cells.
IL = interleukin; MCP-1 = monocyte chemotactic protein-1; RANTES = regulated on activation normal T cell expressed and secreted; TNF-R1 = tumor necrosis factor-receptor 1; ICAM = intracellular adhesion molecule; VCAM = vascular adhesion molecule; TF = tissue factor; PAI = plasminogen activator inhibitor; tPA = tissue plasminogen activator; uPA = urokinase-type plasminogen activator; MMP-9 = matrix metalloproteinase-9; TIMP-1 = tissue inhibitor of metalloproteinase-1; TGFß = transforming growth factor β.

liferation assays are also utilized. Functional assays are numerous, but some of the most commonly employed are shown in detail in Figure 23.2. The list of potential functions to be assayed is growing as our understanding of the biology of the cell types selected evolves. Figure 23.3 illustrates this point by listing many of the known functions of mesothelial cells, from which it becomes obvious that it is necessary to be selective. Selection of appropriate assays should be based upon consideration of the most clinically relevant functions of that cell type. It should be kept in mind that functional assessment, depending upon the cell type, may require evaluation both when unstimulated and stimulated (activated), in order to fully interpret the impact of any given solution on cell function.

Approaches to the design of *in vitro* studies generally can be considered as falling into two categories. The first type of design is one in which cells are exposed for short periods of time, e.g. 30–60 minutes, to the solution in question. This design is often used to evaluate transient factors such as the acidic pH of dextrose based solutions that is known to equilibrate, *in vivo*, to physiological pH within 30 to 60 minutes. This approach is also appropriate for cell functions that can be characterized over short periods of time, e.g. the oxidative respiratory burst of stimulated neutrophils. The cell parameter(s) under study may be measured during the incubation period (co-incubation design), or subsequent to removal from the incubation solution and placement in a physiologically buffered medium (pre-incubation design). The latter approach may also be modified to permit study of longer term effects that a transient insult might have on cell viability and function.

A second general design that is employed is one appropriate for parameters which require study over longer periods of time, e.g. hours to days. A good example is the effect of osmotic agents on mesothelial cell growth. Here cells are continuously cultured under the conditions of choice or conditions while the parameter(s) in question is measured at desired intervals, e.g. intracellular ATP levels. The solution under study can be diluted to some degree with cell culture medium, in order to provide nutrients if the parameter of biocompatibility being measured requires it, e.g. fibroblast proliferation over 72 hours.

In vitro modeling of the in vivo situation.
There has been a tendency for *in vitro* study designs to only loosely simulate *in vivo* conditions of peritoneal dialysis. For instance, as mentioned above, it is now well recognized that the pH of conventional PD solutions, which are formulated at a pH of 5.0–5.5, will be partially neutralized immediately upon infusion due to the presence of a buffering residual peritoneal volume, and will further rise to neutrality over the ensuing 30 to 60 minutes. Simulation of such changes *in vitro* show an amelioration of the effect seen with a constant exposure for 30 to 60 minutes of unadulterated solution. Similarly, Breborowicz and colleagues have observed less severe inhibition of mesothelial cell growth by hyperosmolar solution when *in vivo* osmotic changes are simulated [6]. Thus, in order to avoid inappropriate conclusions, several leading researchers in this field recommend that *in vitro* designs that simulate the clinical picture be adopted wherever possible [7]. Figure 23.4 describes one example of how *in vivo* equilibration of osmolality and pH can be simulated *in vitro* by

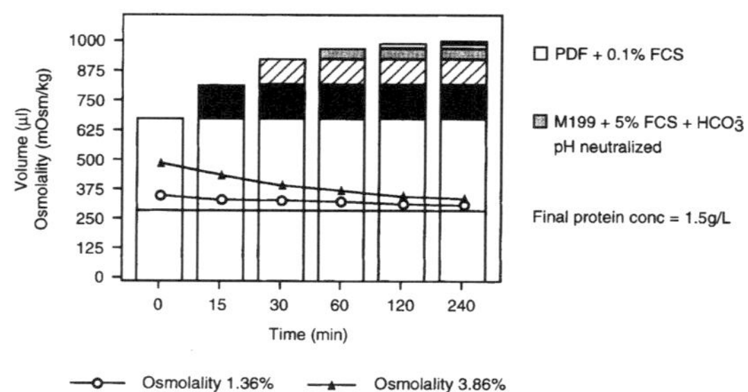

Fig. 23.4. An *in vitro* equilibration system; sequential addition of medium containing fetal calf serum simulates the changes in osmolality, pH, lactate, and protein concentration that occurs *in vivo* during a single CAPD exchange. Reproduced with permission from reference [7].

intermittent and sequential addition of tissue culture medium to a test PD solution. Equilibration methods, however, can be demanding to perform and usually have to be restricted to exposure periods of 4 to 8 hours. Thus, for components of PD solution that are not rapidly changed during the intraperitoneal dwell period and where longer periods of exposure, e.g. days, are preferred, a static incubation design is still a reasonable compromise. A good example is the measure of L929 fibroblast proliferation inhibition as a measure of the cytotoxicity of glucose degradation products (GDP). This assay typically requires 72 hours of incubation, so repetitive equilibration would be difficult to perform, and probably unnecessary, given the chronic exposure pattern *in vivo* of the peritoneum to GDP.

Pitfalls and disadvantages of in vitro test systems
In vitro test systems need to be designed and interpreted carefully to avoid some common pitfalls. For example, it is well known that the chemiluminescence response of neutrophils can be correspondingly stimulated with increasing concentrations of glucose, and likewise can be suppressed with a number of other additives [8]. Consequently, adequate controls always should be run in order to separate true biocompatibility effects from artifacts of the test system that will not occur *in vivo*. A good example of such an artifact was described recently with a study on the

biocompatibility of ascorbic acid for wound management. The authors of this paper reported that autooxidation of ascorbic acid to hydrogen peroxide occurred in their cell culture system, a situation described as unlikely in the *in vivo* environment [9].

Careful selection of cell types and appropriate study design renders *in vitro* testing a useful approach for PD solution biocompatibility testing. However, disadvantages exist with conventional cell culture systems that study a single cell type in a two dimensional format. Studies by Breborowicz using co-culture of mesothelial cells, fibroblasts and peritoneal leukocytes suggest that the response of any one given cell type is dependent upon cell to cell interactions probably mediated by a complex network of cytokines and growth factors [10]. It is also well established in the field of cell biology that interactions between cells and extracellular matrix can affect their growth, metabolism and response to stimuli and suggest that three dimensional matrices be used for cell types such as fibroblasts. Although it is recognized that such refinements may further enhance the relevance of *in vitro* systems, such techniques are beyond the scope of many testing facilities, and it can be argued that investment of additional resources would be better spent moving up the hierarchical ladder of tests.

In Vivo Animal Models

Evaluating the biocompatibility of PD solutions in animals is recommended after *in vitro* assessment is complete and where *in vivo* data are necessary or desirable prior to human exposure. Advantages of using animal models are that they provide an *in vivo* environment where all biological processes are involved and affected in a manner presumably more analogous to the clinical situation. Disadvantages to keep in mind include the inability to also directly extrapolate findings to humans, particularly to ESRD patients, and the resources required for animal surgery, maintenance and care facilities.

In-bred strains of mice, rats and rabbits are frequently used in this field, although Di Paolo utilizes local domestic rabbits, reporting particular resistance to infection and acceptance of long term catheterization (up to 1 year) as advantages [5].

Instillation of test fluids into the peritonea of mice and rats can be achieved by injecting fluid directly transcutaneously under anesthesia, taking care not to perforate the bowel. Custom made miniature peritoneal catheters have been utilized with some success in rats, thereby allowing for easier instillation and removal of fluid. As with most animal studies, antibiotic coverage often is required to minimize the incidence of peritoneal infection. The optimal time for dialysis before outcome parameters are assessed is unclear, but it is becoming more evident that during approximately the first month of dialysis that a period of adaptation to the dialysis fluid and/or implanted catheter occurs in which mesothelial cell desquamation and inflammatory cell infiltration is noted among other observations. Consequently, it is recommended that study be extended beyond this time period.

The list of parameters measured in animal studies of PD solution biocompatibility in the scientific literature continues to expand. Classical histology and morphometry of the peritoneum using both light and electron microscopy has been the mainstay approach of most researchers. Often there is a focus on the response of the mesothelium to the test solution. Gotloib et al. has adapted the imprint technique of Efskind, enabling large areas of mesothelium to be studied relatively simply for many aspects [11]. For instance, they have employed viability, density and surface area of mesothelial cells, mitotic activity and enzymatic activity (e.g. alkaline phosphatase, Na-K-ATPase, 5-nucleotidase, etc.) as biocompatibility parameters.

Animal ex vivo and washout studies
Although uncommon, a few groups have chosen to isolate peritoneal cells (mainly leukocytes) from dialysate effluent of animals and then assay them *in vitro* for cell viability, function, etc. This design of using *in vivo* exposure followed by *in vitro* assessment of viability and function is referred to as an *ex vivo* study. A novel variation to this approach is described by Di Paolo and is coined as the "washout" approach. This technique infuses 0.1% trypsin and 0.1% EDTA in PBS into the rabbit peritoneum for 20 minutes to remove large numbers of mesothelial cells, which can then be isolated for counting, morphometry, flow cytometry, etc. [5].

Human Ex Vivo Studies

It is suggested that human *ex vivo* studies are the next step up the hierarchical ladder of PD biocompatibility testing and the most meaningful in terms of clinical relevance, next to clinical outcomes studies. These studies can be performed in parallel to Phase I to IV clinical trials. Similar to the animal *ex vivo* studies described above, human *ex vivo* designs involve the instillation of solution into the peritoneum, allowing a dwell for a predetermined time, draining of the solution, isolation of peritoneal cells (mainly macrophages) and subsequent study of cell viability, cell function, etc. *in vitro* (Figure 23.5). Additionally, the cell free dialysate can be stored at –70°C and assayed for a variety of inflammatory mediators, such as TNFα, IL-6, MCP-1, or markers of peritoneal membrane status, e.g. CA 125, pro-collagen type I, hyaluronic acid. However, in contrast to cell function, the interpretation of effluent phase molecules can be difficult, so is currently of limited use. For example, although IL-6 is found at high levels in normal uninfected PD effluent, it is unclear as to its exact biological function in this setting. IL-6 is characterized as both an anti-inflammatory cytokine and as a cytokine that is elevated in certain autoimmune and inflammatory diseases. Likewise, although the cancer antigen, CA125, has been proposed as a useful marker of mesothelial cell mass, there is disagreement on the natural course of CA125 appearance over time in PD patients [12, 13].

Clinical Outcome Studies

The ultimate test of the importance of biocompatibility of PD solution will come with demonstration of improved clinical outcomes in long term randomized controlled trials. However, this will be challenging given the logistics and cost associated with such studies, as has been the case in hemodialysis. However, acute clinical symptoms, if they exist, may provide the opportunity to assess some clinically relevant aspects of bioincompatibility. In peritoneal dialysis, for instance, the most obvious is the infrequent observation of pain upon infusion. The latter is believed to be related to the low pH of the solution, and to some extent the presence of glucose degradation products (GDP).

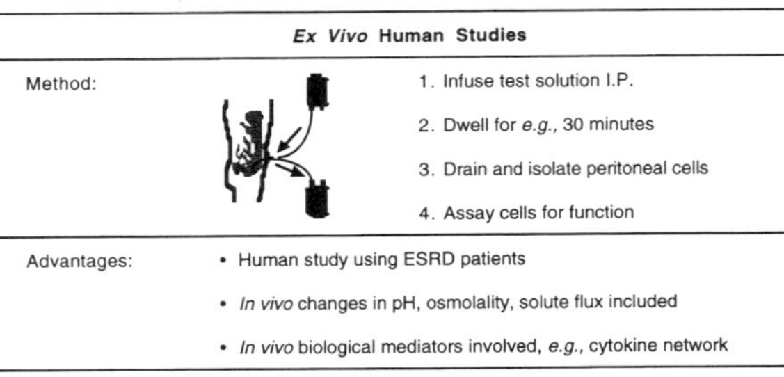

Fig. 23.5. Ex vivo human study design and associated advantages.

Thus, in the specific case of a new product that has a more neutral pH than the conventional product or lower GDP, then a short term clinical study objectively measuring pain would be appropriate.

When to Test for Biocompatibility of PD Solutions

Currently there are no national or international standards or guidelines mandating or describing the approach or need for biocompatibility testing of solutions intended for peritoneal dialysis. However, the medical, scientific and industrial community has voiced a strong interest in the role of biocompatibility in peritoneal dialysis complications, such as ultrafiltration loss, peritonitis and sclerosing encapsulating peritonitis. In this respect, biocompatibility profiling of new formulations is becoming as integral a part of product development as classical toxicology. However, a reasoned approach is required as to when biocompatibility testing is needed and, if it is, what types of tests are appropriate. To illustrate by example, consider the requirements for a new PD solution that is identical to the currently used formulations with the exception that the sodium content is reduced by a few millimoles/L. It is suggested that there is little reason to embark on a biocompatibility study for such a formulation change, as there is little to no scientific logic that can be put forth to argue that this formulation will be more or less biocompatible than the control. In contrast, if the sterilization procedure is significantly altered, or there are new agents included in the formulation, or the formulation is changed significantly in its composition or physico-chemical characteristics, then biocompatibility profiling is prudent.

What to Test for When Biocompatibility Profiling PD Solutions: A Triage Approach

As with device biocompatibility testing, PD solution testing is a comparative exercise and so the inclusion of standards and controls are imperative. In PD solution studies a common standard used is tissue culture medium such as M199 medium supplemented with fetal calf or normal human serum. Controls should include, at a minimum, solutions with known clinical performance, such as Dianeal. Current formulations exist with various calcium, lactate and glucose concentrations, container materials and possibly sterilization cycles, all of which must be considered in the selection of controls.

In previous sections of this chapter, the myriad of testing options for biocompatibility testing have been described. Pragmatically speaking, however, a triage approach, as depicted in Figure 23.6, is recommended. *In vitro* testing using peripheral blood cells is suggested at first, as these are easy to obtain and will often suggest how solutions will perform with other cell systems. Most parameters considered to be bioincompatible in current commercial formulations, such as low pH, hyperosmolality and GDPs, tend to have a basal cytotoxicity effect, in the sense they appear to affect most functions of many cell types. A second line of *in vitro* testing would involve human peritoneal mesothelial cells and fibroblasts, if such clinical material is available. This, however, is not always the case and may necessitate collaboration. Fibroblast cell lines, such as mouse L929, are readily available, easy to manipulate, and offer an alternative to human fibroblasts for inhibition of proliferation testing. Transformed human mesothelial cell lines have been described recently and may prove to be useful in the future [14].

Animal testing, using standard histology and morphometry, would be the next priority, and it is recommended that long term studies are used that avoid the acute changes seen in peritoneal morphology over the first 4 weeks of solution exposure. Rabbit or rat models that utilize indwelling catheters are also preferable. Caution should be taken during the interpretation of any biocompatibility data obtained from animal studies in which peritonitis was a significant problem during the course of the study. Progression to human *ex vivo* studies is highly recommended, as these study designs will provide the most clinically relevant insight into any new formulation. The determination of macrophage function, such as phagocytic index, chemiluminescence response and unstimulated and stimulated cytokine responses, are recommended as first order of assessments. Human *ex vivo* studies require significant resources in terms of expertise, manpower and organizational abilities.

Priority		Approach		
1° *In Vitro*	PMN normal PBMC normal	1°	Equilibration > static conditions	
	HPMC normal HPFB normal/cell line	2°	Viability proliferation and functional assays (stimulated and unstimulated)	
2° Animal Models	Peritoneal histology	• Standard observations:	Mesothelial cell morphology, basement membrane, collagen, fibroblasts, inflammatory cells, etc.	
		• Special observations:	Unusual cell types, etc.	
3° Human *Ex Vivo*	PMØ function	e.g., Unstimulated and stimulated secretion Antimicrobial function; phagocytosis, etc.		

Fig. 23.6. A suggested triage approach for biocompatibility testing.

Special assessments – hypothesis building

Often biocompatibility testing can be structured around a hypothesis that involves the role of a particular component or other aspect of the solution formulation, and which would not be covered by the approaches described so far. For example, in the case of the alternative osmotic agent polyglucose, *in vitro* testing to determine its ability to glycosylate protein and form advanced glycosylated end products (AGE) relative to glucose may be considered as an appropriate form of biocompatibility profiling. The motivation for such work would be based upon the observation that there is a reported association between peritoneal membrane AGE content, time on dialysis and ultrafiltration volumes in PD patients [15]. Additionally, AGE has been shown to play a pivotal role in the induction of cytokine cascades and reactive oxygen species that have been suggested to mediate peritoneal membrane damage and fibrotic changes. Thus, performing an assessment of AGE formation is logical for this particular formulation because of the potential difference in reactivity between polyglucose and glucose in terms of AGE formation. Similarly, there may be other specialized tests for other solutions, depending upon their specific formulation and hypothetical contribution to biocompatibility.

SUMMARY

Biocompatibility testing of PD solutions has become an integral part of new product development. All new formulations should be considered as candidates for biocompatibility profiling, but reasoned comparative analysis of the new formulation versus conventional ones or previously evaluated formulations should dictate the need for testing. Upon embarkation of a profiling exercise, it is recommended that a triage approach be taken by first performing assays using easily obtainable peripheral blood cells, as this will provide a quick and fairly generalizable assessment of performance. Subsequent focus should be on the effect of test solutions on human peritoneal mesothelial cell viability and function. Wherever feasible, studies involving equilibration designs are preferred. Animal models are recommended as the next level of hierarchical testing, followed by human *ex vivo*

study designs. The latter provide evidence that any new solution formulation is exerting an altered biological response *in vivo*. These studies, however, are not substitutes for long term clinical outcome studies. Finally, the importance of the biocompatibility profile of any peritoneal dialysis solution must be considered alongside other clinical advantages and disadvantages that may be associated with its specific formulation.

REFERENCES

1. Anon. ISO-10993: biological evaluation of medical devices – Part I; guidance on selection of tests. London, International Organisation for Standardisation, 1992.
2. Duwe AK, Vas SI and Weatherhead JW. Effects of the composition of peritoneal dialysis fluid on chemiluminescence, phagocytosis and bactericidal activity in vitro. Infect Immun 1981; 33:130–5.
3. Holmes CJ. Biocompatibility of peritoneal dialysis solutions [editorial comment]. Perit Dial Int 1993; 13:88–94.
4. Consensus conference on biocompatibility. Nephrol Dialysis Transplant 1994; 9(2).
5. Di Paolo N, Garosi G, Monaci G and Brardi S. Biocompatibility of peritoneal dialysis treatment. Nephrol Dialysis Transplant 1997; 12:78–83.
6. Breborowicz A, Bolaskas E, Oreopoulos D et al. A new approach in the study of dialysis fluid toxicity on the peritoneal membrane. Perit Dial Int 1991; 11:A29.
7. Topley N. What is the ideal technique for testing the biocompatibility of peritoneal dialysis solutions. Perit Dial Int 1995; 15:205–9.
8. Anderson B and Amirault H. Important variables in granulocyte chemiluminescence. Proceedings of the society for experimental biology and medicine 1979; 162:139–45.
9. Schmidt R, Chung L, Andrews A and Turner T. Toxicity of L-ascorbic acid to L929 fibroblast cultures: relevance to biocompatibility testing of materials for use in wound management. J Biomedl Mat Res 1993; 27:521–30.
10. Breborowicz A, Bolaskas E, Oreopoulos D et al. Co-culture of peritoneal dialysate cells with mesothelial cells and fibroblasts. Perit Dial Int 1991; 11:A31.
11. Gotloib L, Shostak A and Wajsbrot V. Detrimental effects of peritoneal dialysis solutions upon in vivo and in situ exposed mesothelium. Perit Dial Int 1997; 17:13–16.
12. Ho-dac-Pannekeet M, Hiralall J, Struijk D and Krediet R. Longitudinal follow-up of CA 125 in peritoneal effluent. Kidney Int 1997; 51:888–93.
13. Lai K, Lai K, Szeto C, Ho K, Poon P, Lam C et al. Dialysate cell population and cancer antigen 125 in stable continuous ambulatory peritoneal dialysis patients: their relationship with transport parameters. Am J Kidney Dis 1997; 29:669–705.
14. Fischereder M, Luckow B, Sitter T, Schroppel B, Banas B and Schlondorff D. Immortalization and characterization of

human peritoneal mesothelial cells. Kidney Int 1997;
51:2006–12.
15. Nakayama M, Kawaguchi Y, Yamada K, Hasegawa T, Takazoe K, Katoh N et al. Immunohistochemical detection of advanced glycosylation end-products in the peritoneum and its possible pathophysiological role in CAPD. Kidney Int 1997; 51:182–6.

24. The impact of sterilization methods on the quality of peritoneal dialysis solutions

LEO MARTIS

INTRODUCTION

Regulatory agencies around the world granting approvals to market medical products place a great deal of emphasis on assuring that products purporting to be sterile are indeed sterile. In its strictest definition, the term sterile refers to complete absence of viable microorganisms. Therefore, sterility is an abstract concept of negative state, and as such, is not capable of practical demonstration. In practice, however, sterility is defined in a probabilistic term as Sterility Assurance Level (SAL). Because sterility failures are recognized as being among the most critical and dangerous of product defects, the regulatory agencies generally recommend a sterilization process that ensures minimum risk of surviving organisms. In this chapter we will review the primary methods of sterilization, the impact of these methods on the quality of current peritoneal dialysis (PD) solutions, and potential approaches for improving the quality of these fluids.

STERILIZATION METHODS

Terminal sterilization and aseptic processing are the two primary methods available for sterilization of medical products. Terminal sterilization can be performed with steam, dry heat, ethylene oxide, ionizing radiation, or removal of microorganisms by filtration. Aseptic processing involves presterilization of each component of the medical product separately using one of the terminal sterilization methods followed by assembling the final product in an aseptic environment. Modern tech-nological developments have also led to the use of additional procedures such as blow-molding at high temperatures, forms of moist heat other than saturated steam and ultraviolet radiation, and on-line continuous filling in aseptic processing [1]. The choice of the method for sterilization of a medical product or a component of a product depends on economics of the process, effect of sterilization method on the product (design and materials) and package, and attainment and demonstration of required SAL.

Historically, of the two primary methods of making sterile products, aseptic processing was considered to be associated with more sterility failures than terminal sterilization [2]. Also, it was generally accepted that terminally sterilized products attain a 10^{-6} microbial survival probability (i.e. assurance of less than one chance in a million that viable microorganisms are present in the sterilized product), a SAL that was thought not to be possible to achieve with aseptic processing. As a result, the Food and Drug Administration requires all large volume parenterals, defined as single-dose injections with a deliverable volume of 100 mL or more, be terminally sterilized to provide SALs that are at least 10^{-6}. Peritoneal dialysis solutions are considered as large volume parenterals and hence they are required to be terminally sterilized. Of the various methods available for terminal sterilization, only steam sterilization lends itself to the sterilization of PD solutions.

L.W. Henderson and R.S. Thuma (eds.), Quality Assurance in Dialysis, 2nd Edition, 267–273.
© 1999 *Kluwer Academic Publishers. Printed in Great Britain*

STERILIZATION CONSTRAINTS AND DEVELOPMENTS IN PD SOLUTIONS

During the early days of PD in the 1920s and 30s, parenteral solutions readily available at that time such as 0.8% saline [3, 4], 5% glucose [4], and Ringer's solution [5] were used as dialysis fluids. Electrolyte imbalances, pulmonary edema, and acidosis were the common complications observed with these formulations. Subsequent studies, at the end of the 1940's, indicated that the composition of PD fluids must be similar to interstitial fluids and that they must be made hypertonic with respect to blood by addition of an osmotic solute in order to achieve adequate fluid removal [6, 7]. Of the number of chemicals evaluated as osmotic agents, glucose was found to be most safe and effective. Solutions used for intermittent peritoneal dialysis in the early 60's contained glucose as osmotic agent and bicarbonate buffer. These solutions were prepared by terminally sterilizing each component of the solution followed by mixing these components using aseptic techniques [8]. The pH of these fluids was generally around 7.4. Today regulatory agencies around the world require that PD solutions be terminally heat sterilized and achieve SALs that are greater than 10^{-6}. Since calcium, magnesium, dextrose, and bicarbonate are not compatible with each other during steam sterilization, the current PD fluids are formulated at an acid pH of 5.0–5.5 with lactate instead of bicarbonate buffer. Even with these modifications, the current sterilization methods lead to alterations in chemical composition of PD fluids which may compromise the quality of the therapy provided by peritoneal dialysis [9].

CHEMICAL ALTERATIONS OF PD FLUIDS DURING HEAT STERILIZATION

It has been known for a long time that heat sterilization of glucose containing parenteral solutions leads to multiple glucose breakdown products. The nature and extent of degradation depends on glucose concentration, pH of the solution, and sterilization parameters (time and temperature).

Figure 24.1 shows a characteristic ultraviolet absorbance spectrum of a standard PD fluid

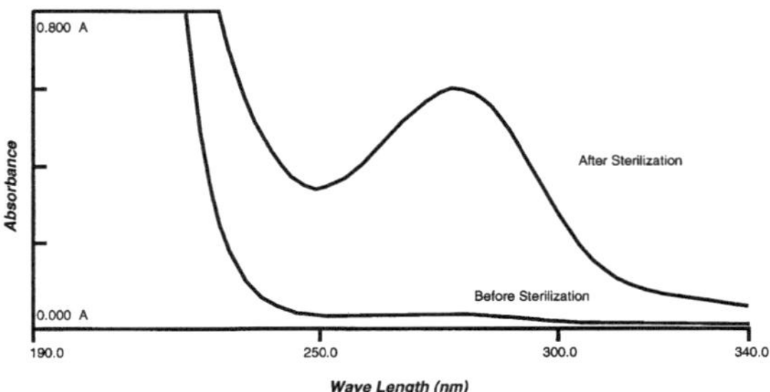

Fig. 24.1. Effect of heat sterilization on ultra violet absorbance of standard PD solution containing 4.25% dextrose.

before and after steam sterilization. One of the main substances formed during sterilization is 5-hydroxymethyl-2-furfural (5-HMF), which has an absorbance maximum at 284 nm. Other breakdown products that have been identified in heat sterilized glucose containing solutions include 2-furaldehyde, formic acid, levulinic acid, 5-hydroxymethylfuroic acid, 2-keto-3-deoxyglucose, and 2-(2'-hydroxyacetyl)furan deoxyglucose, and 2-(2'-hydroxyacetyl)furan [10, 11]. Nilsson-Thorell et al. [11] analyzed different brands of commercial PD fluids and reported the presence of 5-HMF, 2-furaldehyde, acetaldehyde, glyoxal, methylglyoxal, and formaldehyde. In comparison, the concentrations of glucose degradation products were much less in filter sterilized PD solutions (Table 24.1).

CYTOTOXICITY OF GLUCOSE BREAKDOWN PRODUCTS

The first clinical report describing the irritant effect of a PD solution that was ascribed to glucose degradation products was by Henderson et al. [10]. They postulated that the glucose degradation products were responsible for the irritant properties of PD solutions. Wieslander et al. [12, 13] studied in depth the cytotoxicity of glucose degradation products that are found in PD fluids. Commercial dialysis fluids significantly inhibited the growth of a cultured fibroblast cell line, L-929. In addition, these solutions inhibited the release of TNFα from a macrophage cell line and superoxide generation from freshly prepared human leukocytes. The cytotoxicity observed in these studies

Table 24.1. Aldehydes (μmol/L) in different commercial and laboratory-made PD fluids [11]

Test solution	Acetaldehyde	5-HMF	Glyoxal	Methyl-gloyoxal	Formaldehyde	2-Furaldehyde
PD fluid (laboratory made, filtered)	<10	<4	<3	<2	<3	<0.5
PD fluid (laboratory made, heat-sterilized)	290	30	<3.0	23	15	2
Commercial PD fluid	120–420	6–15	<3.0–14	2–12	6–11	<0.05–2

was independent of pH and was absent in dialysis solutions prepared by sterile filtration.

DIALYSATE pH AND ABDOMINAL PAIN

There are several reports in the literature describing abdominal pain in PD patients during infusion of dialysis solution [10, 14, 15]. As many as 10% of patients in some centers have been reported to experience pain on infusion of dialysis solution [10]. If not treated, this problem can lead to patient noncompliance and withdrawal from dialysis therapy. Although there are no well controlled studies documenting the causes and treatment of infusion pain, it is generally accepted that increasing the dialysate pH by the addition of sodium bicarbonate or sodium hydroxide results in relief of pain [14–16]. Yamamoto et al. [16] used PD solutions that were adjusted to pH 6.8 using sodium bicarbonate immediately before each exchange in PD patients over a period of three months. They reported decreased total leukocyte counts in the effluent and increased leukocyte viability with the use of pH adjusted dialysis solutions. Abdominal distension, abdominal pain during instillation, nausea and headache were also reported to be improved. However, adding an alkali to the dialysis fluid prior to infusion further adds to the tediousness of the exchange procedure with the attendant increased risk of bacterial contamination, particularly in visually impaired patients.

DIALYSATE pH AND PHAGOCYTIC CELL FUNCTION

Duwe et al. [17] were the first to recognize the inhibitory effects of peritoneal dialysis solutions on the antibacterial action of normal peripheral blood leukocytes, as measured by chemiluminescence, phagocytosis, and bacterial killing. The ability of peritoneal macrophages to mount a respiratory burst and to produce cytokines also has been shown to be significantly reduced when these cells were exposed to dialysis fluids at pH of 5.2 [17, 18]. Yu et al. [19] reported that exposure of neutrophils to standard lactate containing PD solutions at pH of 5.2 resulted in the development of a prompt and substantial intracellular acidosis (pH declining to 5.7 over a period of 20 minutes). Exposure of macrophages to acidic dialysis solutions was also associated with a rapid and profound reduction in intracellular pH of the macrophages [20]. The NADPH oxidase, the enzyme that catalyzes the reaction of O_2 with NADPH to form NADP and superoxide, has an optimal pH range for activation of 6.8 to 7.9 [21]. Hence, when the macrophage cytoplasmic pH falls well below 6.5, as in the case with the exposure to acidic dialysis solution, one can expect suppressed activity of NADPH oxidase and generation of superoxide. These functional defects of macrophages were corrected by the adjustment of dialysis fluid pH to 7.4 [16, 20, 21].

Alobaidi et al. [22] demonstrated that phagocytic function of peritoneal macrophages was significantly suppressed when the cells were pre-incubated for only 10 minutes in dialysis solution. Incubation for 30 minutes completely abolished phagocytosis even though the cells remained viable. These investigators also provided evidence that the suppressor effect of short exposure to fresh dialysis solution was not reversible even one hour after the macrophages were returned to a more physiological environment. If these findings can be extrapolated to the clinical situation, the initial suppressor effect of dialysis solution may continue despite the gradual normalization of the dialysate (pH, osmolality, glucose, electrolytes, etc.) during its dwell time in the peritoneal cavity. Other investigators have corroborated these findings and have presented evidence that incubation in unused dialysis fluid inhibits the generation of oxygen free radicals by activated peripheral blood leukocytes as well as by peritoneal macrophages [23–25]. It was Topley et al. [18] who conclusively demonstrated that the inhibitory effect on the phagocytic cell function is mainly due to low pH of lactate containing PD solutions.

Several researchers have reported that peritoneal macrophages and lymphocytes appear to be in a state of chronic activation as evidenced by the enhanced expression of surface antigens such as HLA-DR, CD25 (the IL-2 receptor), and CD71 (transferrin receptor) [26–28]. Theoretically, chronic activation of peritoneal leukocytes could result in chronic production of fibrogenic cytokines and oxidative free radicals, which, in turn, could lead to mesothelial cell toxicity and membrane fibrosis [29, 30]. Bos et al. [31] have demonstrated in a rat model that current PD solutions could induce peritoneal mononuclear cell activation. The solution component responsible for activation was not identified in this study, but *in vitro* work by Vachula and colleagues [32] indicated that enhanced expression of CD25 and CD71 on peritoneal mononuclear cells could be initiated by transient exposure to acidic PD solutions. Chronic activation of peritoneal leukocytes and chronic production of fibrogenic cytokines may explain the mechanism of loss of ultrafiltration and peritoneal fibrosis observed in some PD patients.

Low pH in combination with lactate also is shown to inhibit production of IL-1, IL-6 and TNFa by peripheral and peritoneal mononuclear cells [32–35]. These data suggest that cellular host defense is impaired early in the dialysis cycle as a result of pH mediated "stunning" of resident phagocytes. The potential clinical consequence of impaired host defense in the peritoneal cavity would be increased risk of infection or delayed clearing of infection with resultant scarring of membrane.

There have been no large scale clinical studies comparing the effect of pH on peritonitis rates. A recent study compared *in vitro* phagocytic function of peritoneal macrophages isolated from dialysate effluents of patients using peritoneal dialysis solutions with initial pH 5.0 or 7.0 [36]. Peritoneal macrophages derived from pH 7.0 dialysis solution were found to have significantly superior phagocytic function as compared to macrophages obtained following the infusion of dialysis solution at pH 5.0.

DIALYSATE pH AND MESOTHELIAL CELL FUNCTION

There is growing evidence that peritoneal mesothelial cells are not just a passive lining membrane of the peritoneum but are involved in synthesis and secretion of various inflammatory mediators including cytokines, chemokines, and prostaglandins [37]. Because the mesothelial cells are strategically placed in close juxtaposition both to peritoneal macrophages and underlying mesothelial microvascular endothelium, these cells are well suited to regulate the bidirectional interaction between the macrophages and the vascular cells. Thus mesothelial cells are believed to play an important role in the inflammatory response of the peritoneum to both infective agents and toxic components of the solution. Several investigators have shown that current peritoneal dialysis solutions suppress the function of mesothelial cells and the majority of the evidence points to the low pH as the causative factor of cytotoxicity [18, 38–40]. Repetitive, albeit transient, injury to the peritoneal mesothelial cells is also thought to be the initiating event that ultimately leads to loss of ultrafiltration, fibrosis of the peritoneum and therapy failure [41].

WHAT CAN BE DONE TO IMPROVE THE pH AND MINIMIZE GLUCOSE DEGRADATION PRODUCTS OF CURRENT PD FLUIDS?

The quality of current PD fluids can be greatly enhanced by improving the pH and minimizing the glucose degradation products. A number of approaches are available to improve the quality of current PD fluids.

Sterilization at Low pH

Singh et al. [42], demonstrated in 1948 that in unbuffered glucose solutions, a pH of 3 provides the minimum degradation due to heat. Later work by Griffin and Marie [43] showed that, in lactate buffered glucose solutions, a pH of around 5 results in the lowest level of glucose degradation. Recent studies with PD fluids suggest significantly less glucose degradation at pH between 4.0–4.5 compared to a solution at pH of 5.2 [44]. However, reducing the pH of PD fluids below 5.0 is not practical unless it is increased again prior to infusion into the patient.

Sterilization at Higher Temperature and Shorter Duration

The standard process for heat sterilization is 20 minutes at about 121°C. One can obtain similar SALs using higher temperatures for a shorter period of time or lower temperatures for a longer period of time. Glucose degradation could be minimized with sterilization cycles consisting of high temperatures and shorter duration [45, 46]. Implementing these recommendations in practice can be difficult. Even if the temperature in the autoclave can be increased, limits are set by heat transfer and resistance of the bags and tubing materials. However, as small as 5°C increase in sterilization temperature might be valuable in improving the quality of PD fluids [47].

Sterilization with High Glucose Concentration

According to some reports, increased glucose concentration may contribute to a decreased rate of degradation-product formation upon heat treatment. Webb et al. [48], Wing [49], and Wieslander et al. [47] reported that increasing the concentration of glucose reduced the rate of degradation. However, both Singh et al. [42] and Griffin and Marie [43] reported that rate of glucose degradation was unaltered with increasing glucose concentration. This approach has limited practical application since the glucose concentration in dialysate is mainly defined by the ultrafiltration profile required to maintain fluid balance in PD patients.

Two-Chamber Bag Systems

Several variations of two-chamber bag systems have been proposed to improve the pH and reduce the glucose degradation products of current PD

solutions [50–53]. Generally these systems employ similar principles: glucose degradation is minimized by sterilizing dextrose under acidic condition in one chamber of the bag while the electrolytes are placed in the second chamber at an alkaline pH. When the two solutions are mixed after sterilization the pH of the mixed solution is in a more physiologic range. Major drawbacks of such systems are that they are more expensive to manufacture and that they require the patient to mix the contents of the two solutions prior to infusing into the peritoneum.

Aseptic Processing

Several approaches have been proposed for manufacturing PD fluids using aseptic techniques [54–57]. These approaches involve sterilization of each component of the solution using one of the terminal sterilization methods followed by combining these components using aseptic techniques. Aseptic processing allows for manufacturing solutions at physiological pH with much less glucose degradation products than the current PD fluids. In limited clinical studies solutions prepared by aseptic processing are found to be safe and effective [54, 55, 57].

Aseptic processing for making sterile solution products has evolved rapidly over the last two decades. A properly designed and controlled aseptic processing area employing modern high-speed filling equipment, absolute barrier systems for form/fill/seal, robotics, and advanced air purification systems is likely to permit manufacturing of products with SALs approaching 1×10^{-6} [58]. At these SALs, solutions manufactured by aseptic processing and heat sterilization essentially carry similar risks of microbial contamination, while the aseptic processing allows for manufacture of improved quality PD fluids.

SUMMARY

The quality of current PD solutions is compromised by the acidic pH and the presence of glucose degradation products. Both low pH and the glucose breakdown products are a direct result of terminal heat sterilization. The therapy consequences of low pH and glucose degradation products include abdominal pain during infusion of the dialysis fluid and impaired peritoneal cell viability and function. Chronic use of these solutions may cause impaired host defense and hence increased risk of infection, and possibly loss of ultrafiltration, peritoneal fibrosis, and therapy failure. PD solutions prepared at physiologic pH either by aseptic processing or steam sterilization in a two-chamber bag system are devoid of in vitro cytotoxicity and hence may lead to improved quality of therapy provided by peritoneal dialysis. With new technologies permitting aseptic processing to achieve SALs approaching solutions manufactured by terminal steam sterilization, it is possible to produce solutions that are more biocompatible than steam sterilized products without increasing the risk of microbial contamination.

REFERENCES

1. Sterilization and sterility assurance of compendial articles. U.S. Pharmacopeia. 1995; 23:1976–81.
2. Barr DB. FDA's aseptic processing: proposed regulation. J Parenter Sci Technol 1993; 47:57–9.
3. Ganter G. Ueber die Beseitigung giftiger Stoffe aus dem Blute durch Dialyse. Munch med Wschr 1923; 70:1478–80.
4. Balazs J and Rosenak S. Zur Behandlung der Sublimatanurie durch peritoneale dialyse. Wien klin Wschr 1934; 47:851–4.
5. Heusser H and Werder H. Untersuchungen über. Peritoneal dialyse. Beitr klin Chir 1927; 141:38–49.
6. Abbott WE and Shea P. The treatment of temporary renal insufficiency (uremia) by peritoneal lavage. Am J Med Sci 1946; 211:312–19.
7. Odel HM, Ferris DO and Power MH. Peritoneal lavage as an effective means of external excretion. Am J Med 1950; 9:63–77.
8. Boen S. The evolution of peritoneal dialysis. In Atkins RC, Thompson NM and Farrell PC, editors. Peritoneal dialysis. Edinburgh, Churchill Livingston, 1981; 3–11.
9. Martis L and Henderson LW. Impact of terminal heat sterilization on the quality of peritoneal dialysis solutions. Blood Purif 1997; 15:54–60.
10. Henderson IS, Couper IA and Lumsden A. Potentially irritant glucose metabolites in unused CAPD fluid. In Maher J, editor. Frontiers in peritoneal dialysis. New York, Field, Rich, 1985; 261–4.
11. Nilsson-Thorell CB, Muscalu N, Andrén AHG et al. Heat sterilization of fluids for peritoneal dialysis gives rise to aldehydes. Perit Dial Int 1993; 13:208–13.
12. Wieslander AP, Nordin MK, Kjellstrand PTT and Boberg UC. Toxicity of peritoneal dialysis fluids on cultured fibroblasts, L-929. Kidney Int 1991; 40:77–9.
13. Wieslander AP, Nordin MK, Martinson E, Kjellstrand PTT and Boberg UC. Heat-sterilized PD fluids impair growth and inflammatory responses of cultured cell lines and human leukocytes. Clin Nephrol 1993; 39:343–8.
14. Rogamgnoni M, Beecari M, Faiolo S, Granello E, Scalia P and Paleardi F. Abdominal pain with infusion of peritoneal dialysis solutions relieved by alkalization. Perit Dial Bull 1984; 4:188–9.
15. Bunchman TE and Ballal SH. Treatment of inflow pain by pH adjustment of dialysate in peritoneal dialysis. Perit Dial Int 1991; 11:179–80.
16. Yamamoto T, Sakakura T, Yamakawa M et al. Clinical effects of long-term use of neutralized dialysate for continuous ambulatory peritoneal dialysis. Nephron 1992; 60:324–9.
17. Duwe Ak, Vas SI and Weatherhead JW. Effects of the composition of peritoneal dialysis fluid on chemiluminescence, phagocytosis and bacterial activity in vitro. Infect Immunol 1981; 33:130–5.
18. Topley N, Alobaidi HMM, Davies M, Coles GA, Williams JD and Lloyd D. The effect of dialysate on peritoneal phagocyte oxidative metabolism. Kidney Int 1988; 34:404–11.
19. Yu AW, Zhou XJ, Nawab ZM, Gandhi VC, Ing TS and Vaziri ND. Neutrophilic peritoneal dialysis solutions. Int J Artif Organs 1992; 15:661–5.
20. Chaimovitz C, Rapoport J, Konforti A and Douvdevani A. Commercial dialysis fluid causes intracellular acidosis in peritoneal macrophages. J Am Soc Nephrol 1992; 3:407.
21. Rotstein OD, Nasmith PE and Grinstein S. The bacteroids by-product succinic acid inhibits neutrophil respiratory burst by reducing intracellular pH. Infect Immun 1987; 55:864–70.
22. Alobaidi HM, Coles CA, Davies M and Lloyd D. Host defense in continuous ambulatory peritoneal dialysis: the effect of the dialysate on phagocytic function. Nephrol Dial Transplant 1986; 1:16–21.
23. Van Bronswijk M, Verbrugh HA, Heezius HCJM, Van der Meulen J and Oe LP. Dialysis fluids and local host resistance in patients on continous ambulatory peritoneal dialysis. Eur J Clin Microbial Infect Dis 1988; 7:368–73.
24. Bos HJ, Vlaanderen K, van der Meulen J, de Veld JC, Oe LP and Beelen RHJ. Peritoneal macrophages in short dwell time effluent show diminished phagocytosis. Perit Dial Int 1988; 8:199–202.
25. Ing BL, Gupta DK, Nawab ZM, Zhou F, Rahaman MA and Daugirdas JT. Suppression of neutrophil superoxide production by conventional peritoneal dialysis solutions. Int J Artif Organs 1988; 1:351–4.
26. Moughal NA, McGregor SJ, Brock JH, Briggs JD and Junor BJR. Expression of transferrin receptors by monocytes and peritoneal macrophages from renal failure patients treated by continuous ambulatory peritoneal dialysis. Eur J Clin Invest 1991; 21:592–6.
27. Davies SJ, Suassuna J, Ogg CS and Cameron JS. Activation of immuno-competent cells in the peritoneum of patients treated with CAPD. Kidney Int 1989; 36:661–8.
28. Lewis SL, Norris PJ and Holmes CJ. Phenotypic characterization of monocytes and macrophages from CAPD patients. Trans Am Soc Artif Intern Organs 1990: 36:M575–7.

29. Krane SM and Golding MD. Potential role for interleukin A-1 in fibrosis associated with chronic ambulatory peritoneal dialysis. Blood Purif 1988; 6:173–7.

30. Breborowicz A. Free radicals in peritoneal dialysis: agents of damage? Perit Dial Int 1992; 12:194–8.

31. Bos HJ, Meyer F, de Veld JC and Beelen RHJ. Peritoneal dialysis fluid induces change of mononuclear phagocyte proportions. Kidney Int 1989; 36:20–6.

32. Vachula M. Aono F, Kubey W and Holmes C. Effect of peritoneal dialysis fluid on mononuclear cell surface receptor expression. J Am Soc Nephrol 1991; 2:368.

33. Jörres A, Richter D, Hain H et al: Cytokine release from peripheral and peritoneal phagocytes: effect of CAPD dialysate. Kidney Int 1990; 37:329.

34. Jörres A, Jörres D, Gahl GM et al. Leukotriene B4 and tumor necrosis factor from leukocytes: effect of peritoneal dialysate. Nephron 1991;58:276–82.

35. Douvdevani A, Rapoport J, Konforti A, Zlotnik M and Chaimovitz C. The effect of peritoneal dialysis fluid on cytokine release: factors involved and time course. Perit Dial Int 1993; 13:112–17.

36. De Fijiter CWH, Verbrugh HA, Peters EDJ et al. In vivo exposure to the currently available peritoneal dialysis fluids decreases function of peritoneal macrophages in CAPD. Clin Nephrol 1993; 39:75–80.

37. Chaimovitz C. Peritoneal dialysis. Kidney Int 1994; 45:1226–40.

38. Topley N, Mackenzie R, Petersen MM et al. In vitro testing of a potentially biocompatible continuous ambulatory peritoneal dialysis fluid. Nephrol Dial Transplant 1991; 6:574–81.

39. Van Bronswijk H, Verbrugh HA, Bos HJ, Heezius HCJM, Van der Meulen J, Oe LP et al. Cytotoxic effects of commercial continuous ambultory peritoneal dialysis fluids and of bacterial exoproducts on human mesothelial cells in vitro. Perit Dial Int 1989; 9:197–202.

40. Holmes CJ. Biocompatibility of peritoneal dialysis solutions. Perit Dial Int 1993; 13:88–94.

41. Dobbie JW. Pathogenesis of peritoneal fibrosing syndromes (sclerosing peritonitis) in peritoneal dialysis. Perit Dial Int 1992; 12:14–27.

42. Singh B, Dean GR and Cantor SM. The role of 5-(hydroxymethyl)-furfural in the discoloration of sugar solutions. J Am Chem Soc 1948; 70:517–22.

43. Griffin JC and Marie SC. Glucose degradation in the presence of sodium lactate during autoclaving at 121c. Am J Hosp Pharm 1958; 15:893–5.

44. Cooker LA, Luneburg P, Faict D et al. Reduced glucose degradation products in bicarbonate lactate buffered peritoneal dialysis solutions produced in two-chambered bags. Perit Dial Int 1997; 17:373–8.

45. Mannermaa JP, Muttonen E, Yliruusi J et al. The use of different time temperature combinations in the optimization of sterilization of Ringers glucose infusion solution. J Parenter Sci Technol 1992; 46:184–91.

46. Cook AP, MacLeod TM, Appleton JD et al. HPLC studies on the degradation profiles of glucose 5% solutions subjected to heat sterilization in a mecroprocessor-controlled autoclave. J Clin Pharm Ther 1989; 14:189–95.

47. Wieslander AP, Kjellstrand PTT and Rippe B. Heat sterilization of glucose-containing fluids for peritoneal dialysis: biological consequences of chemical alterations. Perit Dial Int 1995; 15:S52–S60.

48. Webb NE, Sperandio GJ and Martin AN. A study of the composition of glucose solutions. J Am Pharm Assoc 1958; 47:101–3.

49. Wing WT. An examination of the decomposition dextrose solution during sterilization. J Pharm Pharmacol 1960; 12:T191–6.

50. Feriani M, Biasioli S, Borin D et al. Bicarbonate buffer for CAPD solutions. ASAIO Trans 1985; 31:668–72.

51. Feriani M, Carobi C, LaGreca G et al. Clinical experience with a 39 mmol/L bicarbonate buffered peritoneal dialysis solution. Perit Dial Int 1997; 17:17–21.

52. Coles GA, Gokal R, Ogg C et al. A randomized controlled trial of a bicarbonate- and a bicarbonate/lactate-containing dialysis solution in CAPD. Perit Dial Int 1997; 17:48–51.

53. Rippe B, Simonsen O, Wieslander A et al. Clinical and physiological effects of a new, less toxic and less acidic fluid for peritoneal dialysis. Perit Dial Int 1997; 17:27–34.

54. Ing TS, Yu AW, Thomson AU et al. Peritoneal dialysis using conventional lactate containing solution sterilized by ultrafiltration. Int J Artif Organs 1992; 15:658–60.

55. Yu AW, Manahan FJ, Filkins JP et al. Peritoneal dialysis using bicarbonate-containing solution sterilized by ultrafiltration. Artif Kidney Dial 1991; 14:463–5.

56. Yatzidis H. A new stable bicarbonate dialysis solution for peritoneal dialysis: preliminary report. Perit Dial Int 1991; 11:224–7.

57. Slingeneyer A, Faller B, Michel C et al. Increased ultrafiltration capacity using a new bicarbonate CAPD solution (abstract). Perit Dial Int 1993; 13:57.

58. Akers JE and Agalloco JP. Aseptic processing – a current perspective. In Morissey RF and Phillips GB, editors. Sterilization technology – a practical guide for manufacturers and users of health care products. New York, Van Nostrand Reinhold, 1993; 283–308.

25. Quality assurance in the treatment of acute renal failure

ANDRE A. KAPLAN

INTRODUCTION

Despite a plethora of information regarding what is or isn't adequate dialysis prescription for end stage renal failure [1–3] there is an amazing paucity of information regarding what is adequate treatment for acute renal failure. Similarly, quality assessment for the dialytic treatment of relatively stable patients with ESRD can be reasonably distilled down to simple mortality [4], an approach which is not easily applicable to acutely ill patients whose mortality risk is already very high and in whom acute renal failure may be an incidental, supplemental insult. Thus, it is still commonly believed that acutely ill patients die *with* renal failure and not *from* renal failure. In agreement with this concept, a recent NIH sponsored conference has suggested that outcome parameters for patients with acute renal failure should be stratified into several levels; by the length of stay, both in the ICU and in the hospital; by the number who recover renal function; by the amount of renal function recovered and, finally, the percentage survival in terms of discharge from the ICU and the hospital [5]. Clearly, considering the initial poor survival of acutely ill patients even before developing ARF, and considering the variability of etiologies and comorbidities, it is exceedingly difficult to obtain such stratified outcome parameters from the experience of a single medical institution. Thus, the same aforementioned NIH conference concluded that evidence based guidelines for the treatment of acute renal failure must be obtained from multicenter trials that use standardized criteria for management and outcomes. Nonetheless, even in the context of a multicenter trial, problems in interpretation of results remain. As convincingly argued by Bellomo and Boyce, the

geographical variability in survival rates, the need for large numbers of patients ($\geqslant 160$) and the differing expertise of the treating physicians present seemingly insurmountable problems [6].

In the current absence of such rigorously obtained guidelines, the purpose of this review will be to consider the available evidence allowing for a definition of adequate dialysis for the patient with acute renal failure. Thus, quality assessment in the treatment of acute renal failure will be defined as the assurance of adequate dialytic care. Furthermore, in order to allow a reasonable depth of discussion, I will forego consideration of fluid removal, electrolyte control and acid base balance and limit the presentation to an evaluation of adequate solute removal as considered in three categories: small, "middle" and large molecular weight toxins.

SMALL MOLECULAR WEIGHT TOXINS

Although many authorities consider urea only as a surrogate marker for small molecular weight toxins, urea kinetic modeling has gained acceptance in the nephrologic community as a means of measuring dialysis adequacy in the ESRD population. For patients with acute renal failure, data exist (vide infra) which identifies a given urea level at which the initiation of prophylactic dialysis provides a benefit to survival. There are also data which suggest a minimally adequate urea clearance. Thus, in the absence of other, better documented criteria, it would appear useful to consider the application of urea kinetics as a means of measuring the adequacy of dialysis for acute renal failure. Given the available information, the first step will be to define the level of urea which can be

L.W. Henderson and R.S. Thuma (eds.), Quality Assurance in Dialysis, 2nd Edition, 275–284.
© 1999 *Kluwer Academic Publishers. Printed in Great Britain*

considered "acceptable" and then determine, using formulae for urea nitrogen appearance, the necessary urea clearance required to maintain blood urea concentrations below that level.

What is an "Acceptable" Urea Level?

It is obvious that the development of uremic symptomatology is an indisputable indication for the initiation of renal replacement therapy. What is less clear is the point at which prophylactic therapy is beneficial to the final outcome. Several studies have attempted to define the level of uremic solute retention which is likely to negatively impact on survival (Table 25.1) [7]. In 1960, Teschan et al. reported on 15 patients who were dialyzed in order to maintain blood urea nitrogen (BUN) levels at approximately 120 mg/dL, demonstrating a substantially improved survival when compared to historical controls [8]. Subsequently, in a study involving a retrospective analysis of 500 patients, Kleinknecht et al. evaluated the results of prophylactic dialysis in patients whose average blood urea nitrogen levels were 93 mg/dL [9]. They found a significantly improved survival when compared to previously treated patients whose dialysis was initiated only after the onset of uremic symptomatology, at a point when their average level of BUN was 163 mg/dL. In the first randomized study of its type, Conger treated 18 Vietnamese war casualties whose dilalytic therapy was initiated at blood urea nitrogen levels of either 120 or 50 mg/dL, finding a significantly increased survival in those undergoing the more rigorous prescription [10]. In a follow-up study, some 10 years later, Gillum et al. investigated two highly intensive dialytic prescriptions, maintaining predialysis blood urea nitrogen levels at or below either 100 or 60 mg/dL, for which no difference in survival could be demonstrated [11]. Although the patient groups and study designs were different, a review of these available data would suggest that improved survival can be achieved if prophylactic dialysis is initiated at blood urea nitrogen levels between 100 and 120 mg/dL. Clearly, however, widespread clinical experience would suggest that a criteria to initiate dialysis based solely on a given urea level should be tempered with a reasonable assessment of the situation at hand. For example, if the renal failure is likely to be rapidly reversible (prerenal azotemia, obstructive uropathy), levels of 150 mg/dL (54 mmol/L) or more may be tolerated in anticipation of the rapid return of endogenous renal function.

Table 25.1. Prophylactic hemodialysis for acute renal failure

Authors/year	No. of patients	Type of study	BUN prior to initiation of treatment (mg/dL)	Survival Total	%	Comments
Teschan et al. 1960 [8]	15	Retrospective Historical Controls	120	10/15	67	Previous survival: 50%
Kleinknecht et al. 1972 [9]	279 221	Retrospective Historical Controls	163 93	170/279 157/221	61 71	Sepsis hemorrhage decreased
Conger 1975 [10]	10 8	Prospective Concurrent Controls	120 50	2/10 5/8	20 64	Sepsis and hemorrhage decreased
Gillum et al. 1986 [11]	17 17	Prospective Concurrent	100 60	9/17 7/17	53 41	No difference with controls

Modified from: Kaplan AA. Extracorporeal blood purification in the treatment of acute renal failure with multiorgan involvement. Blood Purif 1996; 14:86–93 [7]

What is a Minimum Amount of Urea Clearance Required for the Adequate Treatment of Acute Renal Failure?

Given the above conclusions, and considering a simple calculation of urea kinetics (see appendix), one can approximate that a 70 kg patient catabolising 1 g/kg of protein/day would require a minimum urea clearance of 6 mL/min, or 9 L a day, in order to maintain a blood urea nitrogen level at or below 100 mg/dL. In general agreement with this approach, a study designed to compare continuous arteriovenous hemofiltration versus pumped continuous venovenous hemofiltration demonstrated a statistically improved survival as the net delivered urea clearance increased from 7.5 to 15 L/day, regardless of the technique chosen [12].

Two preliminary reports provide further impetus to the idea that urea clearance can be considered as a means of assessing the adequacy of dialysis for acute renal failure. Tapolyai et al. reported that survival of patients with acute renal failure could be retrospectively stratified by the amount of delivered Kt/V, with survivors having received a per treatment Kt/V of 1.09 (urea reduction ratio of 58%) while non—survivors received a Kt/V of 0.89 (urea reduction ratio of 46%) [13]. Although one might argue that the sickest patients are the least likely to receive their fully prescribed dialysis dose, in a follow up assessment from the same institution, involving over 800 patients, Paganini et al. reported that, even after stratification for disease severity, improved survival could still be documented for those receiving a higher delivered Kt/V [14]. Most recently, Schiffl et al. have presented abstracted results claiming a statistically increased survival in patients with acute renal failure receiving daily dialysis versus those receiving dialysis every other day [15]. When stratified by delivered dialysis dose, those patients receiving a weekly Kt/V of less than 3.0 had a mortality of 57% while those receiving a weekly Kt/V of at least 6.0 had a mortality of only 16%. Although there are many unanswered questions regarding these preliminary data, the reported differences in survival are impressive and dwarf those previously reported when outcome in ARF was stratified by other criteria, such as the "biocompatibility" of the dialysis membrane.

Recommendations for Adequate Small Molecular Weight Clearance

In summary, the available data provide us with two goals in regards to nitrogen balance and control of uremia. The combined urea clearance (residual renal function plus that provided by the dialytic therapy) should equal *at least* 15 L/day and urea nitrogen levels should be maintained at or below values of 100 to 120 mg/dL. If the preliminary data by Schiffl et al. [15] are confirmed, these recommendations may require a substantial upward revision. Table 25.2 lists the urea clearance capabilities of the available renal replacement techniques [16]. In perusal of this table it should be kept in mind that the values listed are what are achievable under ideal conditions. Of note is that, as well described in the population with ESRD, critically ill patients are particularly prone to those situations and conditions whereby the prescribed dose of dialysis is not successfully delivered [13, 17]. In a review of this issue, Leblanc et al. underscore the myriad of problems which can reduce the delivered dialysis dose in those patients with acute renal failure [18]. Included in this list is the increased potential for vascular access recirculation because of commonly employed double lumen catheters, the frequent use of a non-heparin technique resulting in the reduced efficiency of a partially clotted dialyzer and the vascular instability of the patient forcing early termination of the treatment.

Assessing the Delivery of the Prescribed Urea Clearance

Although formal urea kinetic modeling may not be easily applied in the patient with acute renal failure and severe hypercatabolism, a minimum check for adequate dialysis should include at least an informal assessment of the delivered dialysis dose. For intermittent hemodialysis performed three times weekly, this should include a pre and post dialysis urea level, with a resultant urea reduction ratio (URR) of at least 65% or a Kt/V of at least 1.2. Many readers will immediately recognize these parameters as those recently published in the NKF sponsored DOQI (dialysis outcomes quality initiative) guidelines for the treatment of ESRD [19] and it is the opinion of this

Table 25.2. Time averaged urea clearance for renal replacement therapies

Technique	Prescription	mL/min	L/day	L/week
Hemodialysis[a]	3 × 4 hr/wk	17.9	26	180
	7 × 4 hr/wk	41.7	60	420
Peritoneal Dialysis	2 l/hr	16.7	24	168
CAVH	14 l/d	6.9	10	70
CAVH (enhanced)[b]	24 l/d	9.7	14	98
CAVHD[c]	1–2 l/hr[d]	19–35	27–51	189–357
CVVH	1–2 l/hr	17–33	24–48	168–336
CVVHD[c]	1–2 l/hrd	19–35	27–51	189–357

[a]Assumes a delivered urea clearance of 250 ml/min
[b]with vacuum suction on filtrate port and predilution infusion
[c]Assumes 3 L/day net filtrate
[d]infused dialysate

Modified from Kaplan AA. Continuous arterio-venous hemofiltration and related therapies. in: Jacobs C, Kjellstrand CM, Koch KM, Winchester JF (editors). Replacement of Renal Function by Dialysis, 4th edition. Kluwer Academic Press, Dordrecht, 1996, pp 390–417.

author that what is considered adequate for the treatment of a relatively stable patient with ESRD should be at least a *minimal* criteria for the replacement of renal function in a patient who is critically ill. In those patients in whom intermittent dialysis is performed more that thrice weekly, comparable criteria derived from the experience with the ESRD population does not exist and a *minimal* criteria for adequacy would be the maintenance of pre-dialysis BUN levels equal to or below 100 to 120 mg/dL. For the continuous therapies, a reasonable estimate of delivered urea clearance can be ascertained by obtaining a daily sample for dialysate/filtrate urea concentration and multiplying by the day's total output.

"MIDDLE MOLECULAR WEIGHT" TOXINS

The above criteria for adequate dialysis are clearly limited to the clearance of small molecular weight toxins using urea as the putative surrogate marker. What about the "middle molecular weight" toxins. The most widely accepted toxin in this category is that of the 11,580 dalton β_2-microglobulin, a substance which has been implicated in the development of dialysis related amyloidosis, a morbidity which requires several years to develop and which is therefore of no concern in the immediate treatment of acute renal failure. In this category, however, is a group of substances which may be considered of much greater importance in the critically ill patient, namely the cytokines.

Cytokine Removal with Dialytic Techniques

The convective based solute transport of hemofiltration based treatments (CAVH, CVVH, continuous arterio-venous hemofiltration and continuous veno-venous hemofiltration) fueled speculation that these modalities might be advantageous in removing middle-molecular weight toxins which were felt to induce the instability and organ failure of the critically ill. In 1984, Coraim et al. studied patients having undergone cardiac surgery and demonstrated the existence of a 1,000 dalton myocardial depressant factor (MDF) which could inhibit *in-vitro* preparations of guinea pig papillary muscle [20]. Chromatographic and pharmacologic studies confirmed the existence of this factor in the filtrate during treatment with CAVH and concurrent assessment demonstrated an improvement in cardiac function. There was, however, no data regarding the serum levels of this substance and the clinical improvement in cardiac function may have been related to a normalization in Starling forces [21]. A follow up study reported, but did not document, a 50% decline in serum levels of the MDF one hour after initiation of CAVH [22]. It is unlikely, however, that this change could be achieved by one hour of filtration and this rapid decrease in the serum level is more suggestive of a decline in production.

Tumor necrosis factor (TNF) is often implicated in the initiation of the inflammatory response and, at least in its monomeric form (17,000 daltons), may be filterable by many CRRT (continuous renal replacement therapy) systems. Bellomo et al. studied twelve septic patients and were able to demonstrate that continuous hemodiafiltration could provide a mean 27 L/day of TNF clearance, but changes in serum levels were minimal [23]. Subsequently Cottrell and Mehta presented preliminary data suggesting that the AN69 polyacrylonitrile membrane was capable of TNF adsorption [24]. Once again, however, their in-vitro system demonstrated little change in "serum" levels.

Using a variety of animal models, several other investigators have attempted to demonstrate the possible advantages of the continuous therapies in the removal of inflammatory mediators [25, 26] and the subject has undergone extensive review [27, 28]. Of the available data, the most convincing is that provided by Grootendorst and colleagues demonstrating that 6 L/hour of zero-balance filtration could remove a myocardial depressant factor from pigs in septic shock [29–31]. These same authors are currently providing filtration rates of up to 100 L/day for their patients with multiorgan failure [32]. Nonetheless, formal documentation of a generalized improvement in survival is lacking and many practical issues remain, such as the net nutrient losses incurred by such high filtration rates.

In a most recent publication, involving trauma patients with multiorgan failure but without ARF, continuous hemofiltration was found to provide a substantial removal of TNF and IL-6, but, as with previous in-vitro and in-vivo studies, serum levels were unaffected and the authors concluded that the removal was clinically insignificant [33]. Unfortunately, despite its sound scientific design, with a concomitantly treated control group, it is difficult to glean definitive conclusions from this study since the mean filtration rates were limited to

only 290 mL/hour, an amount which would be considered trivial by most investigators attempting to treat patients with concomitant ARF.

Recommendations for the Delivery of "Middle Molecular Weight" Clearance

In summary, although inflammatory mediators can be found in the filtrate or dialysate of CRRT systems and can be documented to be adsorbed onto certain membranes, it remains to be demonstrated that this removal results in a significant decline in serum levels or a clinically useful improvement in the inflammatory response. Schetz et al. have provided an in depth review of the subject and make the following conclusions; the endogenous half lives of TNF and IL-1 are so short (6–20 minutes) as to render attempts at extracorporeal removal futile or insignificant; the most active form of TNF is a trimer of about 50,000 daltons, a size which exceeds the sieving capabilities of currently employed hemofiltration membranes; both TNF and IL-1 are partially bound to serum proteins and binding substances which further hinders their removal by hemofiltration [34]. Despite this generalized negative review, the same authors conclude that the available animal studies do suggest clinically relevant removal of a myocardial depressant factor and that clinical studies designed to determine the effect of this removal on survival are warranted.

Thus, given the current state of available information, there is insufficient evidence to support the widespread application of large volume hemofiltration techniques with the expressed purpose of removal of inflammatory cytokines. Although removal and subsequent lowering of myocardial depressant factors may occur, further trials are needed before one can assume a clinically relevant improvement from this treatment strategy.

LARGE MOLECULAR WEIGHT TOXINS

In contrast to strategies designed for the removal of cytokines, treatments designed to remove endotoxins have the theoretical advantage of directing attention to those factors which are considered to be at the top of the inflammatory cascade. The removal of endotoxin represents one of the most appealing and promising roles for extracorporeal blood purification techniques. In essence, the body has only limited means for the removal of these large molecular weight toxins which can include fragments of several hundred thousand daltons or more. Under normal conditions, such as with the cell wall fragments of gut bacteria, these potential toxins are cleared by the reticuloendothelial system, such as by the Kupffer cells of the liver [35]. Under conditions of sepsis, the removal system becomes overloaded and these toxic fragments are trapped in the circulation, stimulating a host of inflammatory processes by way of cytokines, eicosanoids, and nitric oxide [36]. In human experimentation, the role of endotoxin as a primary initiator of the septic syndrome has been difficult to prove since studies were, by design, limited to relatively modest doses of endotoxin. Recently, the detailed description and monitoring of a self inflicted dose of endotoxin has provided strong evidence to support the concept that endotoxin can play a primary role in the initiation of the septic syndrome in humans [37].

Sieving of such large molecular weight substances can not be obtained by any of the renal replacement techniques currently employed, and successful elimination of large endotoxin fragments can only be achieved by plasma exchange or adsorption. The best established indication for this approach is in the treatment of fulminant systemic meningococcemia for which there have been several anecdotal cases and uncontrolled series reporting the successful use of plasma exchange, with or without leucopheresis, for 33 of 40 patients such treated [38–45]. The largest series involved 15 cases with a resulting overall survival of 80%, which was substantially improved over the results obtained in 15 consecutive patients previously treated without plasma exchange [45]. Furthermore, based on the Nicklasson score, a severity of disease score specific for meningococcemia [46] those patients treated with plasma exchange had a predicted mortality of 62% but an actual mortality of only 20%.

Other septic syndromes resulting in ARF may also benefit from extracorporeal removal of endotoxin, either by plasma exchange or adsorption with filters impregnated with polymyxin B [47, 48]. A review of English language publications reveals anecdotal cases and small uncontrolled

series involving 99 patients with an overall survival exceeding 75% [47, 49]. The impressive survival rate documented in these reports is encouraging but one would expect reporting of only the best results. In the least successful of these reports, in which all 4 patients treated with plasma exchange died, post mortem evaluation determined the existence of persistent foci of infection [50]. Similarly, in the most recent report, Stegmayr reported on 25 patients with septic shock and acute renal failure in which 3 of the 5 non-survivors had autopsy evidence of a persistent source of sepsis [51]. Clearly, plasma exchange or adsorption can not be a sole requirement for survival if the nidus of infection persists. Thus, these techniques should be considered only as a means of removing the large molecular weight toxins which may be "artificially" sustaining a systemic inflammatory response, and only as an adjunct to successful irradication of the active infection by the appropriate antibiotics or the eventual surgical drainage.

A most intriguing approach in the overall management of the septic patient with acute renal failure was proposed by Brazilay et al. in which critically ill patients were randomized to receive either continuous renal replacement therapy alone, or in conjunction with plasma exchange [52]. Those receiving the combination treatment had the best survival, suggesting that a combination of treatments offering continuous removal of small, middle and large molecular weight toxins may represent the most advantageous strategy in the extracorporeal management of the patient with multiorgan failure and renal dysfunction.

Recommendations for Large Molecular Weight Clearance

Except for the special case of fulminant meningococcemia, the currently available data does not support the widespread use of techniques designed for large molecular weight toxins. Nonetheless, if future studies determine that large molecular weight substances such as endotoxin play a fundamental, primary role in the ultimate mortality of patients with acute renal failure and sepsis, blood purification techniques designed for large molecular weight toxin removal may become part of the required treatment strategy.

Addendum

Regardless of the desired goals in the delivery of dialytic care for acute renal failure, it is obvious that treatment related complications will limit the success in attaining these goals. In our institution we have initiated a quality control assessment designed to identify problems and allow for their evaluation so as to limit their reoccurrence. An example of our complications assessment sheet is depicted on Figure 25.1. At the end of each dialysis treatment the dialysis nurse completes the assessment by documenting any confirmed or suspected complications. Follow up data is obtained when necessary.

APPENDIX: CALCULATION OF NITROGEN BALANCE FOR PATIENTS WITH ACUTE RENAL FAILURE

In the context of ARF, estimation of nitrogen balance allows for an intelligent choice in proper nutrition, helps identify conditions of hypercatabolism which may be amenable to treatment (gastrointestinal hemorrhage) and allows for the calculation of the minimum amount of urea clearance required to maintain a reasonable level of uremic control and avoidance of uremic complications [53].

Nitrogen balance can be easily evaluated by measuring the rate of urea production, commonly

---

COMPLICATIONS ASSOCIATED WITH HEMODIALYSIS

<u>Vascular Access</u>
Access: Femoral Vein - Subclavian - Internal Jugular
Manufacturer: Quinton - Shiley - Medcom - Other: _________________
Complications:
        A. Thrombosis:
        B. Bleeding:
            Hematoma - Retroperitoneal bleed - Hemothorax -
            Damage/Laceration of Great Vessels
                1. Requiring Transfusion: yes - no
                2. Requiring surgical intervention
                3. Requiring interventional radiology
        C. Infection:
            Erythema - Discharge - Both
            Culture results:________________________________
            Gram stain results: ____________________________
            Catheter tip culture results:_____________________
        D. Pneumothorax
        E. Other:____

<u>Hemodialysis</u>
        A. Hypotension unresponsive to volume replacement:
            1. Cardiogenic shock: pericardial tamponade - arrhythmia - myocardial infarction
            2. Membrane incompatibility (wheezing, hypotension, cuprophane membrane)
            3. Other:___________________________________
        B. Electrolyte abnormality
            1. Tetany (hypocalcemia)
            2. Hypo or hyperkalemia
            3. Hypo or hypernatremia
            4. Acid base disturbance
            5. Other: _______________________________
        C. Air embolism
        D. Pyrogenic reaction:
            1. Immediately upon initiating dialysis (within 15 minutes)
            2. Upon termination of dialysis
            3. During dialysis treatment
            4. Culture results:___________________________
        E. Muscle cramps: 50% dextrose -- Normal Saline --- albumin --- hypertonic saline
        F. Hypoxemia
            1. With acetate dialysis
            2. With bicarbonate dialysis
            3. Other:_________________________________
        G. Hemorrhagic complications
            1. Subdural hematoma
            2. Gastrointestinal hemorrhage
            3. Retroperitoneal hemorrhage
            4. Hemothorax, hemorrhagic pleural effusion
            5. Other_________________________________
        H. Prapism
        I. Dialysis disequilibrium

Fig. 25.1. Clinical protocol of the John Dempsey hospital. Complications associated with hemodialysis.

referred to as urea nitrogen appearance (UNA). The daily UNA can be measured by obtaining a 24-hour urine for urea nitrogen and evaluating the change in blood urea nitrogen occurring at the beginning and end of the 24-hour collection. The UNA can then be calculated using the following formula:

$$UNA\ (g/d) = [BUN_2 - BUN_1]/100 \times total\ body\ water + UUN$$

where UNA equals the daily urea nitrogen appearance in grams/day; BUN_1 and BUN_2 are the levels of blood urea nitrogen in mg/dL at the beginning and end of the 24-hour urine collection; total body water in liters is estimated as 60% of lean body mass plus the amount of any extra edema fluid; and UUN is the 24 hour collection of urine urea nitrogen expressed as grams/day. If there is an ongoing continuous renal replacement therapy, estimation of the net urea removal by that technique is added to the right side of the equation.

Under conditions of neutral nitrogen balance, UNA is dependent on protein ingestion and can be calculated as follows:

$$UNA\ (g/d) = protein\ intake\ (g/d)/6.25 - non\text{-}urea\ nitrogen\ (g/d)$$

It is assumed that every 6.25 grams of protein contains 1 gram of nitrogen and that the production of non-urea nitrogen is 31 mg/kg/day of lean body mass [54].

The minimum amount of urea clearance required to remove a given amount of UNA can be calculated using the following formula:

$$Urea\ clearance\ (L/d) = [UNA\ (g/d)/BUN\ (mg/dL)] \times 100$$

When the above formulas are used, a 70 kg patient receiving 1 g/kg/day of protein will receive 11 grams of nitrogen (70 g/6.25). On balance, approximately 2 grams (70 kg $\times$ 31 mg) of nitrogen becomes nitrogenous wastes other than urea; the remaining 9 grams becomes urea.

In patients with hypercatabolism, urea production is greatly enhanced owing to the breakdown of endogenous proteins and UNA will exceed that predicted from exogenous protein feeding. Under these conditions, endogenous protein breakdown can generate 30 grams or more of urea nitrogen

per day, representing the catabolism of approximately 200 grams of protein. In addition to enhanced proteolysis accompanying hypercatabolism, increased urea production is often the result of gastrointestinal bleeding, with the absorption and breakdown of the blood and its proteins. There is approximately 200 grams of protein/L of whole blood.

REFERENCES

1. Gotch F and Sargent JA. A mechanistic analysis of the National Cooperative Dialysis Study. Kidney Int 1985; 28:526–34.
2. Owen WF, Lew NL, Liu Y et al. The urea reduction ration and serum albumin concentration as predictors of mortality in patients undergoing hemodialysis. N Eng J Med 1993; 329:1001–6.
3. Parker TF, Husni L, Huang W et al. Effects of dose of dialysis on morbidity and mortality. Am J Kidney Dis 1994; 23:670–80.
4. Charra B, Calemard E, Fuffet M et al. Survival as an index of adequacy of dialysis. Kidney Int 1992; 41:1286–91
5. DuBose Jr TD, Warnock DG, Mehta RL, Bonventre JV, Hammerman MR, Molitoris BA et al. ARF in the 21st century: recommendations for management and outcomes assessment. Am J Kidney Dis 1997; 29:793–9
6. Bellomo R and Boyce N. Does continuous hemodiafiltration improve survival in acute renal failure. Semin Dial 1993; 6:16–19.
7. Kaplan AA. Extracorporeal blood purification in the treatment of acute renal failure with multiorgan involvement. Blood Purif 1996; 14:86–93
8. Teschan PE, Baxter CR, O'Brien TF, Freyhof JN and Hall WH. Prophylactic hemodialysis in the treatment of acute renal failure. Am J Med 1960; 53:992–1016.
9. Kleinknecht D, Jungers P, Chanard J, Barbanel C and Ganeval DD. Uremic and non-uremic complications in acute renal failure. Kidney Int 1972; 1:190–6.
10. Conger JD. A controlled evaluation of prophylactic dialysis in post-traumatic acute renal failure. J Trauma 1975; 15:1056–63.
11. Gillum DM, Dixon BS, Yanover MJ, Kelleher SP, Shapiro MD, Benedetti RG et al. The role of intensive dialysis in acute renal failure. Clin Nephrol 1986; 25:249–55.
12. Storck M, Hartl WH, Zimmerer E and Inthorn D. Comparison of pump-driven and spontaneous haemofiltration in postoperative acute renal failure. Lancet 1991; i:452–5.
13. Tapolyai M, Fedak S, Chaff C and Paganini EP. Delivered dialysis dose may influence acute renal failure outcome in ICU patients.(abstract) J Am Soc Nephrol 1994; 5:530.
14. Paganini EP, Tapolyai M, Goormastic M, Halstenberg W, Kozlowski L, Leblanc M et al. Establishing a dialysis therapy/patient outcome link in intensive care unit acute dialysis for patients with acute renal failure. Am J Kidney Dis 1996; 28:S81–9.

15. Schiffl H, Lang SM, Konig A and Held E. Dose of intermittent hemodialysis and outcome of acute renal failure: a prospective randomized study. (abstract) J Am Soc Nephrol 1997; 8:290–1.

16. Kaplan AA. Continuous arterio-venous hemofiltration and related therapies. In Jacobs C, Kjellstrand CM, Koch KM, Winchester JF, editors. Replacement of renal function by dialysis, 4th edition. Dordrecht, Kluwer Academic Press, 1996; 390–417.

17. Evanson JA, Ikizler TA, Schulman G, Knights S, Himmelfarb J and Hakim RM. Delivery of intermittent hemodialysis in acute renal failure patients (abstract). J Am Soc Nephrol 1997; 8:282.

18. Leblanc m, Tapolyai M and Paganini EP. What dialysis dose should be provided in acute renal failure? a review. Adv Renal Replace Ther 1995; 2:255–64.

19. NKF-DOQI clinical practice guidelines for hemodialysis adequacy. Am J Kidney Dis 1997; 30:S15–63.

20. Coraim F, Fasol R, Stellwag F and Wolner E. Continuous arteriovenous hemofiltration after cardiac surgery. In Sieberth HG and Mann H, editors. Contributions to nephrology, vol 93. Continuous arteriovenous hemofiltration. Basel, Karger, 1985; 116–24.

21. Coraim F and Wolner E. Management of cardiac surgery patients with continuous arteriovenous hemofiltration. In Sieberth HG and Mann H, editors. Contributions to nephrology, vol 93. Continuous arteriovenous hemofiltration. Basel, Karger, 1985; 103–10.

22. Coraim FJ, Coraim HP, Ebermann R and Stellwag FM. Acute respiratory failure after cardiac surgery: clinical experience with the application of continuous arteriovenous hemofiltration. Crit Care Med 1986; 14:714–8.

23. Bellomo R, Tippiong P and Boyce N. Tumor necrosis factor clearances during veno-venous hemodiafiltration in the critically ill. Am Soc Artif Intern Org 1991; 37:M322–23.

24. Cottrell AC and Mehta RL. Cytokine kinetics in septic ARF patients on continuous veno-veno hemodialysis (abstract). J Am Soc Nephrol 1992; 3:279.

25. Gomez A, Wang R, Unruh H, Light RB, Bose D, Chau T et al. Hemofiltration reverses left ventricular dysfunction during sepsis in dogs. Anesthesiology 1990; 73:671–85.

26. Stein B, Pfenninger E, Grunert A, Schmitz JE, Deller A and Kocher F. The consequences of continuous hemofiltration on lung mechanics and extravascular lung water in a porcine endotoxic shock model. Int Care Med 1991; 17:293–8.

27. Grootendorst AF and van Bommel EFH. The role of hemofiltration in the critically-ill intensive care unit patient: present and future. Blood Purif 1993; 11:209–23.

28. Journois D and Silvester W. Continuous hemofiltration in patients with sepsis or multiorgan failure. Semin Dialysis 1996; 9:173–8.

29. Grootendorst AF, Bommel EFH van, Hoven B van der, Leengoed LAMG van and Osta ALM van. High volume hemofiltration improves hemodynamics of endotoxin-induced shock in the pig. J Crit Care 1992; 7:67–72.

30. Grootendorst AF, van Bommel EFH, van der Hoven B, van Leengoed LAMG and van Osta ALM. High volume hemofiltration improves right ventricular function of endotoxin-induced shock in the pig. Int Care Med 1992; 18:235–40.

31. van Bommel EFH, Grootendorst AF and van Leengoed LAMG. Influence of high-volume hemofiltration on hemodynamics in porcine endotoxic shock (abstract). Blood Purif 1992; 10:88.

32. Grootendorst AF and van Saase JL. The role of continuous renal replacement therapy in sepsis and multiorgan failure. Am J Kidney Dis 1996; 28:S50–7.

33. Riera JASI, Vela JLP, Quintana L, Lopez EA, de Solo BO and Checa AA. Cytokines clearance during venovenous hemofiltration in the trauma patient. Am J Kidney Dis 1997; 30:483–8.

34. Schetz M, Ferdinande P, Van den Berghe G, Verwaest C and Lauwers P. Removal of pro inflammatory cytokines with renal replacment therapy: sense or non-sense? Int Care Med 1995; 21:169–76.

35. Vallance P and Moncada S. Hyperdynamic circulation in cirrhosis: a role for nitric oxide? Lancet 1991; 337:776–8.

36. Parrillo JE. Pathogenetic mechanisms of septic shock. N Eng J Med 1993; 328:1471–7.

37. Travera Da Silva A, Kaulbach HC, Chuidian FS, Lambert DR, Suffredini AF and Danner RL. Shock and multiple organ dysfunction after self administration of Salmonella endotoxin. N Engl J Med 1993; 328:1457–60.

38. Osterud B. Meningococcal septicemia: the use of plasmapheresis or blood exchange and how to detect severe endotoxin induced white cell activation. Scand J Clin Lab Invest 1985; 45:47–51.

39. Bjorvatn B, Bjertnaes L, Fadnes HO, Flaegstad T, Gutteberg TJ, Kristiansen BE et al. Meningococcal septicaemia treated with combined plasmapheresis and leucapheresis or with blood exchange. Br Med J 1984; 288:439–41.

40. Brandtzaeg P, Sirnes K, Folsland B, Godal HC, Kierulf P, Bruun JN et al. Plasmapheresis in the treatment of severe meningococcal or pneumococcal septicaemia with DIC and fibrinolysis: preliminary data on eight patients. Scand J Clin Lab Invest 1985; 45:53–5.

41. Brandtzaeg P, Kierulf P, Gaustad P, Skulberg A, Bruun JN, Halvorsen S et al. Plasma endotoxin as a predictor of multiple organ failure and death in systemic meningococcal disease. J Infect Dis 1989; 159:195–204.

42. Westindorp RGJ, Brandt A, Thompson J, Dik H and Meinders AE. Experiences with plasma and leucapheresis in meningococcal septicaemia (abstract). Int Care Med 1990; 16:S102.

43. McClelland P, Williams PS, Yaqoob M, Mostafa SM and Bone JM. Multiple organ failure a role for plasma exchange? Int Care Med 1990; 16:100–3.

44. Drapkin MS, Wisch JS, Gelfand JA, Cannon JG and Dinarello CA. Plasmapheresis for fulminant meningococcemia. Pediatr Infect Dis J 1989; 8:399–400.

45. van Deuren M, Santman FW, van Dalen R, Sauerwein RW, Span LFR and van der Meer JWM. Plasma and whole blood exchange in meningococcal sepsis. Clin Infect Dis 1992; 15:424–30.

46. Niklasson PM, Lundbergh P and Strandell T. Prognostic factors in meningococcal disease. Scand J Infect Dis 1971; 3:17–25.

47. Stegmayr BG. Plasmapheresis in severe sepsis or septic shock. Blood Purif, 1996; 14:94–101.

48. Hanasawa, K, Aoki H, Yoshioka T, Matsuda K, Tani T and Kodama M. Novel mechanical assistance in the treatment of endotoxic and septicemic shock. Am Soc Artif Intern Organs Trans 1989; 35:341–3.
49. Kaplan AA. Therapeutic plasma exchange for non-renal disease. Semin Dialysis 1996; 9:265–75.
50. Hauser W, Christmann FJ, Klein T and Traut G. Therapeutic plasma exchange in septic shock. In Bambauer R, Malchesky PS and Falkenhagen D, editors. Therapeutic plasma exchange and selective plasma separation. Stuttgart-New York, Schattauer, 1987; 287–93.
51. Stegmayr BG. Plasma exchange in patients with septic shock including acute renal failure. Blood Purif 1996; 14:102–8.
52. Barzilay E, Kessler D, Berlot G, Gullo A, Geber D and Zeev IB. Use of extracorporeal supportive techniques as additional treatment for septic induced multiple organ failure patients. Crit Care Med 1989; 17:634–8.
53. Kaplan AA. Renal problems in critically ill patients. In Bongard FS and Sue DY, editors. Current diagnosis and treatment in critical care. Lange-Appleton, 1994; 88–116.
54. Maroni BJ, Steinman TI and Mitch WE. A method for estimating nitrogen intake of patients with chronic renal failure. Kidney Int 1985; 27:58–65.

26. Quality assurance in renal transplantation

ROBERT W. STEINER

INTRODUCTION

The basics of quality assurance for renal transplant programs are as follows: (1) *regular meetings* of relevant transplant program personnel at which there are (2) brief *reviews of the general scope* of the committee's responsibilities, (3) identification of *specific problems*, (4) *monitoring* of transplant program performance in those areas, (5) *initiation of changes* to improve performance, (6) *evaluation of those changes*. Confidentiality of proceedings is a practical requirement for transplant quality assurance meetings to insure that program deficiencies will receive full and frank analysis. Any quality assurance activity must be focused on *selected issues* and rely on the judgment of the transplant team to direct and prioritize its efforts. As the purpose of all quality assurance activities is patient benefit, it should be relatively easy to integrate meaningful quality assurance activities into a renal transplant program.

Optimal quality assurance efforts recognize each individual's desire to contribute to better outcomes, thereby maintaining morale as performance is improved. The process defines the broad goals of the organization and helps to meet those goals by systematically addressing the activities and structure of the organization to improve performance.

The worst in quality assurance activity results in paperwork and other clerical efforts which consume resources and produce little improvement. The staff focuses narrowly on statistical goals or other descriptive activity, e.g. motivated by fear either of criticism or of regulatory sanctions; the staff primarily attempts to collect data to document lack of deficiency – overall system improvement and innovation are not directly addressed. Program changes which are made are not well planned or evaluated retrospectively for efficacy.

APPROACHES TO QUALITY ASSURANCE

A number of approaches to quality assurance in renal transplantation are presented below with illustrations of the potential pitfalls of each process.

1. *Quality assurance is addressed through medical or surgical case discussion conferences.* The case discussion format provides an easy way to place quality assurance on the hospital agenda. Unfortunately, these conferences are often focused on medical education rather than critical, systematic evaluation of transplant program activities. Many potentially important individuals (nurses, administrators) do not attend. There is often no closure – no ultimate, formalized consensus as to how program activities might change in response to perceived goals, and there is no method of evaluating a change in policy or procedure.

A similar problem exists when quality assurance activities are confined to producing reports for the medical literature from transplant program experience, as systematic program review is not mandated, particularly to identify unrecognized opportunities for improvement or to propose or evaluate solutions. These two formats (medical M & M, and reports to the literature) also do not provide the confidentiality needed to address honestly many quality assurance issues.

L.W. Henderson and R.S. Thuma (eds.), Quality Assurance in Dialysis, 2nd Edition, 285–297.
© 1999 *Kluwer Academic Publishers. Printed in Great Britain*

2. *Quality assurance is incident-driven.* A key incident prompts an investigation and a change in policy based on that incident. For example, a patient develops pulmonary edema and requires intubation after OKT3 therapy. Guidelines are then established for control of volume status prior to OKT3 administration. Incident-driven quality assurance has the advantage of dealing with a motivating, often serious occurrence. It does not involve systematic review of program activities to detect less obvious areas where change would be beneficial. At the worst, changes in response to incident-driven quality assurance can be impulsive and may cause further unanticipated problems.

3. *Quality assurance is concerned with collection of data on program activities.* For example, quality assurance is concerned with meeting statistical performance standards which may be internally or externally imposed. This approach is prospective, but not likely to contribute to an improvement in quality of care, as data tabulation is an end in itself. When statistical quotas are not met, only the way data are interpreted or classified may be changed, which is not real quality improvement. For best results, data collection is selective and meaningful and only the beginning of productive quality assurance activity.

4. *Quality assurance is approached via data collection relative to selected problems.* For example, several observed cases of inadequate delivery of aerosol pentamidine for pneumocystis carinii pneumonia (PCP) prophylaxis, and observation of two cases of post transplant PCP prompts a tabulation which suggests ineffective delivery of pentamidine, and then consideration of a change to trimethoprim/sulfamethoxazole prophylaxis, which is then evaluated for efficacy. This approach is likely to produce relevant data as it derives from consensus of experienced personnel about important program goals. It focuses on making explicit a consensus on a detected deficiency in care, rather than on improving care in general.

None of the above approaches fully conform to current quality assurance theory, although some of the features of each are necessary in any quality assurance effort. All of these approaches are presented to illustrate potential limitations or deficiencies in the quality assurance process.

5. *The process of continuous quality improvement* when correctly formulated [1] is intended to be an efficient, productive approach to program evaluation and change. It goes beyond the consensus-on-deficiency approach just described above. In this process, relevant members of the transplant team meet to identify various *goals* of the program. Meeting these designated goals becomes the focus of quality assurance efforts. Individuals who are served by various aspects of the program are also identified. For example, transplant coordinators serve transplant nephrologists and surgeons by providing information on patients admitted for transplantation. Transplant physicians serve referring nephrologists in caring for their patients. All aspects of the program ultimately serve the patients who are in various phases of transplantation. The emphasis on goal identification enables all concerned to focus on general program improvement. Continuous quality improvement postulates that most highly functioning transplant personnel are motivated and responsible and will become even more so when given a chance to contribute to overall program improvement. However, the posture of the quality assurance team is to attempt to improve *all* aspects of the program, even when "acceptable" performance is documented.

It is also important that quality indicators and quality analysis extend to the evaluation of medical care by transplant physicians and surgeons. This aspect of center quality assurance may be best considered by a subset of the entire committee. Significant patient morbidity and especially postoperative mortality *must* be reviewed for possible program quality improvement, and physicians play a central role in preventing these unfortunate outcomes.

As previously stated, continuous quality improvement shares features of the several previously described quality assurance approaches. Consideration of program goals is still driven in part by perceived deficiencies and successes. Data collection is necessary, and the experience of others can be used to suggest ways to improve care and to define the general standard. All quality assurance activity in the final analysis must still be selectively focused and rely on the experience and consensus of the transplant team to prioritize effort.

EVALUATION OF CURRENT PROGRAM EXPERIENCE

Published transplant experience provides a background against which a program can identify possible areas of deficiency and suggestions for overall improvement in quality, even in areas where a reasonable standard of care has been achieved. The large body of experience in medical journals forms an obvious basis for program evaluation but has several inadequacies. (a) A good experience is more often published than are poor results. A program that has a high rate of certain postoperative surgical complications may address the problem internally but not report these data to the medical community. (b) Quality assurance is not directly addressed in many reports. Detailed analysis of complications and possible improvements in care may not concern many clinical investigators. (c) Patient care protocols (and therefore categories for data comparison) are not uniform. For example, the incidence of postoperative cardiac events can be expected to vary inversely with the rigor of a program's preoperative cardiac evaluation. Lower dose postoperative maintenance immunosuppression may increase the number of reversible mild rejections. (d) Published experience can be quickly out of data. For example, changes in immunosuppression (Neoral, mycophenolate, tacrolimus) and newer antiviral agents (acyclovir, ganciclovir) make some earlier experience in post transplant infection less relevant to present practice. (e) Statistical comparisons of published experience from different programs can be difficult. Utilizing the conventional definition of statistical significance, an incidence of one postoperative ureteral obstruction in a program doing fifty transplants per year is no different than an incidence of five occurrences in fifty transplants (p-value by chi square > 0.05), nor is an incidence of zero versus three events per year in a program doing twenty-five transplants a year.

A more fundamental criticism of statistical analysis of quality assurance data in this era of medical malpractice awareness is that the conventional scientific standard of statistical significance ($p < .05$) is arbitrary and does not necessarily conform to a lay "common sense" appreciation of probable cause and effect. It may be productive to investigate a problem identified with odds of only nine of ten ($p = 0.1$) or four out of five ($p = 0.2$) that a numerical difference in collected data does not occur by chance alone. Thus, statistical comparisons for assessing program performance have limitations.

PRESENT REGULATION AND MONITORING

Several regulatory bodies require that renal transplant programs participate in certain quality assurance activities or report selected data on a regular basis. The Joint Commission on Accreditation of Healthcare Organizations (JCAHO) requires quality assurance via a hospital-wide process which is required to (a) establish the most important aspects of care (b) identify indicators for monitoring care, both trends and important single events, (c) evaluate care when problems are suggested, and (d) implement and evaluate corrective action in response to those problems. In addition to inpatient care, some of the relevant areas which are to be monitored are diagnostic radiology, diabetic services, ambulatory care services, nuclear medicine, nursing, pathology, pharmacy, other hospital patient care support services, and infection control. The JCAHO requires monthly meetings of clinical departments or services, medical record review, surgical case review, blood and drug usage review, and monitoring of the clinical performance of all individuals who are involved in patient care, including those not permitted by the hospital to practice independently [2]. There is no specific quality assurance requirement for a renal transplant program as such, but the requirement for monthly meetings of clinical services appears to apply to the transplant team as a clinical entity.

The United States is divided into sixteen regional End Stage Renal Disease (ESRD) Networks, administered by the Health Care Finance Administration. Reporting requirements to one's network involves an ESRD patient status report signed by the nephrologist, surgeon, and other members of the health care team, which indicates dialysis modality, transplant status (active, inactive, under evaluation) and rationale for same. The network also requires a report at the time of transplantation on numerous recipient characteristics, including HLA typing, MLC response, PRA, history of previous transplants, nephrectomy, splenectomy, HBAG and CMV status, transfusion history, and early graft function. Donor (living related or cadaver) information includes presence of cytomegalovirus (CMV) antibody, hepatitis B surface antigen (HBAG), neoplasm, warm and cold allograft ischemia time, cadaver donor pretreatment, and renal function preharvest.

The United Network for Organ Sharing (UNOS) requires follow up data from each renal transplant recipient at the time of transplant, at six months, and then annually. Historical data which are requested pertain to (a) health status (e.g. working, homebound, hospitalized, HIV status), (b) medication (cyclosporine, azathioprine, prednisone, intravenous Solu-Medrol, ALG, OKT3), (c) graft status (quality of graft function, graft nephrectomy, need for dialysis, biopsy, cause of graft loss), and (d) patient status (alive or dead, autopsy).

Data which are collected and reported by these various regulatory bodies can be useful as a general standard for comparison to program performance, but these data are not sufficient for detailed analysis of program performance. Overall program performance data are found in the Annual Report of the United Network for Organ Sharing (UNOS) [3].

SCOPE OF POSSIBLE QUALITY IMPROVEMENT INITIATIVES

The overall goal of a renal transplant program can be stated simply: to maximize long term patient and allograft survival with a minimum of patient morbidity. The scope of related quality assurance activity can be divided into eleven areas: (a) preoperative recipient screening, (b) management of the living donor, (c) cadaver kidney quality, (d) surgical care, (e) postoperative medical care, (f) immunosuppression, (g) long term graft survival, (h) long term post transplant care, (i) patient education and psychological well-being, (j) the managed care interface, and (k) human subjects research. At present, good programs often differ significantly in many protocols and practices relative to the above categories.

The following sections will attempt to set out

important areas for renal transplant quality assurance. To document fully, or take a position on the numerous and important controversies which are addressed, is beyond the scope of this chapter. In many cases, the precise risks and benefits associated with many of the alternative approaches which are discussed below have not been quantified. Quality indicators for various deficiencies are presented in the text and in tables at the end of this chapter. *The occurrence of such an "indicator" event does not mean that a quality problem exists.* However, if the indicator event occurs *often enough*, a quality problem *may* be present. By the same token, it is naive to think that all bad outcomes or less-than-perfect situations can be eliminated, even if resources are unlimited. However, such realities should not limit the identification of quality deficiency indicators or the establishment of quality goals. Only in this way will centers consistently improve. The quality indicators suggested in this chapter are not the only ones which centers might consider. Quality improvement committees may find other indicators which are appropriate to the center and the area of concern.

Preoperative Screening

The number of possible screening procedures and protocols for preoperative disease is almost unlimited, and preoperative screening must be selective and oriented to procedures which are relatively likely to promote patient well-being. Requirements for extensive preoperative screening may discourage the patient from seeking transplantation or may result in long delays. Long delays may also result from disorganization in the center intake process, e.g. lack of communication with referring nephrologists as to the testing required before the center will declare the patient acceptable for transplantation. Screening procedures such as gastroesophageoduodenoscopy, colonoscopy, cystoscopy, and arteriography have a low but definite morbidity and add to patient inconvenience. These procedures also add to the cost of transplantation. It is difficult to evaluate the utility of admittedly low yield screening procedures which are recommended to rule out unlikely and/ or inapparent problems in dialysis patients. For example, the possible occurrence of an undetected preoperative bladder carcinoma in a transplant recipient may not justify a protocol to cystoscope candidates routinely. Broad recommendations for pretransplant recipient screening have been published by the American Society of Transplant Physicians and reflect the variation in practices of many centers [4].

The fundamentals of preoperative screening can be divided with some overlap into: (a) achieving a complete and current history and physical examination, (b) cardiac evaluation, (c) detecting chronic infection, (d) detecting occult neoplasm, (e) characterizing patients immunologically and identifying immunologically high risk patients, (f) anticipating anatomic problems, (g) anticipating special medical problems, and (h) assessment of patient compliance.

A physician knowledgeable in renal transplantation (usually a member of the transplant team) should generate or review the basic *intake patient profile:* medical history, physical examination, and laboratory testing, which should include detailed head and neck examination, pelvic and rectal examination, EKG, chest X-ray, and frequently Pap testing and mammography. There should be a way to keep waiting list patient information current at the transplant center. The discovery of e.g. a previously unreported history of active duodenal ulcer, an unexplained change in a cardiogram, or a new deep-seated foot infection in a diabetic potential recipient just prior to cadaveric transplantation will often disqualify that recipient, add to graft cold ischemia time, and unnecessarily strain staff resources or contribute to inappropriate preoperative decisions. These last minute surprises may be unavoidable to some extent, but their occurrence should prompt a review of preoperative evaluation and communication. Postoperative events which may bear on the quality of the renal transplant candidate evaluation process (i.e. potential quality indicators) are listed in Table 26.1.

Cardiac disease is a major cause of morbidity and mortality for dialysis patients [5, 6] and for transplant recipients [7]. Many patients may require no further screening beyond a routine EKG. Patients with cardiac risk factors should have noninvasive testing with a stress, stress thallium or persantine-thallium study. Many dialysis patients do not have the endurance to complete cardiac exercise testing [8, 9]. Usually patients with

Table 26.1. Quality assurance indicators which may suggest deficiencies in preoperative recipient screening

- Delays between initial referral to the center and activation for transplantation.

- Previously unappreciated medical problems discovered in patients called in for cadaveric renal transplant.

- Postoperative medical or surgical complications.

- Active coronary artery disease in the first post transplant year.

- Solid neoplasm in the first post transplant year.

- Death from any cause in the first post transplant year.

- Occurrence of possibly pre-existing infection, e.g. (dental abscess, tuberculosis) or recurrent urinary tract infections.

- Post transplant noncompliance with appointments or medications.

- Patients found unacceptable for transplantation by center who undergo successful transplantation elsewhere.

positive noninvasive testing go on to angiography and possible coronary bypass grafting or angioplasty. Global (but not segmental) myocardial hypokinesis may improve dramatically with transplantation and is not a reason to reject a patient [10]. The occurrence of significant cardiac morbidity post-operatively should suggest a review of intake protocols and physician communication. Cardiac events such as myocardial infarction or sudden death in the first post transplant year may also be a reflection of failure of pretransplant cardiac screening.

Immunosuppression will exacerbate preexisting *chronic infections* such as otitis media, dental abscesses, prostatitis, chronic pyelonephritis, occult tuberculosis, and osteomyelitis. These abnormalities are usually detected by intake physical examination and must be corrected before transplantation. Preoperative cholecystectomy for asymptomatic cholelithiasis or sigmoidectomy for diverticulosis are not required in most programs [4]. The identification of infection postoperatively that could have been a chronic pretransplant condition should be viewed as a possible failure of pretransplant screening. Individual pretransplant counseling in patients with hepatitis may be indicated. Chronic hepatitis B may be exacerbated by immunosuppression, but this condition is often not generally considered to be a contraindication to transplantation [11, 12]. Increasingly, programs are requiring patients with hepatitis C to undergo pretransplant liver biopsy. Those patients with significant cirrhosis are not offered transplantation [13]. Generally, the progression of hepatitis C is slow and variable from patient to patient whether on dialysis or after transplantation; interferon treatment is often not curative in either setting and can cause rejection post transplant [14]. Thus, the risks of transplantation for many willing patients with hepatitis are not prohibitive, and quality outcomes must be assessed both with the uncertainties in predicting outcome and patient autonomy in mind.

The presence of *malignant neoplasm* in the recipient is an absolute contraindication to renal transplantation. Basic screening for neoplasm includes chest X-ray, stool guaiac test, Pap smear, mammogram, and PSA titer. Abnormalities such as a thyroid or prostatic nodule should be pursued. A variety of neoplasms may develop in long term dialysis patients [15], including renal neoplasm [16] but screening ultrasound or CT studies of native kidneys are not required by many transplant programs. Neoplasms arise *de novo* with increased frequency in renal transplant recipients [17], but the emergence of nonhematologic neoplasm in the first year post transplantation suggests a failure in preoperative screening.

Patients must be accurately *tissue typed for HLA and DR antigens,* and the presence of preformed antibody to those antigens quantified (% panel reactive antibody or PRA). Patients who are at increased *immunologic risk* for acute or accelerated rejection are those with increased PRA, e.g. greater than 50%, and those who are candidates for repeat transplants, especially when previous transplant survival has been brief [18]. The field of tissue typing is changing rapidly, and DNA based methods are increasingly used [19]. High risk patients should be identified prospectively. Many programs treat these patients with "induction" therapy, e.g. with OKT3 or ALG. Early acute rejection may indicate a deficiency of either cross-matching or immunosuppression.

Preoperative assessment of *anatomic problems* must be carried out by transplant surgeons. Factors include small recipient size, previous surgery in the iliac fossa (including vascular procedures), large polycystic kidneys which preclude seating of the allograft, and severe iliac vascular disease that may make arterial implantation difficult, or may produce a steal syndrome and exacerbate distal arterial insufficiency. The patient with recurrent urinary infection may require nephrectomy or repair of reflux into the native kidney.

Another goal of the intake procedure is *anticipating special postoperative medical problems.* These may occur with marked obesity [20], hypercoagulable states [21], psychological sensitivity to corticosteroids, marked hypertension, drug allergies, aversion to blood products (Jehovah's Witnesses), and the occasional case of hypercalcemia and tertiary hyperparathyroidism [22], to name several. Many significant postoperative medical complications are to some extent foreseeable and their occurrence should prompt an evaluation of preoperative screening and preparation.

Prospective assessment of *patient compliance* can be extremely difficult. Poorly compliant dialysis patients may be highly motivated to avoid a return to that modality, so a past history of noncompliance may not be predictive. The opinions of medical and psychosocial personnel who know the patient well are of primary importance. The two major compliance questions are (a) will the patient take his medicines, and (b) will the patient keep his medical appointments and follow basic medical advice? Patients who are homeless or otherwise lack basic support systems are at high risk for noncompliance, as are patients who cannot communicate adequately with medical personnel, e.g. due to a language barrier. Patients who cannot afford medicines pose obvious risks. A demented patient presents special compliance and ethical questions. Graft failure post discharge – whether in the first year or later – is significantly influenced by patient compliance [23]. Compliance problems postoperatively therefore should prompt review of preoperative psychosocial evaluation.

Management of the Living Donor

Living donorship has become an even more attractive alternative for transplant programs with growing waiting lists and a shortage of cadaveric donors [24]. Quality goals of living donorship (related or unrelated) are (a) a safe nephrectomy,

(b) the absence of current and future renal disease in the donor, (c) no disease communicated via the allograft, (d) living kidney donation which is informed and uncoerced, and (e) excellent long term graft function. Living donors must understand the nature and likelihood of benefit of living donor transplantation for the end stage renal disease patient. Donors must also understand the benefits and drawbacks of cadaveric transplant and dialysis. Donor evaluation protocols have been recently reviewed and suggest some differences of opinion as to donor risk and suitability among centers [25].

Living donor evaluation protocols differ among programs but include a thorough history and physical, laboratory screening (including HIV, CMV, hepatitis C and B testing), IVP, and renal arteriography. Cardiac stress testing should be undertaken in older donors and should be at least as complete as for recipients with similar risk factors. In general, the presence or likelihood of significant renal disease rules out donorship. The presence of, e.g. low grade hematuria which has been completely evaluated in a young potential donor can present a difficult decision, as it often has a benign prognosis [26]. The finding of borderline hypertension also presents a difficult decision as to donor acceptability. Potential donors can often be allowed to donate in borderline cases after detailed discussion, provided that they understand the risks and benefits. Occasionally, psychosocial evaluation can uncover unacceptable family dynamics involving coercion or other unusual incentives to a potential donor. Suggested quality indicators for living donor counselling are listed in Table 26.2.

Cadaver Kidney Quality

Cadaver kidney quality will become more of an issue as cadaveric waiting lists lengthen. Cadaver kidneys will increasingly be taken from older donors, donors with hypertension, and donors with possible acute ATN [27]. UNOS and regional organ procurement agencies may at times offer cadaveric kidneys from donors of marginal quality, to be accepted for transplantation at the discretion of the individual program. Poorer cadaveric kidney quality may result in a higher postoperative dialysis rate, a lower one year graft

Table 26.2. Suggested quality indicators for counselling potential living kidney donors

- Is donor counselling structured and uniform?

- Are the alternatives of dialysis and cadaveric transplantation presented as viable?

- Is the small but definite personal health risk with donation recognized?

- Is the 5–10% chance of unsuccessful or short-lived transplant presented?

- Does the center recognize its conflict of interest and its duty to provide balanced donor information?

survival, and poor quality of graft function long term [28, 29]. These same complications may of course arise from factors which are independent of cadaver kidney quality: deficient preservation techniques, increased warm or cold ischemia time [30], cyclosporine toxicity, postoperative ATN, early allograft rejection, inadequate immunosuppression, anatomic problems from the surgery itself, and poor patient compliance. Complications from allograft recovery which are related to the recovery procedure include shortened or traumatized renal arteries, veins, or ureters, inadequate preservation of ureteral blood supply, failure to identify or preserve multiple renal arteries, and prolonged warm ischemia time. Centers may be deficient in transplanting cadaveric kidneys of poor quality, but centers may also inappropriately reject good cadaveric kidneys. Kidneys which are rejected and are then successfully transplanted by other centers are indicators for this quality problem.

Surgical Care

Postoperative surgical complications in renal transplantation are generally uncommon and include bleeding, allograft arterial and venous thrombosis, ureteral anastomotic leakage, or necrosis, wound infection or dehiscence, and lymphocele [31–33]. Rarely, the bowel may be traumatized or arterial insufficiency of the ipsilateral leg may be exacerbated. Postoperative ileus can occur with refeeding and occasionally can lead to bowel perforation. Early surgical complications that affect graft function can be misdiagnosed and mistreated as rejection. Allograft needle biopsy very occasionally can be complicated by bleeding or arteriovenous fistulae [34]. Ultrasound guidance helps avoid overlying bowel or large vessels. The possibility of bleeding should be anticipated before each biopsy so that transfusion, angiography, and even urgent surgery are facilitated.

Postoperative Medical Care

The chief goals in postoperative medical renal transplant care are (a) management of known preoperative risk factors, (b) effective dialysis support, (c) infection management, (d) management of immunosuppression, and (e) patient psychological well-being. Preoperative risk factors can be divided into general risks and patient-specific factors. General risks stem from the prevalence of cardiac disease in the dialysis population [5, 6], the effect of age on post transplant mortality and morbidity [35, 36], and the expected risks of fluid, electrolyte, and hemorrhagic complications. Postoperative complications should be reviewed to see if they are consequences of failure of preoperative planning.

Prophylaxis and treatment for infection that arises in the immediate post transplant period involve several areas. Cytomegalovirus (CMV) infection is particularly common and can be particularly severe in seronegative recipients who receive kidneys from seropositive donors and in patients who receive increased immunosuppression [37, 38]. CMV prophylaxis is indicated in high risk groups [39] and is employed by some centers in all patients in the postoperative period. Acyclovir (or valacyclovir), ganciclovir, or immune globulin are used for CMV prophylaxis [39]. Acyclovir is effective prophylaxis and treatment for herpes simplex infection [40]. Other factors which influence the occurrence and severity of infection are delays in diagnosis and management of immunosuppression once infection is present. Significant – even fatal – viral infection post transplant is not always preventable with current prophylaxis and treatment.

Bacterial infection arises from common postoperative sources: wound, lungs, intravenous access, and urinary tract [41]. Many programs prophylax with daily oral antibiotics for urinary

tract infection either permanently or for several months post transplant [42]. Perioperative pulmonary care, surgical technique, and intravenous and bladder catheterization techniques are obvious risk factors for bacterial infections. Opportunistic infections from nocardia, candida, other fungal agents (blastomycosis, aspergillus and coccidioidomycosis), and PCP are strongly influenced by the total amount of immunosuppression, especially with OKT3 or ALG [38, 41], and environmental variables [41]. PCP prophylaxis can be accomplished with daily trimethoprim-sulfamethoxazole [43] for several months post transplant. Post transplant infection with tuberculosis, coccidioidomycosis and at times other fungi can represent a failure of pretransplant surveillance and/or treatment for preexisting infection. Perhaps more importantly, significant infection should be reviewed to see if it could have been detected earlier, e.g. gradually worsening pulmonary infiltrates due to aspergillus. At present, infection control remains a major area of concern in transplant quality assurance.

Immunosuppression

The overall goals of immunosuppressive management are to maximize graft survival but to minimize complications of therapy. Immunosuppression protocols differ in many respects among renal transplant centers. The intensity and timing of postoperative immunosuppressive therapy markedly influences early graft survival, but the latter is also a function of the number of both immunologically high risk recipients and medically high risk recipients in whom immunosuppression may be more likely to be curtailed when intercurrent medical problems arise.

There are many new drugs available or about to become so for postoperative and long term immunosuppression. We now have available an effective rabbit ATG [44] and will have a variety of new monoclonal agents [45]. A variety of new drugs for chronic immunosuppression may also become available [46]. IVIG may have some utility in prophylaxis or treatment of rejection [47]. Cyclosporine or tacrolimus-based regimens are utilized currently, and target level protocols should be established for these drugs [64]. In the last few years, target postoperative cyclosporine levels have tended upward and tacrolimus levels downward, and prednisone is tapered more rapidly. The center should also decide which monoclonal or polyclonal agents it will use. It is probably best to learn to use a few agents well but to have a number of immunosuppressive strategies available; this area should be addressed by all programs periodically.

Long-Term Graft Survival

Many renal programs share care or return patients after transplant to a referring nephrologist who is not affiliated with the transplant center. Therefore there may be difficulty in monitoring and effecting long term allograft survival, which nevertheless is a quality concern of every renal transplant program. Suboptimal chronic immunosuppressive regimens in inexperienced hands can shorten graft survival [48]. Average effective maintenance chronic CSA dosing has been in the range of 4–5 mg/kg/day [49] but due to wide variation in individual pharmacokinetics, therapy must be guided by CSA levels. Chronic therapy with microemulsion CSA could justify doses in a slightly lower range [50]. Steroids seem to add to the overall effectiveness of CSA immunosuppression [51], but selected patients may tolerate gradual prednisone withdrawal [52]. A reliable cyclosporine or tacrolimus blood assay with which referring physicians are familiar is essential for good long-term graft survival. Although trough CSA levels may not be as relevant as earlier post-dose levels or the area under the concentration-time curve [53], they are easier to obtain on a routine, outpatient basis. Long term graft survival will be influenced by patient compliance both in taking medication and in obtaining accurate timing of "trough" CSA levels. "Rescue" therapy with FK506 in patients who initially receive CSA may be effective [54]. Education of the referring nephrologists as to current immunosuppressive practices is a major factor in long term graft success.

Long-Term Medical Care

Long-term medical care of the renal transplant recipient involves a unique constellation of problems [55]. Who is responsible for overall health maintenance versus immunosuppression management alone should be established. Often the patient may only see the transplant nephrologist for all post transplant care, and the nephrologist must therefore be aware of health maintenance issues. With managed care, the non-nephrologist "gatekeeper" must be aware of immunologic issues and should not delay biopsy when a rising creatinine is first detected or unwittingly manipulate drugs which alter CSA metabolism. Cardiac disease is responsible for an increasing percentage of long-term post transplant mortality [7, 56]. As most patients with preexisting coronary artery disease are transplanted uneventfully [8, 9], initially asymptomatic coronary artery disease will be present in many transplant patients and can be expected to progress. Periodic cardiac assessment and treatment of hyperlipidemia [57] are essential. Diagnosis of transplant renal artery stenosis leading to progressive hypertension and azotemia can be difficult [58]. Calcium channel blockers offer some advantages for management of hypertension and may improve allograft function [59]. Low dose antibiotic prophylaxis for urinary tract infection [42] is indicated in many female patients and all post transplant patients who have had post transplant UTI to avoid allograft pyelonephritis, which can seriously impair graft function. Renal transplant patients are at increased risk for neoplasm, particularly cutaneous neoplasms, lymphoma, and renal tumors [17]. The multiple nonimmunologic complications of steroid therapy (osteopenia, cataracts, hyperlipidemia) should prompt dosing prednisone on a strict mg/kg basis. For many programs, the quality of long term medical care is approached only through dialogue with referring nephrologists concerning these specific health care issues. Quality indicators for long term care are suggested in Table 26.3.

Patient Education and Psychological Assessment

Patient education is performed in association with the center's intake process; prospective recipients should be made familiar with the possibilities of a prolonged, complicated hospital course, early graft failure, and perioperative mortality. Patients should know that lifelong physician follow up and lifelong medication will be necessary even with the most successful transplant. They should be famil-

Table 26.3. Quality indicators which may indicate deficiencies in long term post transplant medical care

- Responsibilities for health maintenance and immunosuppression are not assigned.

- Other involved physicians are ignorant of center's long term immunosuppressive protocols.

- Vascular and myocardial disease occur frequently (poor control of lipids and blood pressure).

- Infection is frequent , especially urinary tract infection and transplant pyelonephritis.

- Neoplasm is diagnosed late, e.g. metastatic disease.

- Patients exhibit marked weight gain posttransplantation.

iar with the expected complications and side effects of immunosuppressive medicines. Other issues which may be discussed are likelihood of recurrent disease [60] and exacerbation of chronic hepatitis by immunosuppression.

Patient psychological well-being immediately post transplantation should receive direct attention from the transplant program. Patient perception of medical events and resultant stress may not correspond to the clinical reality. Patient expectations are also frequently high due to pretransplant patient denial and encouragement from many sources. Psychological reactions to steroids, cyclosporine, and OKT3 can sometimes be anticipated and discussed prospectively. At times, a preoperative trial of prednisone or CSA is helpful to assess effects on mental status. Patient perception of hospital and staff cleanliness, infection control protocols, and medical sophistication of center personnel may produce postoperative stress. Some programs may decide to use a patient questionnaire in the first two or three months post transplantation to assess quality of outcome regarding counselling and psychological issues. Psychological events postoperatively may also reflect inadequacies in preoperative psychological screening.

Managed Care and Quality Assurance

The emergence of managed care entities does not change the fundamental purposes or methods of renal transplant quality assurance. Some cost consciousness has always been a part of medical care, but managed care programs bring it to the fore. The quality assurance issues in managed care first concern adequate input to the managed care entity from experienced center personnel at all stages of the transplantation process. Managed care organizations can generate intake criteria which are inappropriately restrictive and can also make insufficient use of nephrologists who are experienced in transplantation in long term follow up. With "gatekeepers" and "primary caregivers", health maintenance is less of a problem. Considering that the difference in cost between a patient with a well-functioning transplant and a patient who requires dialysis is conservatively over $30,000 per year, the enlightened managed care organization should not oppose quality assurance review. At bottom, managed care entities are new "customers" which centers must serve, and centers must make themselves aware of the specific needs of the managed care entity. The center should define its quality goals relative to the managed care organization, and the quality of that service should be evaluated by the center. At the same time, the other quality goals of the center regarding good patient service and good outcomes must remain intact.

Human Subjects Research

A number of academic and private centers have become involved in post transplant drug studies. These studies are often well supported by pharmaceutical companies and provide financial benefit to those companies and to centers involved in the studies. Many studies of drugs in the post transplant period have provided crucial information on the efficacy and side effects of new drugs, to the benefit of future patients [44, 61–63]. As with any new center activity, drug studies create new center quality goals and "customers" – in this case, the study sponsor. Drug studies also need to be evaluated in light of ongoing center commitment to quality care and protection of patients from coercion or deception which might arise from the center's self interest in enrolling patients. Possible quality indicators for evaluating drug studies are presented in Table 26.4.

Table 26.4. Quality indicators which suggest deficiencies in post transplant human subject drug study practices

- No prioritization of studies by scientific importance or possible immediate benefit to patient.

- Lack of involvement of long term caregivers in patient entry.

- No predetermined criteria from the center for excluding patients from the study.

- Patient accrual rate too high for degree of risk ("over-selling").

- No predetermined criteria from the center for removing patients from the study.

- High rates of subject withdrawal from the study or non-adherence to the study protocol by center or patient.

Organizing Quality Assurance Activity in a Renal Transplant Program

The amount of time and effort spent on quality assurance activities varies widely among renal transplant programs in the United States. Financial considerations or lack of overt program commitment to quality assurance may limit quality assurance activities. The present standard of practice in this area is somewhat broad. A proposed basic plan for the organization and activity of a renal transplant quality assurance program is outlined in Table 26.5. The categories for possible quality analysis closely relate to the eleven areas outlined in the section *"Scope of possible program evaluation"* above. The emphasis given by such a quality assurance committee to data from each area would vary from program to program and would depend on individual program strengths

Table 26.5. Organizing a quality assurance program

A. Committee members: medical and surgical staff members and transplant coordinators, floor nursing or administration where appropriate.

B. Meet regularly (monthly or bimonthly).

C. Review the following scope of potential quality assurance activity, discuss incidents and suggestions for change, select problem areas, gather data:

1. Pretransplant recipient evaluations (testing requirements reasonable, patient information current).
2. Postoperative medical complications (cardiac, infection, and dialysis related, related to inadequate pretransplant evaluation, physician or communication, or to postoperative care).
3. Surgical complications (arterial or venous thrombosis, ureteral breakdown or stenosis, wound infection or dehiscence, bleeding, biopsy complications).
4. Early allograft dysfunction (efforts to diagnose, cadaver donor selection).
5. Rejection (incidence, efficacy of baseline immunosuppression, diagnosis, treatment, complications of treatment in role of newer immunosuppressive agents in center practices).
6. Patient psychological status.
7. Long term complications (neoplastic, cardiac, infections, patient compliance).
8. Long term allograft function.
9. Living donor counselling and evaluation.
10. Managed care interface.
11. Post transplant human subject drug studies.

D. Prioritize problems and institute changes where appropriate.

E. Evaluate effect of changes.

and weaknesses and designated priorities. Although the process of continuous quality improvement postulates that *all* areas of a transplant program are subject to review and improvement by the transplant team, emphasis and priority depend on available resources and perceived needs in these different areas.

REFERENCES

1. Berwick DM. Sounding board. Continuous improvement as an ideal in health care. New Engl J Med 1989; 320:53–6.
2. Accreditation Manual for Hospitals. The Joint Commission on Accreditation of Healthcare Organizations. Chicago, 1990.
3. 1996 Annual Report of the U.S. Scientific Registry for Transplant Recipients and the Organ Procurement and Transplantation Network – Transplant Data: 1988–1995, UNOS, Richmond, VA, and the Division of Transplantation, Bureau of Health Resources Development, Health Resources and Services Administration, U.S. Department of Health and Human Services, Rockville, MD.
4. Kasiske BL, Ramos EL, Gaston RS et al. The evaluation of renal transplant candidates: clinical practice guidelines. JASN 1995; 6:1–34.
5. Parfrey PS, Harnett JD and Barre PE. The natural history of myocardial disease in dialysis patients. J Am Soc Neph 1991; 2:2–12.
6. Rostand SG, Gretes JC, Kirk KA et al. Ischemic heart disease in patients with uremia undergoing maintenance hemodialysis. Kidney Int 1979; 16:600–11.
7. Hill MN, Grossman RA, Feldman HI et al. Original investigations. Changes in causes of death after renal transplantation, 1966 to 1987. Am J Kidney Dis 1991; 17:512–18.
8. Philipson JD, Carpenter BJ, Itzkoff J et al. Evaluation of cardiovascular risk for renal transplantation in diabetic patients. Am J Med 1986; 81:630–4.
9. Holley JL, Fenton RA, Arthur RS et al. Thallium stress testing does not predict cardiovascular risk in diabetic patients with end stage renal disease undergoing cadaveric renal transplantation. Am J Med 1991; 90:563–70.
10. Burt RK, Gupta-Burt S, Suki WN et al. Reversal of left ventricular dysfunction after renal transplantation. Ann Int Med 1989; 111:635–40.
11. Parfrey PS, Forbes RDC, Hutchinson TA et al. The clinical and pathological course of hepatitis B liver disease in renal transplant recipients. Transplantation 1984; 37:461–6.
12. Huang C, Lai M and Fong M. Hepatitis B liver disease in cyclosporine-treated renal allograft recipients. Transplantation 1990; 49:540–4.
13. Fishman JA, Rubin RH, Koziel MJ et al. Hepatitis C virus and organ transplantation. Transplantation 1996; 62:147–54.
14. Pereira BJG and Levey AS. Hepatitis C virus infection in dialysis and renal transplantation. Kidney Int 1997; 51:981–99.
15. Port FK, Ragheb NE, Schwartz AG et al. Neoplasms in dialysis patients: a population-based study. Am J Kidney Dis 1989; 14:119–23.
16. Ishikawa I, Saito Y, Shikura N et al. Ten-year prospective study on the development of renal cell carcinoma in dialysis patients. Am J Kidney Dis 1990; 16:452–8.
17. Penn I. The changing pattern of posttransplant malignancies. Transplantation Proc 1991; 23:1101–3.
18. Almond PS, Matas AJ, Gillingham K et al. Risk factors for second renal allografts immunosuppressed with cyclosporine, Transplantation 1991; 52:253–8.
19. Bunce M, Young NT and Welsh KI. Molecular HLA typing – the brave new world. Transplantation 1997; 64:1505–13.
20. Holley JL, Shapiro R, Lopatin WB et al. Obesity as a risk factor following cadaveric renal transplantation. Transplantation 1990; 49:387–9.
21. Knight RJ, Schanzer H, Rand JH et al. Renal allograft thrombosis associated with the antiphospholipid antibody syndrome. Transplantation 1995; 60:614–15.
22. Garvin PJ, Castadeda M, Linderer R et al. Management of hypercalcemic hyperparathyroidism after renal transplantation. Arch Surg 1985; 120: 578–83.
23. Dunn J, Golden D, Van Buren CT et al. Causes of graft loss beyond two years in the cyclosporine era. Transplantation 1990; 49:349–53.
24. Bertolatus JA. Renal transplantation for the nephrologist: living donor kidney transplantation: what did we learn during the 1980s? What should we learn during the 1990s? Am J Kid Dis 1991; 17:596–9.
25. Bia MJ, Ramos EL, Danovitch GM et al. Evaluation of living renal donors. Transplantation 1995; 60:322–327.
26. Mohr DN, Offord KP, Owen RA et al. Asymptomatic microhematuria and urologic disease. A population-based study. J Am Med Ass 1986; 256:224–9.
27. Rosenthal JT, Miserantino DP, Mendez R et al. Extending the criteria for cadaver kidney donors. Transplantation Proc 1990; 22:338–9.
28. Rao KV, Kasiske BL, Odlund MD et al. Influence of cadaver donor age on posttransplant renal function and graft outcome. Transplantation 1990; 49:91–5.
29. Leunissen KML, Bosman FR, Nieman FHM et al. Amplification of the nephrotoxic effect of cyclosporine by preexistent chronic histological lesions in the kidney. Transplantation 1989; 48:590–3.
30. Finn WF. Prevention of ischemic injury in renal transplantation. Kidney Int 1990; 37:171–82.
31. Tilney NL and Kirkman RL. Surgical aspects of kidney transplantation. In Garavoy MR and Guttmann RD, editors. Renal transplantation. Edinburgh, Churchill Livingstone, 1986; 93–123.
32. Belzer FO, Glass N and Sollinger H. Technical complications after renal transplantation. In Morris PJ, editor. Kidney transplantation, 3rd edition. Philadelphia, W.B. Saunders, 1988; 511–32.
33. Starzl TE, Broth CG, Putman CW et al. Urological complications in 216 human recipients of renal transplants. Ann Surg 1973; 172:609.

34. Wilszek HE. Percutaneous needle biopsy of the renal allograft. Transplantation 1990; 50:790–7.

35. Roza AM, Gallagher-Lapek S, Johnson CP et al. Renal transplantation in patients more than 65 years old. Transplantation 1989; 48:689–725.

36. Pirsch JD, Stratta RJ, Armbrust MJ et al. Cadaveric renal transplantation with cyclosporine in patients more than 60 years of age. Transplantation 1989; 47:259–61.

37. Dunn DL, Mayoral JL, Gillingham KJ et al. Treatment of invasive cytomegalovirus disease in solid organ transplant patients with ganciclovir. Transplantation 1991; 51:98–106.

38. Munda R, Hutchins M et al. Infection in OKT3-treated patients receiving additional antirejection therapy. Transplantation Proc 1989; 21:1763–5.

39. Davis CL. In-depth review. The prevention of cytomegalovirus disease in renal transplantation. Am J Kidney Dis 1990; 16:175–88.

40. Wade JC, Newton B, Flournoy N et al. Oral acyclovir for prevention of herpes simplex virus reactivation after marrow transplant. Am Intern Med 1984; 100:823.

41. Rubin RH and Tolkoff-Rubin NE. Infections: the new problems. Transplantation Proc 1989; 21:1440–5.

42. Maddux MS, Veremis SA, Bauma WD et al. Effective prophylaxis of early posttransplant urinary tract infections (UTI) in the cyclosporine (CSA) era. Transplantation Proc 1989; 21: 2108–9.

43. Higgins RM, Bloom SL, Hopkin JM et al. The risks and benefits of low-dose cotrimoxazole prophylaxis for pneumocystis pneumonia in renal transplantation. Transplantation 1989; 47:558–60.

44. Tesi RJ, Kano JM, Horn HR et al. Thymoglobulin reverses acute renal allograft rejection better than ATGAM – a double-blinded randomized clinical trial. Transplantation Proc 1997; 29:S21–3.

45. Soulillou JP. Relevant targets for therapy with monoclonal antibodies in allograft transplantation. Kidney Int 1994; 46:540–53.

46. First MR. An update on new immunosuppressive drugs undergoing preclinical and clinical trials: Potential applications in organ transplantation. Am J Kid Dis 1997; 29:303–17.

47. Peraldi MN, Akposso K, Haymann JP et al. Long-term benefit of intravenous immunoglobulins in cadaveric kidney retransplantation. Transplantation 1996; 62:1670–3.

48. Cho YW and Cecka JM. Organ procurement organization and transplant center effects on cadaver renal transplant outcomes. In Cecka KM and Terasaki PI, editors. Clinical transplants 1996. Los Angeles, UCLA Tissue Typing Laboratory, 1997.

49. Helderman JH, Van Buren DH, Amend WJC et al. Chronic immunosuppression of the renal transplant patient. JASN 1994; 4:S2-S9.

50. Keown P, Landsberg D, Halloran P et al. A randomized, prospective multicenter pharmacoepidemiologic study of cyclosporine microemulsion in stable renal graft recipients. Transplantation 1996; 62:1744.

51. St Sinclair NR. Low-dose steroid therapy in cyclosporine-treated renal transplant recipients with well-functioning grafts. Can Med Assoc J 1992; 147:645–57.

52. Hricik DE, Kupin WL and First MR. Steroid-free immunosuppression after renal transplantation. JASN 1994; 4:S10–16.

53. Lindholm A and Kahan BD. Influence of cyclosporine pharmacokinetics, trough concentrations, and AUC monitoring on outcome after kidney transplantation. Clin Pharmacol Ther 1993; 54:205.

54. Woodle ES, Cronin D, Newell KA et al. Tacrolimus therapy for refractory acute renal allograft rejection. Transplantation 1996; 62:906–10.

55. Bruan WE. Long-term complications of renal transplantation. Kidney Int 1990; 37:1363–78.

56. Mahony JF, Caterson RJ, Pollock CA et al. Coronary artery disease is the major late complication of successful cadaveric renal transplantation. Clin Transplantation 1990; 4:129–32.

57. Kasiske BL, Tortorice KL, Heim-Duthoy KL et al. Lovastatin treatment of hypercholesterolemia in renal transplant recipients. Transplantation 1990; 49:95–100.

58. Glicklich DG, Tellis VA, Quinn T et al. Comparison of captopril scan and doppler ultrasonography as screening tests for transplant renal artery stenosis. Transplantation 1990; 49:217–19.

59. Palmer BF, Dawidson I, Sagalowsky A et al. Improved outcome of cadaveric renal transplantation due to calcium channel blockers. Transplantation 1991; 52:640–5.

60. Mathew TH: In-depth review. Recurrence of disease following renal transplantation. Am J Kidney Dis 1988; 12:85–96.

61. Mayer AD, Dmitrewski J, Squifflet JP et al. Multicenter randomized trial comparing tacrolimus (FK506) and cyclosporine in the prevention of renal allograft rejection. Transplantation 1997; 64:436–43.

62. The Tricontinental Mycophenolate Mofetil Renal Transplantation Study Group. A blind, randomized clinical trial of mycophenolate mofetil for the prevention of acute rejection in cadaveric renal transplantation. Transplantation 1996; 61:1029–37.

63. Vincenti F, Kirkman R, Light S et al. Interleukin-2-receptor blockade with daclizumab to prevent acute rejection in renal transplantation. NEJM 1998; 338:161–6.

Index

299

L.W. Henderson and R.S. Thuma (eds.), Quality Assurance in Dialysis, 2nd Edition, 299–301.
© 1999 *Kluwer Academic Publishers. Printed in Great Britain*

Developments in Nephrology

Developments in Nephrology

Kluwer Academic Publishers – Dordrecht / Boston / London